Conditioning Young Athletes

Tudor O. Bompa, PhD

Michael Carrera

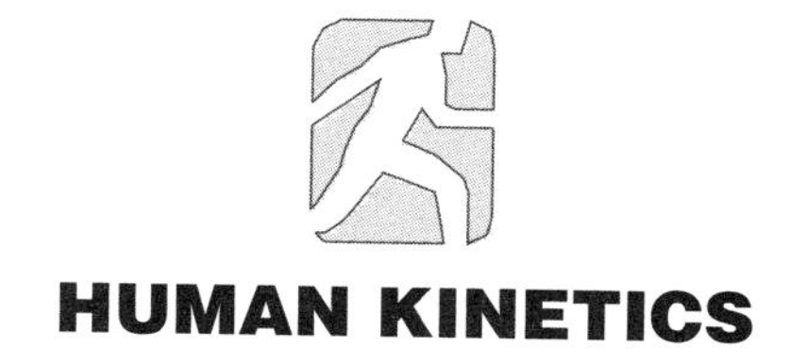

HUMAN KINETICS

Library of Congress Cataloging-in-Publication Data

Bompa, Tudor, 1932-
Conditioning young athletes / Tudor Bompa, Michael Carrera.
pages cm
Includes bibliographical references and index.
1. Physical fitness for children. I. Carrera, Michael, 1975- II. Title.
GV443.B619 2015
613.7'042--dc23
2014045516

ISBN: 978-1-4925-0309-5 (print)

This book is a revised edition of *Total Training for Young Champions,* published in 2000 by Tudor O. Bompa.

The web addresses cited in this text were current as of February 2015, unless otherwise noted.

Acquisitions Editor: Justin Klug; **Senior Managing Editor:** Amy Stahl; **Associate Managing Editor:** Nicole Moore; **Copyeditor:** Amanda M. Eastin-Allen; **Proofreader:** Jim Burns; **Indexer:** Dan Connolly; **Permissions Manager:** Martha Gullo; **Graphic Designer:** Tara Welsch; **Cover Designer:** Keith Blomberg; **Photograph (cover):** Jason Allen; **Photographs (interior):** Jason Allen, except where otherwise noted; **Photo Asset Manager:** Laura Fitch; **Visual Production Assistant:** Joyce Brumfield; **Photo Production Manager:** Jason Allen; **Art Manager:** Kelly Hendren; **Associate Art Manager:** Alan L. Wilborn; **Illustrations:** © Human Kinetics; **Printer:** Sheridan Books

We thank St. John Lutheran School in Champaign, Illinois, for assistance in providing the location for the photo shoot for this book.

Printed in the United States of America 10 9 8 7 6 5 4 3 2 1

The paper in this book is certified under a sustainable forestry program.

Human Kinetics
Website: www.HumanKinetics.com

United States: Human Kinetics
P.O. Box 5076
Champaign, IL 61825-5076
800-747-4457
e-mail: humank@hkusa.com

Canada: Human Kinetics
475 Devonshire Road Unit 100
Windsor, ON N8Y 2L5
800-465-7301 (in Canada only)
e-mail: info@hkcanada.com

Europe: Human Kinetics
107 Bradford Road
Stanningley
Leeds LS28 6AT, United Kingdom
+44 (0) 113 255 5665
e-mail: hk@hkeurope.com

Australia: Human Kinetics
57A Price Avenue
Lower Mitcham, South Australia 5062
08 8372 0999
e-mail: info@hkaustralia.com

New Zealand: Human Kinetics
P.O. Box 80
Mitcham Shopping Centre, South Australia 5062
0800 222 062
e-mail: info@hknewzealand.com

E6398

This book is dedicated to all the hard-working coaches, athletes, and parents who strive to achieve excellence in sport performance. May you also form lasting relationships and positive experiences in pursuit of your goals.

Dr. Tudor O. Bompa and Michael Carrera

To my wife, thank you for your love, guidance, and sacrifice throughout the completion of this project. You are always there to support me, and this book was no different. To my four children, thank you for the gift of fatherhood. What an amazing journey. To Dr. Tudor Bompa, thank you for your friendship and unbridled support over the many years.

Michael Carrera

Contents

Preface

Childhood is the most physically active stage of human development. Children like to play games and participate in physical activity and sports, and they certainly love to compete. In today's society, sport has become a way of life. Parents plan their vacations and days off work around hockey and soccer tournaments, and children dream about developing into professional athletes, buying jerseys, hats, stickers, and even video games that promote their favorite players. Coaches are bombarded with various training philosophies, equipment, and scrutiny from parents, administrators, other coaches, and athletes! Rarely is an off-season or transition period used to reset the athlete physically, mentally, and emotionally from a tough season. Today athletes transition from play to training and back to play. It is no surprise that burnout is rampant in many sports. Today's sporting environment is highly competitive and time consuming. Competition is important, but so is proper training and time devoted to rest, play, and other nonsporting activities. *Conditioning Young Athletes* is not about building the best athlete; rather, it's about designing the best program so that your athletes can grow, prosper, and reach their personal best in all aspects of sport, competition, and health.

Parents, coaches, and administrators search for the best training programs to increase children's athletic potential. Coaches often become role models, and children dream of surpassing the achievements of Peyton Manning, Gracie Gold, Usain Bolt, Sidney Grosby, or Serena Williams. It is, however, a grave mistake to submit children to the training programs of adults. After all, children are not simply little adults. Each child is unique at each stage of development. The physical and psychological changes (at times abrupt) that occur at each stage are accompanied by critical behavioral transformations. It is important for anyone working with children to be well informed regarding all the physical, emotional, and cognitive changes occurring during the development stages and to structure training that is best suited for each stage.

As coaches and parents we need to keep in mind that informal training and preparation for sport begin in early childhood, when kids should be encouraged to run, jump, play with balls, and enjoy all the activities on the playground and in the backyard. Many years are available for focusing on a particular sport or physical activity.

Of the great number of books devoted to training, the majority refer to elite athletes, and few discuss training programs specifically for children. Along with many specialists and researchers on the specifics of training for young athletes, through both experience and in-depth study, we have gathered information and experience regarding the best possible approach to training children. The intent of *Conditioning Young Athletes* is to bridge the gap between research and application and between a hit-and-miss and a long-term approach to children's training.

For each developmental stage there is a corresponding phase of athletic training: Initiation takes place in prepuberty, athletic formation occurs in puberty, specialization happens in postpuberty, and high performance occurs in maturation. While each developmental stage roughly corresponds to a typical age range, it's important to understand that training programs must be designed according to an athlete's stage of maturation rather than chronological age because individual needs and demands vary among athletes. Children of the same chronological age may differ by several years in their level of biological maturation. Moreover, while an early-maturing child may show dramatic improvements initially, often a late maturer will be the better athlete in the long run. Current research in athletic training substantiates such a claim; thus, it's important to look beyond the short-term achievements and let children develop at their own pace.

The training models in *Conditioning Young Athletes* focus solely on the three major stages of development: prepuberty, puberty, and postpuberty. The first two chapters provide information about the anatomical, physiological, and psychological aspects children experience at each stage. In chapter 3, we discuss the importance of assessment—not so much to compare the athlete to others but rather to set points of improvement and fitness goals. We chose assessment techniques that are easy to apply to many team and individual sports. Chapters 4 through 8 discuss training for flexibility, speed, agility and quickness, strength and power, and endurance, respectively. Each of the training chapters includes suggestions for structuring workouts, periodization models for each stage of development, and illustrated or photographed exercises and activities. Of the vast number of exercises for developing coordination, flexibility, speed, agility, endurance, strength, and power, we have selected those that are most accessible and that anyone can perform without sophisticated machines. Our model is very simple: You don't have to do what is new, just what is necessary for success in sport. Fancy and expensive equipment is not the key to successful athletic development. Rather, the key is to design and implement a plan that focuses on the proper stage of athletic development and provides an opportunity for the athletes to mature in all areas of fitness, including strength, speed, flexibility, and endurance. Specialization should occur in the later years of athletic development, so coaches and parents should be patient and take the time to properly assess and slowly progress young athletes in all training goals. We also urge you to consider the exercises and programs only as a guideline. As you become more familiar with the training stages, you can add to or change any exercise or program to accommodate individual needs, specific training conditions, and environment.

Chapter 9 discusses appropriate timing for participating in organized competition and ways in which parents and coaches can guide competition and training to ensure athletes have a positive experience. In chapter 10 we discuss proper nutrition for young athletes, in particular the five fueling habits. We also discuss the importance of a balanced diet that consists of primarily whole foods and what to eat before, during, and after a competition or training session. Chapter 11 puts all of the information from the previous chapters together in specific, long-term training plans for various team and individual sports. The final chapter discusses training myths that are often propagated and marketed to parents, coaches, and trainers. While many forms of equipment and gadgets can be useful in conditioning young athletes, there are also pieces of equipment that not only fail to improve strength, speed, or power, but can actually decondition the exact variable of fitness the equipment claims to improve.

A positive experience in sports and competition is key to ensuring children will enjoy an active lifestyle for years to come. Doing too much too soon, however, can result in overtraining or injury, and it might also lead children to lose interest and drop out of sports before ever fully developing their talents. An organized long-term training program such as presented here greatly increases the chance that athletes will stay with their sports and enjoy long-term excellence rather than short-term burnout. And that's what makes a well-conditioned athlete.

Acknowledgments

It is a great pleasure to once again work with Michael Carrera as coauthor of this book. Mike is an exceptional specialist with a prosperous future in sport training and, in particular, with junior athletes. His knowledge base is exemplary, and he has contributed greatly in writing this book. My sincerest thanks.

Dr. Tudor O. Bompa

Together we would like to thank Justin Klug, Amy Stahl, and the entire Human Kinetics staff for all their hard work, patience, and dedication in publishing this book. The editing process was seamless, guided by a professional group of people who came together to produce a thoughtful and focused book. Thank you all for sharing your experience and talents.

Dr. Tudor O. Bompa and Michael Carrera

chapter 1

Training Guidelines for Young Athletes

Success in any arena is usually the result of planning, hard work, and commitment, and athletic training is no exception. All successful athletes are trained individuals who excel in a particular physical activity and usually have followed a well-designed, long-term training program over several years. In sport, training is the process of executing repetitive, progressive exercises or work that improves the potential to achieve optimum performance. For athletes, this means long-term training programs that condition the body and mind to the specifics of competition and lead to excellence in performance.

Although many coaches and instructors are competent at designing seasonal training programs, it is essential to look beyond this short-term approach and plan for the athlete's long-term development. Proper athletic training should start in childhood so the athlete can progressively and systematically develop both the body and the mind to achieve long-term excellence rather than immediate success that is followed by burnout.

Far too often, the sport programs of children imitate the programs of well-known elite athletes—those who, through their national or international achievements, have captivated the imaginations of young athletes and their coaches. The followers of such programs often say, "If the program worked for Kobe Bryant or Sidney Crosby, it should work for my kids too!" Coaches commonly employ these programs in detail without evaluating the degree to which they serve the interests of young athletes and with no guiding concepts, such as training principles. With the stroke of a key, coaches and parents can download complex programs from a website or article and begin to blindly train their athletes with little consideration of the child's current physical needs. Of course, these coaches and parents don't intend to hurt or damage the athlete's development. Rather, they want to give their kids a fighting chance to excel in the overly competitive sporting environment—sometimes at the detriment of initiating and maintaining a clear focus on development. For instance, it is very common for parents to streamline their children into a particular sport or competition. Johnny wants to play in the NHL, or Julie wants to be a professional soccer player and bring home an Olympic gold medal. In both cases, parents can misinterpret a child's early love for a sport as an opportunity to focus programs, coaching, and skill development on one particular sport. We have witnessed children as young as six years of age whose entire physical development is geared around the particular movements of a sport. In reality, children should be encouraged to play games, activities, and multiple sports in order to optimize athletic development, muscle strength, and neural programming. Children are not just little adults. They have complex, distinct physiological characteristics that must be taken into account.

Reversing the Coin

On one end of the spectrum are child athletes who are doing too much, training excessively, and specifically training for one sport or particular drills while neglecting much-needed multilateral development. Unfortunately, on the other end of the spectrum are children who are overweight, overfed, undernourished, and detrimentally sedentary.

Childhood obesity gradually increased in the 1980s through the 1990s (Ogden et al., 2010) both in the United States and worldwide (Ebbeling et al., 2002). Data from 2003 and 2004 show that of U.S. children and adolescents between the ages of 6 and 19 years, more than 33% were at risk of being classified as overweight and 17% were, in fact, overweight (Wang and Beydoun, 2007). Trends in obesity and weight gain do vary by sex, race, and ethnic group; however, of primary significance is that children are getting fatter, unhealthier, and less active. For these children, the program does not focus on what type or intensity of activity is best but rather emphasizes that any type of consistent activity, especially in the form of cardiovascular exercise such as walking, running, or cycling, can decrease health risks and improve health outcomes into adulthood.

Building the Foundation

A mantra commonly heard in locker rooms and gyms as athletes reunite after a short sabbatical from competition or training is "Build the foundation." Following a hard-fought season or training phase, an athlete's body is tired, worn out, and in need of relaxation and—most important—regeneration. Once the body heals from the thralls and strains of competition, it is essential that athletes take the time to rebuild the foundation of strength, power, endurance, speed, agility, and all the motor abilities that are important to their sport. A strong foundation ultimately leads to optimal performance and less injury.

There was a time when children began at an early age to build a foundation of motor skills. Skills such as running, jumping, skipping, and performing push-ups or chin-ups were not taught in multimillion-dollar gyms or athlete development centers but rather on the street corner, local park, or backyard. Kids were once just kids and not aspiring professional athletes. Today, with the advent of gaming, 24/7 video on demand, smartphones, and smart TVs and a decreased emphasis on physical activity in schools, kids who don't have access to recreational play or organized sporting activities or who aren't encouraged to run, jump, and skip simply sit in front of the TV or computer for hours on end. Human bodies are designed to move. A sedentary body will lead to obesity, sickness, and disease. Researchers at the University of South Australia analyzed the change in running speed and cardiovascular endurance in children between the ages of 9 and 17 years from data collected between 1964 and 2010. Results show that running speed and endurance gradually declined as the years progressed (American Heart Association Scientific Sessions, Tomkinson, 2013). In essence, kids today are less fit than their parents. This can be attributed to many reasons, including the prevalence of gaming and other sedentary habits and the overconsumption of sugar-filled drinks (Ludwig et al., 2001). Although the jury is out on the precise effect of obsessive gaming on health, any activity that limits one's ability to engage in regular physical activity will negatively affect cardiovascular health.

The overall health trend for kids does not look good. Kids are getting fatter and becoming less active. A host of technological advances and behavioral changes such as no longer walking or cycling to school have contributed to our current health crisis. Kids need to get active. We are not talking about long-term athletic development or upper-level sporting camps; we are simply discussing the need for greater movement opportunities. Numerous governing bodies in the United States, including the Centers for Disease Control and Prevention (2015), recommend that children get 60 to 90 minutes of physical activity every day in the form of running, jumping, skipping, cycling, and muscle strengthening.

No one will argue that life is easy. In fact, the demands and expectations of balancing work and family life have become more difficult and burdensome over the past few decades. A sedentary lifestyle makes us unhealthy, tired, and, many times, sick. We as a society need to get healthier, and sometimes the best start is getting more active. Parents may struggle to find a suitable physical outlet for their children. Cracking down on the time kids spend in front of the TV or gaming is difficult enough, let alone trying to get them outside to play a game of pick-up street hockey, basketball, or old-fashioned tag. In previous years, kids would expend at least some energy walking to a friend's house or hanging out at the park. Today, they "hang out" at social media sites or on their cell phones and never have to leave their bedrooms. Times have changed. What hasn't changed is the accessibility of organized team sports—regular house-league organized sports. Numerous organizations provide an opportunity for kids to play basketball, soccer, football, hockey, and many other sports for the pure love of exercise and team spirit and without the burden of advancing to a higher league, getting a scholarship, or becoming a professional athlete. If you are a parent who is struggling to encourage your child to become more active and want a suitable form of exercise that will improve strength and endurance and help build relationships, look to house-league organizations in your area. There is no finer way to get kids active, engaged, and moving and instill the value of being active for a lifetime.

Here are some benefits of organized sport:

- It promotes healthy living with an emphasis on building skills, strength, and endurance.
- It improves mental health and focus.
- It teaches important life skills, including self-respect and respect for others, in a safe environment. As the saying goes, there is no *I* in *team*.
- It teaches important life lessons about winning, losing, and striving to give one's best effort.
- It provides positive role models in coaches, parents, organizers, and other athletes.
- It emphasizes fitness and fun because each player gets equal playing time.
- It provides a great introduction to sport and exercise in a nonthreatening environment, which may motivate participation, growth, and involvement in further levels of sport and activity.

When it comes to training and athletic development for youngsters, it is evident that some kids are overly active and focused on improving and growing in sport. Other kids are active and enjoy sport but prefer to remain in a noncompetitive and safe environment. Some kids are reluctant to participate in any kind of sport or exercise altogether and rarely achieve the basic recommended levels of physical activity.

The focus of this book is to provide the tools necessary for conditioning young athletes—tools that coaches, parents, and athletes can use to better understand the physical necessities of their sport and how to properly train for optimal performance in both the short term and the long term. More than 35 million young athletes in the United States play organized sport every year (Nettle and Sprogis, 2011). A proper training philosophy is of the utmost importance if athletes are to streamline their training from multilateral development and general conditioning to sport-specific training and specialization. Training philosophy is important for preparing the plan, working the plan, and avoiding burnout. The remainder of this chapter discusses four training guidelines for young athletes: developing a long-term training program, adding training variety, understanding individual characteristics, and increasing training load appropriately.

Developing a Long-Term Training Program

For a long time, some coaches suggested that performing sport-specific exercises from an early age was the optimal way to train for a sport. Some sport physiologists took this concept, which some coaches still use today, and developed it into a principle of training. They suggested that to yield the fastest results a training program must do the following:

- Stress the energy system that is dominant in a given sport. For instance, a sprinter must do only sprints, and a long-distance athlete must train only the aerobic energy system.
- Follow motor skill specificity, meaning that athletes must select exercises that mimic the skill patterns used in the sport and that involve only the muscle groups used to perform a technical skill.

Even though laboratory research demonstrates that specificity training results in faster adaptation and leads to faster increments in performance, this does not mean that coaches and athletes have to incorporate specificity training from an early age. In this narrow approach to children's sport, the only scope of training is achieving quick results irrespective of what may happen in the future of the young athlete. In an attempt to achieve fast results, coaches expose children to highly specific and intensive training without taking the time to build a good base. This is like trying to erect a high-rise building on a poor foundation. Such a construction error clearly will result in the collapse of the building. Likewise, encouraging athletes to narrowly focus on their development in one sport before they are ready physically and psychologically often results in the following problems:

- It can lead to unilateral, narrow development of the muscles and organ functions.
- It can disturb harmonious physical development and biological equilibrium, which are prerequisites of physical efficiency, athletic performance, and the development of a healthy person.
- Over the long term, it can result in overuse, overtraining, and even injuries. In fact, young athletes should not be encouraged to push through injuries with the misunderstanding that their young bodies can take any kind of stress and eventually bounce back. That may not be the case.
- It can have a negative effect on the mental health of the children involved because this type of training and participation in many competitions can create high levels of stress.

- It can interfere with children developing social relationships because of the many hours associated with intensive training. For example, children may fail to make friends outside of sport.
- It can affect the motivation of children because the program can be too stressful, boring, and lacking in fun. Often young athletes quit the sport before they experience physiological and psychological maturation. Consequently, a talented young person may never find out how talented she could have become.

Multilateral Development

It's important for young children to develop a variety of fundamental skills and to become good general athletes before they start training in a specific sport. This is called multilateral development, and it is one of the most important training principles for children and youths.

Multilateral, or multiskill, development is common in Eastern European countries, where some sport schools offer a basic training program. Children who attend these schools develop fundamental skills such as running, jumping, throwing, catching, tumbling, and balancing. The children become extremely well-coordinated and acquire skills that are fundamental to success in a variety of individual and team sports, such as track and field, basketball, and soccer. Most programs also have a swimming component, as swimming helps children develop aerobic capacities while minimizing the physical stresses placed on their joints. Proper understanding of the need to fully diversify programs for child athletes and offer multilateral skill development has spurred the opening of many sport schools—schools dedicated to academic achievement with a heightened emphasis on sport development—throughout North America.

If we encourage children to develop a variety of skills, they will probably experience success in several sporting activities, and some will have the inclination and desire to specialize and develop their talents further. When children demonstrate interest in further developing their talents, we must provide the necessary guidance and opportunities. It takes years of training to become a world-class athlete, and we must provide those young athletes striving for excellence with a systematic, long-term plan based on sound, scientific principles.

Figure 1.1 illustrates the sequential approach to developing athletic talent over several years. Although the ages will vary from sport to sport and from individual to individual,

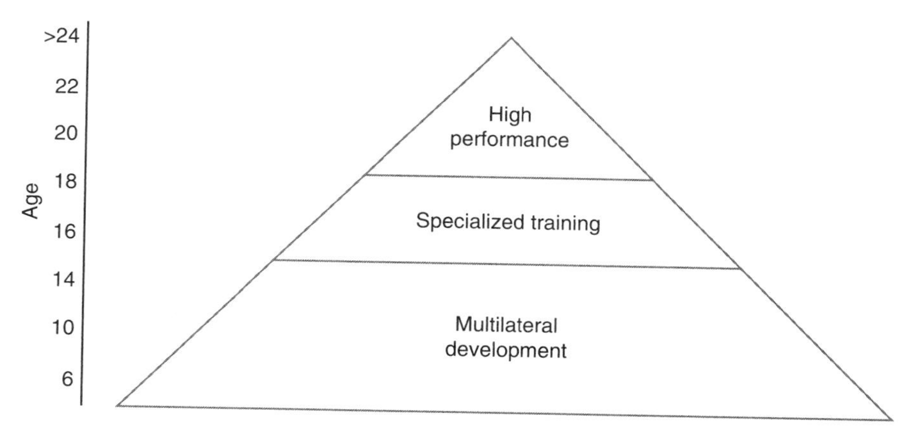

Figure 1.1 The suggested long-term approach to specificity of training includes a base of multilateral development.

Reprinted, by permission, from T.O. Bompa, 1999, *Periodization training for sports* (Champaign, IL: Human Kinetics), 39.

the model demonstrates the importance of progressive development. The base of the pyramid, which we may consider the foundation of any training program, consists of multilateral development. When the development reaches an acceptable level, athletes specialize in one sport and enter the second phase of development. The result will be a high level of performance.

The purpose of multilateral development is to improve overall adaptation. Children and youths who develop a variety of skills and motor abilities are more likely to adapt to demanding training loads without experiencing stresses associated with early specialization. For example, young athletes who specialize in middle-distance running may be able to further develop their aerobic capacities by running, but they are also more susceptible to overuse injuries. Athletes who are capable of swimming, cycling, and running can exercise their cardiorespiratory systems in a variety of ways and significantly reduce the chance of injuries. Just because a young athlete wants to become a professional baseball player does not mean that running is the only cardiovascular movement he should perform. On the contrary, other skills such as jumping, skipping, climbing, and cycling help strengthen the development of muscles at varying angles, encourage neuromuscular focus, and help the athlete enjoy a variety of skills that are necessary before the body can begin to specialize in specific movement patterns. Furthermore, emphasizing cable or dumbbell movements intended to help the baseball swing (which are often touted as sport-specific movements) at such a young age is not necessary, especially if athletes are struggling to perform fundamental exercises such as push-ups or chin-ups.

Focus on the fundamentals and the specifics will take care of themselves. As a society we tell our children to slow down and not be in a rush to grow up—"Just be a kid," we say, knowing that they will have many years to be adults. The same applies to sport. As an athlete matures in age and physiological function, specificity in training will inevitably become the focal point. Sport-specific training programs and the stress of repeating movements that are essential to the desired sport will become a must. The athletic conditioning required to safely transition to and recover from the intensity of sport-specific training will depend on the athlete's overall strength development and coordination and the preparedness of her nervous system—the key components of multilateral training.

We should encourage young athletes to develop the skills and motor abilities they need for success in their chosen sport and other sports. For example, a well-rounded sport program for children and youths would include low-intensity exercises for developing aerobic capacity, anaerobic capacity, muscular endurance, strength, speed, power, agility, coordination, and flexibility. A multilateral training program that focuses on overall athletic development along with sport-specific skills and strategies will lead to more successful performances at a later stage of development. As table 1.1 demonstrates, a multilateral program provides many benefits. If we are interested in developing successful, high-performance competitors, we must be prepared to delay specialization and sacrifice short-term results. The following two studies demonstrate this.

In a landmark longitudinal (14-year) study performed in the former East Germany (Harre, 1982), children aged 9 to 12 years were divided into two groups. The first group participated in a training program that entailed early specialization in a given sport and incorporated exercises and training methods that were specific to the needs of the sport. The second group followed a generalized program that incorporated specific drills as well as a variety of other sports and skills and overall physical training. As table 1.1 illustrates, the results prove that a strong foundation leads to athletic success.

An important Soviet survey (Nagorni, 1978) that analyzed the progression of sport-specific training reported similar findings. Among the conclusions of the study were the following:

Table 1.1 Comparisons Between Early Specialization and Multilateral Development

Early specialization	Multilateral program
Quick performance improvement	Slower performance improvement
Best performance achieved at 15-16 years of age because of quick adaptation	Best performance at age 18 years and older (the age of physiological and psychological maturation)
Inconsistent performance in competitions	Consistent performance in competitions
Many athletes burn out and quit the sport by age 18 years	Longer athletic life
Prone to injuries because of forced adaptation	Few injuries

- The vast majority of the best Soviet athletes had a strong multilateral foundation.
- Most athletes started to practice the sport at 7 or 8 years of age. During the first few years of activity, they all participated in various sports, such as soccer, cross-country skiing, running, skating, swimming, and cycling. Between the ages of 10 and 13 years the children also participated in team sports, gymnastics, rowing, and track and field.
- Specialized programs started at 15 to 17 years of age without compromising sport performance and activities performed at earlier ages. The athletes achieved their best performances after 5 to 8 years in the specialized sport.
- The athletes who specialized at a much earlier age achieved their best performances at a junior age level. These performances were never duplicated when they became seniors (over 18 years). Quite a few athletes had retired from sport before reaching senior levels. Only a minority of the athletes who specialized early on were able to improve performance at the senior age.
- Many top-class Soviet athletes started to train in an organized environment at the junior age level (14 to 18 years). They had never been junior champions or held a national record. At the senior age, however, many achieved national- and international-class performances.
- Most athletes believed that their success was facilitated by the multilateral foundation they had built during childhood and the junior age.
- The study concluded that specialization should not start before the age of 15 or 16 years in most sports.

Research over the past 30 years about the consequences of early specialization has yielded similar results. With emphasis on universal sporting competitions, athletes are subtly encouraged to specialize at an earlier age (Capranica and Millard-Stafford, 2011). Young athletes are now taking on rigorous training schedules that are similar to adult training models. Such schedules can include more than 10 hours of training per week and can lead to many negative consequences, including physical, mental, and emotional problems. In an article published in *British Journal of Sports Medicine*, Mostafavifar and colleagues (2013) argue that early specialization in one sport can lead to numerous practical and physiological implications, including the following:

- A decrease in motor skill development because focus shifts from general development to sport-specific programming

- Increased risk of injury to the cardiovascular and musculoskeletal systems because of the intensity and volume of training
- Improper recovery due to a lack of knowledge about nutrition and proper macro- and micronutrient ratios
- Early burnout due to hours of dedication
- Early injury due to overuse

The intent of this chapter is not to discourage a discussion on the viability of early specialization. Rather, the intent is to highlight the adverse effects of prematurely nudging an athlete to train beyond the body's ability to heal and recover. The debate between early and late specialization continues, but the priorities—the long-term mental and physical health of the young athlete and the formula for achieving one's greatest potential with minimal risk of injury—should remain the same.

Although multilateral training is most important during the early stages of development, it should also be part of the training regimen for advanced athletes. Figure 1.2 illustrates that although the ratio between multilateral development and specialized training changes significantly throughout the long-term training process, athletes need to maintain throughout their careers the multilateral foundation they established during their early development. Take, for instance, the case of Jane, a 12-year-old tennis player. Every week Jane engages in 10 hours of tennis training and 4 to 5 hours of other physical and multilateral training such as flexibility, basic strength (using medicine balls and dumbbells), and agility exercises. A parent or a coach might feel that more tennis drills would make Jane a more-skilled player. However, increasing her tennis training is possible only at the expense of reducing her multilateral training. In the short term Jane's tennis skills may improve, but the lack of training in basic physical abilities such as strength, agility, and flexibility would thwart her playing abilities in the long term. A lack of good physical qualities at the age of 18 would result in weaker strokes, slower movement on the court, and decreased agility and quickness, thus lowering Jane's overall tennis-playing potential.

Figure 1.2 suggests a long-term ratio between specific and multilateral development. The latter slightly decreases as Jane matures. If Jane is doing 4 to 5 hours of multilateral

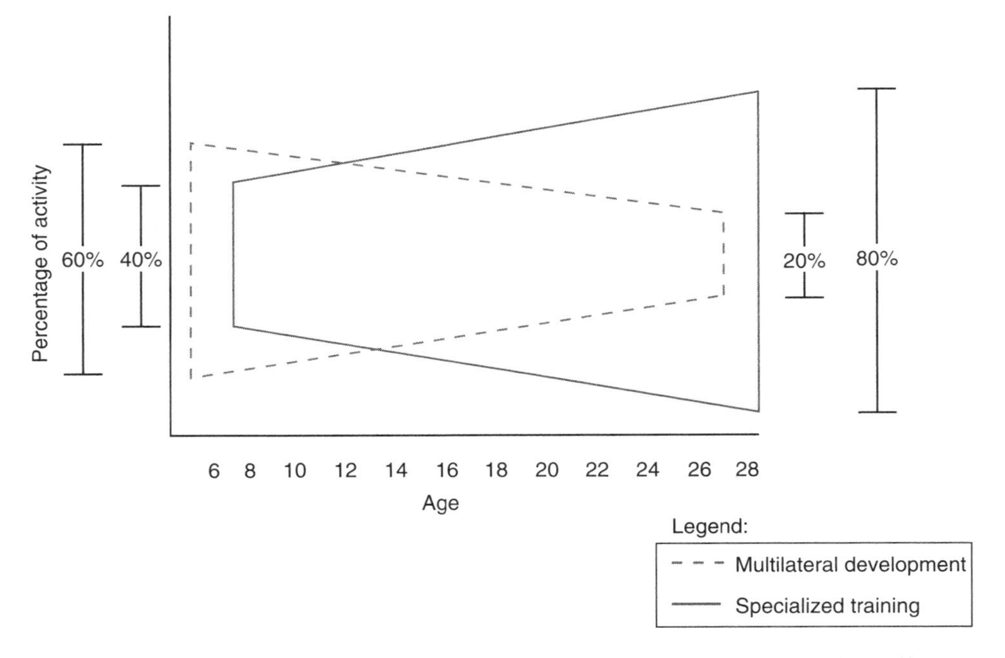

Figure 1.2 Ratio between multilateral development and specialized training for different ages.

training per week at age 12, she might do 3.5 to 4 hours per week at age 16. At the same time, her tennis-specific training may increase from 10 hours per week at age 12 to 14 to 16 hours per week at age 16.

Specialized Development

Specialization takes place after athletes have developed a solid multilateral foundation and when they have the desire to specialize in a particular sport or a position in a team sport. Specialization is necessary for achieving high performance in any sport because it leads to physical, technical, tactical, and psychological adaptation. It is a complex process. From the onset of specialization, athletes have to prepare for ongoing increments in training volume and intensity.

Once specialization takes place, training should include both exercises that enhance development for the specific sport and exercises that develop general motor abilities. However, the ratio between the two forms of training varies considerably from sport to sport. For example, consider the difference between long-distance runners and high jumpers. The training volume for long-distance runners will consist mostly of running drills or activities that enhance aerobic endurance, such as cycling and swimming, whereas a program for high jumpers will consist of approximately 40 percent high jump-specific drills and exercises and 60 percent exercises that develop particular motor abilities (e.g., plyometrics and weight training for developing leg strength and jumping power).

As table 1.2 demonstrates, there are general ages at which athletes should start developing skills and specializing in a given sport with the hope of eventually reaching a high-performance standard. It is important to understand, however, that even during the specialization stage of development, athletes should dedicate only 60 to 80 percent of their total training time to performing sport-specific exercises. They should spend the balance of their time on multilateral development and improving specific biomotor abilities.

Table 1.2 Guidelines for the Road to Specialization

Sport	Age to begin practicing the sport (yr)	Age to start specialization (yr)	Age to reach high performance (yr)
Archery	12-14	16-18	23-30
Athletics			
Sprinting	10-12	14-16	22-26
Middle-distance run	13-14	16-17	22-26
Long-distance run	14-16	17-19	25-28
Jumps	12-14	16-18	22-25
Triple jumps	12-14	17-19	23-26
Long jumps	12-14	17-19	23-26
Throws	14-15	17-19	23-27
Badminton	10-12	14-16	20-25
Baseball	10-12	15-16	22-28
Basketball	10-12	14-16	22-28
Biathlon	10-13	16-17	23-26
Bobsled	12-14	17-18	22-26
Boxing	13-15	16-17	22-26
Canoeing	12-14	15-17	22-26

(continued)

Table 1.2 *(continued)*

Sport	Age to begin practicing the sport (yr)	Age to start specialization (yr)	Age to reach high performance (yr)
Continental handball	10-12	14-16	22-26
Cycling	12-15	16-18	22-28
Diving			
Women	6-8	9-11	14-18
Men	8-10	11-13	18-22
Equestrian	10-12	14-16	22-28
Fencing	10-12	14-16	20-25
Field hockey	11-13	14-16	20-25
Figure skating	7-9	11-13	18-25
Football	12-14	16-18	23-27
Gymnastics			
Women	6-8	9-10	14-18
Men	8-9	14-15	22-25
Ice hockey	6-8	13-14	22-28
Judo	8-10	15-16	22-26
Modern pentathlon	11-13	14-16	21-25
Rowing	11-14	16-18	22-25
Rugby	13-14	16-17	22-26
Sailing	10-12	14-16	22-30
Shooting	12-15	17-18	24-30
Skiing			
Alpine	7-8	12-14	18-25
Nordic (under 30K)	12-14	16-18	23-28
Nordic (over 30K)	10-12	17-19	24-28
Jumping	—	14-15	22-26
Soccer	10-12	14-16	22-26
Speed skating	10-12	15-16	22-26
Squash/handball	10-12	15-17	23-27
Swimming			
Women	7-9	11-13	18-22
Men	7-8	13-15	20-24
Synchronized swimming	6-8	12-14	19-23
Table tennis	8-9	13-14	22-25
Tennis			
Women	7-8	11-13	17-25
Men	7-8	12-14	22-27
Volleyball	10-12	15-16	22-26
Water polo	10-12	16-17	23-26
Weightlifting	14-15	17-18	23-27
Wrestling	11-13	17-19	24-27

Once athletes have decided to specialize, they must prepare to use specific training methods for adapting to the physical and psychological demands of the sport. The training demands increase significantly, formalized testing begins, and coaches plan and schedule organized competitions on a yearly basis.

Specialization takes place at different ages depending on the sport. In sports that require artistry of movement, complex motor skill development, and a high degree of flexibility, such as gymnastics, diving, and figure skating, athletes should specialize at a young age. For sports in which speed and power dominate, such as football, baseball, and volleyball, athletes can start practicing the fundamental sport techniques at a young age. Specialization, however, should take place only once athletes are capable of effectively coping with the demands of high-intensity training. In most speed and power sports, specialization should take place toward the end of the adolescent growth spurt. For sports in which success depends on the ability to cope with maximal endurance efforts, such as long-distance running, cross-country skiing, and cycling, athletes can specialize at the time that they develop speed and power or later. Some endurance athletes are capable of achieving outstanding performance results at 30 years of age or older.

Adding Training Variety

Throughout the long process of developing young athletes, children and youths experience thousands of hours of training and complete exercises and drills many thousands of times to develop their abilities. If training programs are not closely monitored and varied, many athletes will have difficulty coping with the physical and psychological stresses. Including diverse exercises and developing a range of skills in the training program at every stage of the developmental process not only helps athletes develop new abilities but also prevents injury, boredom, and burnout.

Most team sports expose athletes to a variety of training methods. To strive for excellence in sports such as hockey, baseball, and basketball, athletes must become competent in many skills and exercises. They develop this competence most effectively through training diversity. In other sports, especially individual sports such as swimming and cycling, there is less diversity. For example, swimmers rarely participate in other sports and often perform the same exercises, technical elements, and drills for 2 to 3 hours a day, 4 to 7 days a week, 45 to 50 weeks a year, for 20 years. This type of repetitive training may lead to overuse injuries and psychological problems, particularly the emotional difficulties associated with monotony and boredom.

To overcome these problems, coaches should incorporate a variety of exercises into each practice session. Using a variety of technical movements from other activities can enrich a coach's list of drills. Coaches can also include exercises that develop the motor abilities specific to the sport, such as speed, power, and endurance. For example, middle-distance runners who experience excessive muscular fatigue or overuse injuries may benefit more by completing an interval workout while running in the water than by running on a hard track surface. Cross-country skiing also helps develop endurance without placing the same strain on the joints of the legs. A coach who is creative and knowledgeable has a distinct advantage because he can design each workout to use a variety of exercises and drills. If possible, periodically conducting a session away from the normal training environment will keep young athletes stimulated, interested, and, in some cases, more motivated.

Coaches can also vary training sessions by holding part of the practice, such as the warm-up, with athletes from other sports. For instance, football players can warm up with track athletes, whose warm-up activities incorporate more agility. Or basketball players can warm up with middle-distance runners on the grass, where some interval training can also be performed (e.g., 6 × 60 seconds at 60 to 70 percent velocity, with an easy jog of 4 to 5 minutes between). Similarly, baseball players can warm up with track and field throwers using medicine balls. It is also possible to design sessions that encourage athletes to train particular motor abilities by participating in other sports during the off-season. For example, distance runners could develop their endurance through cross-country skiing, cycling, or swimming.

Performing a variety of exercises also develops muscles other than those the athlete uses specifically in the chosen sport. Too much specificity training may result in overuse injuries. Moreover, it may cause imbalances between the agonistic muscles (those specifically used in a sport) and the antagonistic muscles (those that oppose to movement of the agonistic muscles). When a strong imbalance exists between these two sets of muscles, the pull of agonistic muscles is so strong that it may cause an injury to the tendons and muscle tissue of the antagonistic muscles. Therefore, incorporating a variety of exercises that use many muscles of the body can decrease the incidence of injury. Similarly, variations of movement, including practicing other sports, will improve coordination and agility. A well-coordinated and agile athlete will quickly learn difficult skills later.

Coaches who are creative and incorporate variety into their training programs will see the benefits. Athletes will remain highly motivated and will be less likely to experience overuse injury.

Understanding Individual Characteristics

Every athlete has unique personality traits, physical characteristics, social behaviors, and intellectual capacities. Designing an individual training program is an important step in determining an athlete's strengths and limitations by using both subjective and objective measures. The limited working capacity of athletes varies significantly. To effectively design training programs for athletes, coaches must consider individual strengths and limitations, individual differences (e.g., stage of development, training background, and experience), health status, recovery rate between training sessions and following competitions, and sex particularities.

Also, it is no longer suitable or acceptable to categorize children and youths strictly based on chronological age because children of the same age can differ in anatomical maturation by several years. Considering anatomical age, biological age, and athletic age is crucial.

Anatomical Age

Anatomical age refers to the several stages of anatomical growth that we can recognize by identifying particular physical characteristics. Table 1.3 summarizes the developmental stages of children and youths. Note, though, that many individual differences exist regarding characteristics.

Anatomical age clearly demonstrates the complexities of growth and development and helps explain why some children develop skills and motor abilities faster or slower than others do. A child who is more developed anatomically will learn many skills faster than a child who is less developed. Although many children follow similar growth patterns, variations exist. For example, climate, latitude, terrain (mountainous vs. flat), and living environment (urban vs. rural) can significantly affect the rate at which youths develop. For instance, children in countries with hot climates mature much faster sexually, emotionally, and physically. As a result, athletic performance in these youths can

Table 1.3 Stages of Anatomical Age

Phase of development	Chronological age (yr)	Stage	Anatomical age	Developmental characteristics
Early childhood	0-2	Newborn Infant Crawling Walking	0-30 days 1-8 mo 9-12 mo 1-2 yr	Fast organ development
Preschool	3-5	Small Medium Big	3-4 yr 4-5 yr 5-6 yr	Unequal rhythm of development when important and complex changes occur (functional, behavioral, personality)
School years	6-18	Prepuberty	6-11 yr (girls), 7-12 yr (boys)	Slow and balanced development when the functions of some organs become more efficient
		Puberty	11-13 yr (girls), 12-14 yr (boys)	Fast growth and development in height, weight, and the efficiency of some organs; sexual maturation with change in interests and behaviors
		Postpuberty, adolescence	13-18 yr (girls), 14-18 yr (boys)	Slow, balanced, and proportional development; functional maturation
Young adult	19-25	Maturity	19-25 yr	Maturation period doubled by perfecting all functions and psychological traits; athletic and psychological potentials are maximized

increase faster between the ages of 14 and 18 than in youths who live in countries with colder climates. Similarly, children living at high altitudes tend to be more effective in endurance sports than children living at low altitudes. Runners from Kenya, for example, dominate distance running in track and field. Living at a high altitude, where oxygen is available in lower proportions than at sea level, has made these individuals adjust to performing with less oxygen. Consequently, the genetics of individuals from this region are superior for endurance. They use oxygen more effectively, giving them an advantage over athletes coming from low plains.

From the perspective of athletic development, the third phase (16-18 years) is the most important. During this phase, athletes may be at many different levels of physical and skill development. In some sports, such as hockey or football, athletes will be developing a variety of skills and motor abilities and establishing a foundation for future development. In other sports, such as gymnastics, they will be maximizing their performances. During the latter part of the school years, many athletes who have developed a solid foundation and desire to pursue excellence in a particular sport will be able to specialize.

Biological Age

Biological age refers to the physiological development of the organs and systems in the body that help determine the physiological potential for reaching a high performance level in both training and competition. When categorizing and selecting athletes, coaches must consider biological age. Using a rigid classification system based on chronological age will frequently result in misjudgments, faulty evaluations, and poor decisions.

Two athletic children of the same anatomical age who are the same in height, weight, and muscular development could be of different biological ages and possess different abilities to perform a training task. A tall child who looks strong is not necessarily a faster athlete. Similarly, a slightly smaller youngster may be more agile in certain positions in team sports. Whereas anatomical age is visible, biological age is not: One cannot see how efficient an athlete's heart is or how effectively an athlete utilizes oxygen. A less impressive physique may hide a powerful and efficient heart, which is so important in endurance sports. To find a child's training potential, you must assess biological age objectively through simple tests.

Without considering biological age, it is difficult to determine whether certain children are too young to perform particular skills or to tolerate specific training loads. It is also difficult to assess the potential of older athletes, who many consider to be too old to achieve high performance. Unfortunately, in many sport programs, coaches still use chronological age as the major criteria for classification. For example, many studies have demonstrated that children born in December are less likely to experience success in sport programs than those who were born in January of the same year. In many cases, when divisions are determined by chronological age, children born in the same calendar year are placed in the same category. As a result, children born early in the year will likely have an anatomical and biological advantage over children born later in the year.

It is important to consider individual differences in biological age. The following list illustrates some tremendous differences in the biological ages of international sport champions.

- Constatina Tomescu-Dita, from Romania, was a gold medalist in the marathon at the 2008 Beijing Olympic Games at the age of 38. She is also the oldest Olympic marathon champion in history.
- At the 1964 Olympic Games in Tokyo, M. Takemoto, from Japan, received a silver medal in gymnastics at the age of 44.
- At the 1998 Winter Olympic Games in Nagano, Tara Lipinski, a 15-year-old from the United States, won the gold medal in figure skating.
- Ellina Zvereva, from Belarus, received a gold medal in discus at the 2001 World Championships at the age of 40.
- In 1988, 15-year-old Allison Higson, from Canada, broke the world record in the 200-meter breaststroke.
- In 1991, 12-year-old A. Yeu, from China, was a world champion in diving.
- Gordie Howe, from Canada, was still playing hockey in the National Hockey League at the age of 52. (He played from 1946 to 1971 and again from 1979 to 1980.)

This list, which represents only a small percentage of the athletes who have achieved remarkable performances in sport, demonstrates that chronological age does not always represent an athlete's level of biological potential.

Athletic Age

Coaches often determine anatomical age and biological age subjectively because conducting accurate assessments is difficult. As a result, it is difficult to determine when children and youths are ready to participate in high-caliber competitions. Many national and international sport organizations have closely examined scientific research regarding biological potential at a given age. Although controversy often surrounds such decisions, many organizations have stipulated minimum age requirements for competition. Table 1.4 presents some minimum age requirements for international competitions, such as world championships or the Olympic Games.

Table 1.4 Ages for Participation in International Competitions

Sport	Minimum age (yr)	Designated age (yr)	
		Junior	Senior
Track and field	14	18	>19
Boxing	—	18	>19
Canoeing	—	19	>20
Diving	14	—	—
Equestrian	—	18	>19
Fencing	—	20	>21
Gymnastics	14		
Women	12	14	>19
Men	14	18	22
Ice hockey	—	18	>21
Modern pentathlon	16	19	>20
Rowing	16	18	>19
Skiing (Nordic)	—	19	>20
Swimming	—	15	>16
Tennis	—	18	>19
Volleyball	—	18	>19
Weightlifting	16	19	>20

Athletic age, especially the minimum age and the designated age for senior-level competition, has important implications on the design of long-term training plans. In most sports, training programs have to be structured so that the focus for children and youths is on overall development and not early specialization. If coaches focus on developing athletes over several years, they will likely produce some great international champions.

Increasing Training Load Appropriately

Understanding the methods used to increase training load is essential for creating a good training program. The amount and quality of work that children and youths achieve in training directly affects the amount that their physical abilities will improve. From the early stages of development through the high-performance level, athletes must increase the workload in training gradually, according to their individual needs. During adaptation to a particular training load, athletes increase their capacities to cope with the stresses and demands of training and competition. Athletes who develop gradually will likely be more capable of performing work over a long period.

The rate at which young athletes improve their performance depends on the rate and method they use to increase the training load. If they maintain the load at approximately the same level for a long time (i.e., standard load), improvements in performance are barely visible. If they increase the load too much, some immediate benefits may be visible but the likelihood of injuries substantially increases. It is important, therefore, for young athletes to slowly increase the training load. Although immediate, short-term results will be difficult to attain, the long-term potential for improved performance is much greater.

During the early stages of development it is difficult to monitor training loads in some young athletes because performance improvements in strength, speed, and endurance may be the result of normal growth and development. However, it is important to progressively increase training loads. Athletes aged 10 to 15 years who participate on a baseball team that practices twice a week and plays a game each weekend all season (i.e., standard load) likely will not experience significant improvements during the season as a result of training. They may improve as a result of their growth and development, but without an increase in overall training volume it will be difficult to further develop baseball skills and specific motor abilities. You can progressively increase training programs for young, developing athletes in the following areas.

Duration of Training Sessions

The length of each training session can increase from the beginning of the season to the end—for example, from one hour to two hours, as table 1.5 suggests.

As the duration increases to an hour and a half, it is important to maintain the children's interest by choosing a variety of drills and activities. Coaches should also include longer rest intervals between drills and exercises so the children may more easily cope with fatigue. (Note that a training session performed in hot and humid conditions should always be much shorter than a regular session because children become fatigued more quickly.)

Number of Exercises

To progressively increase the training load, athletes can also expand the number of exercises and drills they perform per training session over the weeks and years. Increasing the number of repetitions of technical drills or exercises for physical development will certainly improve an athlete's performance. As the number of exercises and drills increase, however, the instructor must carefully monitor the rest interval between them. Longer rest intervals will give children more energy to perform all the work planned for that training session.

Frequency of Training Sessions

To constantly and progressively challenge the bodies of young athletes toward performance improvement, you must regularly increase the frequency of training sessions, or the number of training sessions per week. This is essential because skills develop during training sessions, not during games and competitions. For young athletes to constantly master the skills of the sport and to develop the motor abilities needed for future competitions, they must have more training sessions than games. Therefore, parents should require that instructors and coaches, especially in team sports, have a ratio of two to four training sessions to one game. Such an approach will pay off later in an athletic career because athletes will properly acquire skill fundamentals at the ideal age.

Table 1.5 Progression of Training Session Length for a Soccer Team

Month	Duration of sessions (min)
April	60
May	75
June	90
July	90
August	Off

Coaches who extend their season so there are more weeks to prepare before competition begins will likely see positive results. This is true more for individual sports, such as track and field and swimming, than for team sports. In team sports such as soccer, baseball, and football, children often experience few weeks of training before games start.

The ideal situation is to practice for most months of the year, as this will lead to better development of skills and motor abilities. Coaches and parents can take advantage of a long preseason training period to work with the athletes on skill acquisition without the pressure of playing games on weekends. The issue with today's training schedule is that athletes are not given an opportunity for down time—a chance to recover from the season and simply engage in fun activities. Parents and coaches are quickly shifting their kids from season play to off-season, sport-specific training camps or to indoor or outdoor leagues with weekend games, depending on the sport. There seems to be an inherent fear that skill development will stop if the athlete allows the body to transition to a lower workload or adds variety in training. On the contrary, the body uses such downtime to strengthen the integrity of the cardiac, neuromuscular, and other vital systems and to refresh the athlete for when training frequency increases. Instead of adding more games or increasing an athlete's workload, coaches should organize general training sessions for the athletes at the end of the regular season.

If coaches and instructors cannot organize such a training program, parents should do so. A basement, a garage, an open field, or the backyard are all great places for training simple skills, especially motor abilities. To develop basic strength or endurance one does not need the most sophisticated facilities.

Young children may commit only a few months to practicing a specific sport, and often these are the months of the competitive season. As young athletes become older and more experienced, however, they should commit more months to training in a specific sport if they desire high performance results. When young athletes make the commitment to specialize in a particular sport, they will likely be training 10 months or more a year.

We also suggest a progression in the frequency of training. At first the duration of training can increase from two times per week at 60 minutes to two times per week at 75 minutes, then to two times per week at 90 minutes. If you consider this the upper level of the child's tolerance, the frequency of training sessions can then increase from two times per week at 90 minutes to three times per week at 90 minutes. In a later stage of developing the athlete's potential, the frequency can increase to four or five training sessions per week (or even higher for some sports).

As the frequency reaches an upper limit (e.g., three times at 90 minutes) for that developmental stage, the number of exercises and drills per training session can increase. Consider two methods:

1. Increase the number of exercises before taking rest (e.g., from 1 set of 8 ball passes, drills, or exercises to 1 set of 10, 12, or even 14).
2. Decrease the rest interval between sets (e.g., from 2 minutes to 1.5 minutes to 1 minute).

Step Loading

It is important to progressively increase training loads because athletes who experience standard loads, even at a young age, will likely stop improving. The most effective way to increase the training load is to understand and use the step method. With this method, the load increases for two or three weeks and then decreases for one week to allow regeneration, or recovery. Figures 1.3 and 1.4 illustrate two options. We recommend the option shown in figure 1.3 for young children and the option shown in figure 1.4

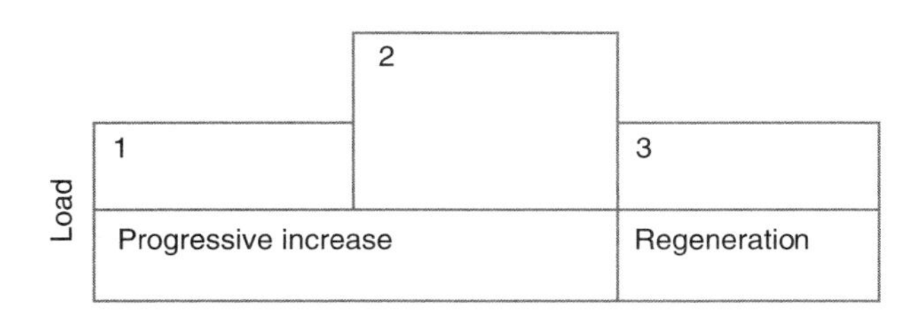

Figure 1.3 Step loading for young children.

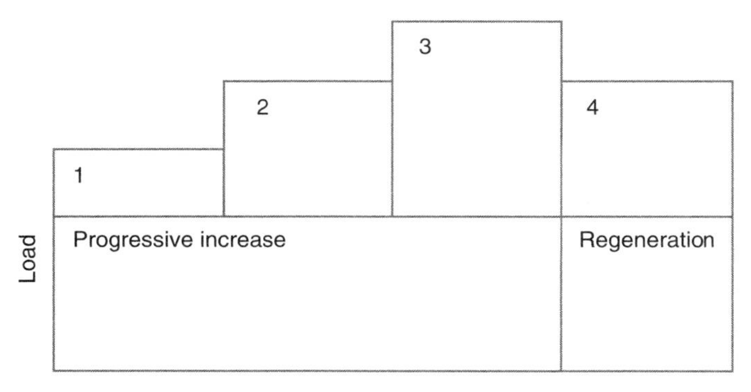

Figure 1.4 Step loading for late teens and advanced young athletes.

for athletes in their late teens and young athletes who are advanced in a particular sport. Both models refer to the training weeks when athletes are not in competition.

As figure 1.3 suggests, the training load should increase progressively. During the first two steps, each representing a week, the increased load challenges young athletes to adapt to a greater amount of work. As the athletes become fatigued, the load slightly decreases in the third week to allow for recovery before it again increases further.

As figure 1.4 demonstrates, athletes in their late teens and advanced young athletes are expected to cope with a more challenging program. During the first three weeks of training the load increases from week to week, which leads to higher adaptation levels and, ultimately, superior performances. The fatigue level will be high by the end of the third step, so the load slightly decreases in step 4 to allow for recovery. To continue increasing the training load after the third week will result in greater fatigue, which may lead to a critical level of fatigue or, over time, overtraining. If a regeneration week is not incorporated into the training plan when athletes are experiencing fatigue, some may get injured, and they may lose interest in training and eventually drop out.

Table 1.6 suggests training elements that you can use to increase the load from step to step or decrease the load for the regeneration week of the four-week cycle. Table 1.6 does not list all of the training elements. For instance, others, such as distance, speed, or the number of drills and repetitions, must be increased in the same fashion.

Note that in table 1.6 the number of training sessions peaks in step 3 to four per week. If you use the three-week step method for children (figure 1.3), then the progression may be two training sessions for the first step and three training sessions for the second step. The number of hours of training increases in the same way. Regarding the rest interval, *standard* means the normal periods the instructor uses. After step 3 (figure 1.4) or step 2 (figure 1.3), the instructor can use a slightly shorter rest period to further challenge the bodies of the young athletes.

Table 1.6 How Training Elements Increase in the Step Method

Training element	Step 1	Step 2	Step 3	Step 4
Training sessions/wk	2-3	3	4	3
Duration of training sessions (min)	75	90	90-120	75-90
Rest interval between sets of drills or exercises	Standard	Standard	Shorter	Standard

The regeneration week is crucial to the step method. The athletes are tired at the end of the highest step, and to continue training at the same level of demand is a mistake. For the well-being of the young athletes, the training demand should decrease during this week. This will remove fatigue from the body, relax the mind, and replenish overall energy. Toward the end of this week the athletes will feel rested and ready for one or two more weeks of increased load increments.

As the regeneration week ends, the step method can be applied again but at a slightly higher training demand. At the beginning of the preseason phase, you can increase the workload by 5 to 10 percent. As the athletes adjust to this workload, especially in the second part of the preseason phase, the load increment can be increased from step to step by 10 to 20 percent.

The step method is most valid during the preseason, when athletes train for upcoming competitions. It is not valid during the competitive season, especially for team sports, when athletes play games at the end of the week. During the season, therefore, the load of training per week is steady and a regeneration period is scheduled to remove fatigue after a game. Athletes perform most training during the middle of the week and plan light training for the one day (or maximum of two days) before a game so that they will not experience fatigue that could impair their performance on game day (table 1.7).

Certainly, other options for organizing the weekly program exist. A coach may organize only two training sessions per week (e.g., Tuesday and Thursday), each one of steady intensity. Each session may, however, be of lighter intensity if the children look tired. Remember that rested children always play better games.

Training young athletes must be viewed as a long-term proposition in which the load and the overall physical, technical, tactical, and mental demands are increased gradually during the stages of growth and development. Laying the foundation of sound training during childhood through multilateral development rather than narrow, sport-specific training will give young athletes a better foundation for high performance. Providing variety in training, accounting for individual differences among athletes, and appropriately planning the load progression from stage to stage will also result in a more effective training program.

Chapter 2 discusses how to apply the concepts in this chapter to the three stages of children's athletic development: initiation, athletic formation, and specialization. The physical and emotional characteristics of each stage largely dictate a young athlete's training potential and therefore must be taken into account when designing a training program.

Table 1.7 Structure of Training per Week During the Season

Monday	Tuesday	Wednesday	Thursday	Friday	Saturday	Sunday
Off	Light training	Intense training	Intense training	Light training	Game training	Off

chapter 2

Stages of Athletic Development

Sport scientists and coaches claim that athletes who experience well-organized and systematic training programs as children and youths usually accomplish the best performances. Impatient coaches who pressure children to achieve quick results usually fail because the athletes often quit before attaining athletic maturation. By employing correct training principles (discussed in chapter 1) and dividing the training of children and youths into systematic stages of development with clearly defined objectives, coaches and parents will more likely produce healthy and outstanding athletes.

It is important, however, to keep in mind that children evolve at different rates. The growth rates of children's bones, muscles, organs, and nervous systems differ from stage to stage, and these developments largely dictate a child's physiological and performance capabilities. This is why a training program *must* consider individual differences and training potential. Even in a team sport with, for example, 14-year-old players, the differences between the players may be so great that some have the athletic potential of 16-year-olds (early developers), whereas others have only the physical capabilities of 12-year-olds (late developers). To neglect such large differences could mean that an early developer might be undertrained, whereas the late developer is overstressed.

One benefit of organized play in the form of house-league sports is that athletes are able to comfortably develop at their own pace in accordance with their physiological tendencies. In our experience, parents and coaches alike are quick to move their children to higher levels of play. This is not a surprise, as all parents want to give their children the best possible opportunity and challenge them to be the best they can be. Sometimes, however, moving a child too quickly to a more advanced league or competition can stress the body and, more important, provide a negative experience of isolation, insecurity, and distress. No one thrives when they feel like the small fish in a big sea. House-league sports, which limit the amount of stress placed on the athletes and truly endorse fun as the primary objective, give late bloomers an opportunity to improve skill, mental proficiency, and fitness while waiting for nature to catch up. At times, taking a step back and providing a nurturing, supportive environment is the best plan for producing an outstanding athlete and healthy individual.

A gradual, progressive program with no abrupt increases in intensity greatly increases training efficiency and reduces the chance of frustration and injury. This process is called periodization of long-term training. The term *periodization* is derived from the word *period*, meaning a certain time or phase of training. Periodization is the process of dividing training programs of all athletes, from entry level to elite class, into small segments of time, or short phases, so training is more effective. Periodization also refers to the long-term progression of the motor abilities necessary for an athlete to excel in the sport of her choice. In short, periodization is a holistic approach to athletic development that takes into account training, psychological, and sociological factors. Comprehensive periodization models for several sports are provided at the end of chapter 11.

It is essential for anyone involved in children's sports to incorporate periodization principles into each child's training. Figure 2.1 demonstrates that all athletes, regardless of their high-performance potential, should participate in a multilateral phase and a specialized phase of training. The concepts, discussed in chapter 1, now must be applied to the specifics of each stage of development. The effectiveness of a training program and the workload planned in training must carefully take into account the physical and mental characteristics of each child. The athletic potential of a child is strictly dependent on his physical and mental development. To disregard this means discomfort, stress, and even the possibility of injuring the young athlete. In the multilateral phase, gradually introduce athletes to sport-specific training (initiation) and progressively form their athletic talents (athletic formation). The primary purpose of the multilateral phase is to build the foundation upon which the athlete can effectively develop complex motor abilities, resulting in a smooth transition to the specialized phase.

There are two stages in the specialized phase: specialization and high performance. During the specialization stage, athletes choose which sport, and which position in the chosen sport, they would like to play. Once athletes begin to specialize, the intensity and volume of training can increase progressively, and you can individualize conditioning programs. The final stage of the specialized phase focuses on high performance in the chosen sport.

Although figure 2.1 outlines ages associated with each stage, it is important to understand that this model can shift considerably depending on the sport. For example, in sports such as women's gymnastics and diving, the ages at each stage may be two to four

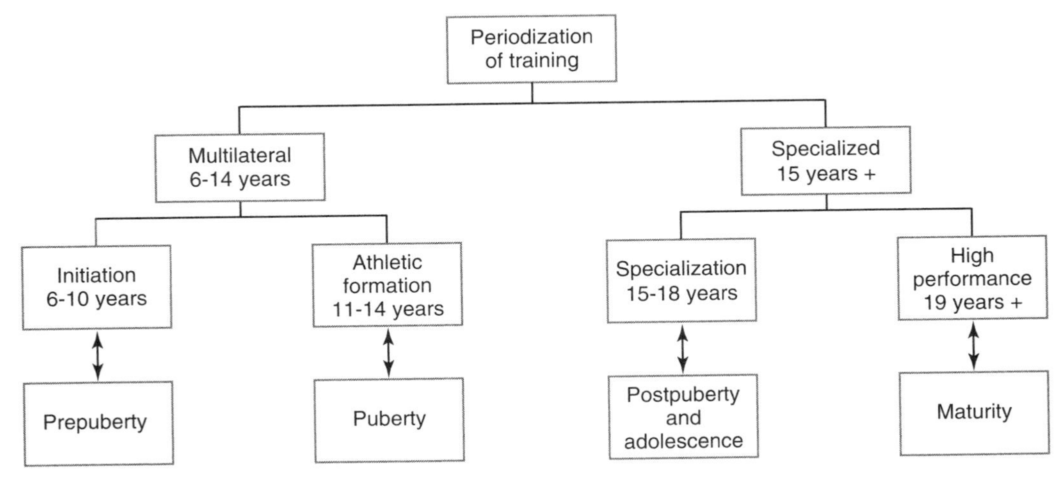

Figure 2.1 Ratio between multilateral development and specialized training for different ages.

Adapted, by permission, from T.O. Bompa, 1999, *Periodization: Theory and methodology of training*, 4th ed. (Champaign, IL: Human Kinetics), 258.

years earlier. It is also critical to understand that the rate at which children develop varies greatly, and you must consider the maturation differences of each athlete. The training programs in this book are based on the average rate of growth and development of a typical young athlete. Although the training guidelines and suggested programs refer to chronological age, they should be applied according to the specific characteristics of each young athlete. In other words, in setting a training program for a group of children, you should consider the children's state of readiness for that kind of work rather than chronological age and adjust training and competitive programs accordingly. Familiarity with the physical, mental, and social characteristics of athletes in the initiation, athletic formation, and specialization development stages will allow you to establish a training program that will enhance athlete development, resulting in high performance.

Setting the Foundation for Motor Skills Training

Motor skill development, which begins at infancy, sets the stage for the development of more complex tasks, fluidity of movement, and muscular strength and power. Children develop both gross motor skills and fine motor skills concurrently. Gross motor skills involve large movements that rely on the coordination of the large muscles of the body. Movements such as running, jumping, climbing, and catching are all gross motor skills that children develop at an early age and continue to perfect as years pass. Fine motor skills involve very small or more precise movements, such as picking up a Cheerio with the thumb and index finger. These movements improve at the same time as gross motor skills and are often learned and practiced in a school or day care setting. It is important to learn and practice motor skills. Beginning in the initiation phase (discussed later in this chapter), children should be encouraged to run, play tag, throw, and catch a ball and participate in various sports to strengthen their motor skills—both gross and fine. The least-active child usually demonstrates the lowest number of quality motor skills. Also, by practicing various exercises that improve motor skills, children can improve their confidence and decrease their chances of experiencing anxiety and depression as a result of not fitting in (Skinner and Piek, 2001).

Motor skill development begins very early in life, becomes more pronounced during the initiation stage (6-10 years of age), is enhanced during the athletic formation stage (11-14 years of age), and is perfected during the specialization stage (15-18 years of age) and into the high-performance stage. The development of motor skills leads to advanced coordination of all fitness components, including strength, aerobic endurance, flexibility, and speed development. What appears to be a simple movement, such as the discus or hammer throw or a slap shot in hockey, is actually a skillful coordination of various muscles and neural patterns that work together to produce a complex movement. There are always hours and years of training behind the statement "He makes it look so easy." At times, athletes and parents focus on training body parts instead of movement patterns. For example, after a short athletic development camp, a young athlete approached us saying how much he enjoyed the discus and shot put events. He always regarded himself as a strong athlete and beat all his friends in arm-wrestling matches. He vowed that the following year he would try out for the track and field team at his school and win the regional championship. Intrigued by his enthusiasm and with his father standing at his side, we asked him what he would do to physically prepare for the events. He responded as expected: "I am going to dedicate myself to building the strongest arms that I can." To the eye, both the shot put and discus throw appear to rely on brute arm strength. In reality, safely and effectively propelling the objects a great distance relies on the strength and power of the legs, hips, and core and on coordinating the precise contraction and relaxation of all muscle groups involved. Such a coordinated motor skill is learned and patterned during hours of dedicated practice.

Coordination is a complex motor skill necessary for high performance. Strength, speed, flexibility, and endurance make up the fitness foundation of high performance, and good coordination is necessary for skill acquisition and perfection. A well-coordinated child will always acquire a skill quickly and be able to perform it smoothly. Compared with a child who might perform a movement with stiffness and difficulty, a well-coordinated young athlete will expend less energy on the same performance. Therefore, good coordination results in more skill effectiveness.

Agility refers to an athlete's ability to quickly and smoothly change directions, move with ease in the field, or fake actions to deceive her direct opponent. Balance is an athlete's ability to maintain and control a body position or steadiness while performing an athletic skill. This is vital not only in gymnastics but also in most team sports, in which the balance of the body and limbs is important in deceiving an opponent or avoiding being deceived by fake actions in the field.

Although these motor skills are largely genetically determined, they are highly trainable. We have designed the games and exercises in this chapter to help young athletes improve coordination, agility, and balance. A young athlete who repetitively performs these skills will over time show better accuracy, timing, and precision and an improvement in overall performance.

The time to train for improved coordination is during the early years, when athletes learn everything quickly. Participating in a well-designed multilateral program during the initiation and athletic formation stages can help young athletes improve their coordination, balance, and agility. Unlike specificity training, a multiskill program will create a solid foundation that will enrich skills and abilities later in one's athletic career, leading to superior performance.

Recognizing the close relationships between strength, speed, and endurance as well as coordination and agility allows both instructor and athlete to understand the multilateral process. The greater an athlete's strength, speed, and endurance, the easier the development of coordination and agility. For example, strength improvement helps athletes to quickly move limbs and change directions. Leg strength, or the ability to powerfully apply force against the ground, will increase speed. Achieving a good strength level will also help young athletes learn skills in sports such as gymnastics, baseball, and skiing. For example, mounting a gymnastics apparatus or learning a skill in which one lifts the whole body is impossible without improving strength. Athletes will also learn batting, pitching, and throwing more quickly if their strength is greater. Most team-sport athletes will greatly benefit from improved strength, coordination, and agility.

Regardless of the level of inherited coordination, one cannot expect consistent gains in this important ability without giving special attention to improvement throughout childhood and adolescence. Multilateral development—the exposure to a variety of skills and exercises—will result in visible coordination gains. The higher the coordination level, the easier it is to learn new and complicated technical and tactical skills. As a result, an athlete will quickly and efficiently adjust to the unusual circumstances of athletic competition.

Initiation Stage—6 to 10 Years of Age

Children in the initiation stage should participate in low-intensity training programs that emphasize fun. Most young children are not capable of coping with the physical and psychological demands of high-intensity training or organized competitions. Training programs for these young athletes must focus on overall athletic development and not sport-specific performance.

During this stage, the body is growing at a steady rate and larger muscle groups are more developed than smaller ones. The cardiorespiratory system is developing and aerobic capacity is adequate for most activities. Anaerobic capacities, however, are limited at this stage as children have low tolerance for lactic acid accumulation. Body tissues are susceptible to injury. Ligaments are becoming stronger, but the bone ends are still cartilaginous and calcifying.

Attention span is short at this age and children are action oriented; thus, they cannot sit and listen for long periods of time. It is especially important for training at this stage to be varied and creative. Participation and fun should be emphasized over winning.

The following guidelines will help an instructor design training programs that are suitable for young athletes in this stage.

- Emphasize multilateral development by introducing a wide variety of skills and exercises, including running, jumping, catching, throwing, batting, balancing, and rolling.
- Provide every child with enough time to adequately develop skills and with equal playing time in games and activities.
- Positively reinforce children who are committed and self-disciplined. Reinforce improvements in skill development.
- Encourage children to develop flexibility, coordination, and balance.
- Encourage children to develop various motor abilities in low-intensity environments. For example, swimming is a terrific environment for developing the cardiorespiratory system while minimizing the stresses on joints, ligaments, and connective tissues.
- Select a suitable number of repetitions for each skill, and encourage children to perform each technique correctly.
- Modify the equipment and playing environment to a suitable level. For example, children do not have the strength to shoot an adult-size basketball into a 10-foot-high (3 m) basket using correct technique. The ball should be smaller and lighter and the basket should be lower.
- Design drills, games, and activities to maximize children's opportunities for active participation.
- Promote experiential learning by giving children opportunities to design their drills, games, and activities. Encourage them to be creative and use their imaginations.
- Simplify or modify rules so children understand the game.
- Introduce modified games that emphasize basic tactics and strategies. For example, if children have developed basic individual skills such as running, dribbling a ball with the feet, and kicking a ball, they will likely be ready to successfully play a modified game of soccer. During the game, you could introduce the young athletes to situations that demonstrate the importance of teamwork and position play. House leagues where kids are able to play with other children their age are ideal for this age group, as the children learn to practice their skills in a team environment.
- Encourage children to participate in drills that develop attention control to prepare them for the greater demands of training and competition that occur in the athletic formation stage of development.
- Emphasize the importance of ethics and fair play.
- Provide opportunities for boys and girls to participate together.
- Make sure that sport is fun.
- Encourage participation in as many sports as possible.

The initiation stage is the most important phase in developing coordination. This is why it is also called the rapid gain phase. This occurs irrespective of whether a child participates in organized and supervised sport activities or simply plays with peers. At this developmental stage, children who are involved in a variety of activities make greater gains in coordination compared with those who participate in one sport that applies only sport-specific training. Multilateral training that exposes children to numerous skills, drills, games, relays, and other exercises enriches their skill experience and, as a result, improves their coordination dramatically.

During prepubescence, children develop basic skills and movements through play and games. As they participate in various physical activities, they also develop the ability to distinguish between simple and complex skills and exercises. For instance, prepubertal children will learn to dribble a basketball with their better hand. As they grow and become more comfortable with this skill, they also learn to dribble with the opposite hand. The next step in highly coordinated and agile dribbling is to dribble between the legs with both the left and right hands. As skill improves, the player will also learn how to defend against a highly coordinated opponent or how to get the ball from someone whose skills might not be as good as his own.

Athletes also improve other elements of coordination during prepubescence, such as the feel and perception for an activity, thus enhancing their learning potential. Similar gains are visible in developing rhythm—reproducing a series of movements with regularity and pacing—as in dance and artistic sports. Visible improvements also occur in timing, or the ability to time reactions to the moves of a partner or an opposing player. These actions also benefit from improvement in visual orientation to the surrounding environment, which allows the athlete to sense the actions and maneuvers of teammates and the opposition.

Athletic Formation—11 to 14 Years of Age

It is appropriate to moderately increase the intensity of training during the athletic formation stage of development. Although most athletes are still vulnerable to injuries, their bodies and capacities are rapidly developing. During this stage, the cardiorespiratory system continues to develop and tolerance to lactic acid accumulation gradually improves.

It is important to understand that variances in individual performance may be the result of differences in growth. Some athletes may be experiencing a rapid growth spurt, which can explain why they lack coordination during particular drills. To account for this, emphasize developing skills and motor abilities rather than performing and winning.

The following guidelines will help an instructor design training programs that are appropriate for the athletic formation stage.

- Encourage participation in a variety of exercises from the specific sport and from other sports, which will help the athletes improve their multilateral base and prepare them for competition in their selected sport. Progressively increase the volume and intensity of training.
- Design drills that introduce athletes to fundamental tactics and strategies and that reinforce skill development.
- Help athletes refine and automate the basic skills they learned during the initiation stage and learn skills that are slightly more complex.
- Emphasize improving flexibility, coordination, and balance.
- Emphasize ethics and fair play during training sessions and competitions.

- Provide all children with opportunities to participate at a challenging level.
- Introduce the athletes to exercises that develop general strength. Athletes should begin developing the foundation for future strength and power during this stage. Emphasize developing the core sections of the body—in particular the hips, lower back, and abdomen—as well as muscles at the extremities—shoulder joints, arms, and legs. Most exercises should involve body weight and light equipment, such as medicine balls, resistance bands, and light dumbbells. Refer to chapter 7 for multilateral strength programs.
- Continue developing aerobic capacity. A solid endurance base will enable athletes to cope more effectively with the demands of training and competition during the specialization stage.
- Introduce athletes to moderate anaerobic training, which is new to athletes in the athletic formation stage. This will help them adapt to high-intensity anaerobic training, which takes on greater importance in most sports during the specialization stage. Athletes should not compete in events that place excessive stress on the anaerobic lactic acid energy system, such as the 200-meter sprint and 400-meter dash in track and field. They are usually better suited for short sprints of less than 80 meters, which involve the anaerobic alactic energy system, and endurance events of longer distances (e.g., 800 meters and longer) at slower speeds, which test aerobic capacities.
- Avoid competitions that place too much stress on the body. For example, most young athletes do not have sufficient muscular development to perform a triple jump with the correct technique. As a result, some may experience compression injuries from the shock that the body must absorb somewhere during the stepping and hopping segments of the jump.
- To improve concentration, introduce athletes to more complex drills. Encourage them to develop strategies for self-regulation and visualization. Introduce formalized mental training.
- Introduce athletes to a variety of fun competitive situations that allow them to apply various techniques and tactics. Young athletes like to compete; however, it is important to de-emphasize winning. Structure competitions to reinforce skill development. For example, base the objective of a javelin-throwing competition on accuracy and technique rather than on how far athletes can throw the javelin.
- Provide time for play and socializing with peers.

The fast improvement in coordination that occurs during prepubescence sometimes slows or even slightly regresses during pubescence. Growth spurts of up to four or five inches (10-12 cm) per year, specific to this stage of children's development, normally occur with disturbances in coordination. This is mostly because limb growth, especially in the legs, changes the proportions between body parts and their leverage and, consequently, the ability to coordinate their actions proficiently.

Although these trends are evident in all children, those who practice sport continue to gain in the quality of coordination compared with those who do not. During pubescence, balance and the accuracy and timing of physical actions continue to improve in these children. Girls tend to improve visual orientation and rhythm of motions better than boys because of sex differences and because girls have a more natural talent for dance and artistic sports.

Differences in coordination abilities are also visible between early- and late-maturing children. Early maturers go through a slight coordination crisis, which may temporarily affect the fine coordination of physical actions (Sharma and Hirtz, 1991). Consequently, because of their fast rhythm of physical growth, early maturers need more exercises for coordination improvement than do late maturers. The key is to introduce a variety of exercises that require balance, changes in rhythm, and spatial orientation. The athletes should feel that they are in control of the exercise if improvements are to be made. Choosing exercises that are too easy or too difficult for the athletes will stunt progress. The best program for improving coordination includes a variety of exercises and games that are at the skill level of the individual athletes or groups of athletes.

Specialization—15 to 18 Years of Age

Athletes in the specialization stage are capable of tolerating greater training and competition demands compared with those in earlier stages. The most significant changes in training take place during this stage. Athletes who have been participating in a well-rounded program emphasizing multilateral development will now start performing more exercises and drills aimed specifically at high performance development in one sport. Closely monitor the volume and intensity of training to ensure that athletes improve dramatically with little risk of injury. Toward the end of this athletic development stage the athletes should have no major technical problems. Thus, the coach can move from a teaching role to a coaching and training role.

The following guidelines will help an instructor design training programs that are suitable for athletes who specialize in a particular sport.

- Closely monitor the development of athletes during this stage. They will be developing strategies for coping with the increased physical and psychological demands of training and competition. They are also vulnerable to experiencing physical and psychological difficulties from overtraining.
- As competition and the demands of the sport increase, so will the athletes' self-awareness. Top-level athletes in the league may develop a superiority complex, whereas those who struggle to keep up with the demands of competition may begin to isolate themselves and undermine their skills. It is important that coaches provide an environment that enables team cohesiveness and ensures that all players understand the unique abilities each brings to the team. This provides an opportunity for the skilled players to mentor those who are struggling and allows the late bloomers to find their groove. Given the opportunity, those who struggled early on can become the superstars.
- A coach who feels that an athlete needs more practice in a particular skill or dominant motor ability can suggest that the athlete practice a couple of extra hours per week. Parents are more than willing to do what it takes to help their children reach full potential in sport.
- Check for progressive improvements in the dominant motor abilities for the sport, such as power, anaerobic capacity, specific coordination, and dynamic flexibility.
- Increase the training volume for specific exercises and drills to facilitate improvement in performance. The body must adapt to specific training load increments to effectively prepare for competition; therefore, now is the time to stress specificity.
- Then, increase training intensity more rapidly than volume, although volume must still increase progressively. Prepare athletes to perform a particular skill, exercise, or drill with the appropriate rhythm and speed. Training should closely simulate the actions that take place during competition. Although fatigue is a normal outcome

of high-intensity training, it is important that athletes do not reach the state of exhaustion.

- Involve athletes in the decision-making process whenever possible.
- Continue to emphasize multilateral training, particularly during the preseason. However, it is more important to emphasize specificity and to use training methods and techniques that develop a high level of sport-specific efficiency, particularly during the competitive season.
- Encourage athletes to become familiar with the theoretical aspects of training.
- Emphasize exercising the muscles that athletes primarily use when performing technical skills (i.e., prime movers). Strength development should start to reflect the specific needs of the sport. Athletes who are weight training can start performing exercises that require fewer repetitions and a heavier weight. Avoid maximum strength training, in which athletes perform fewer than four repetitions of an exercise, particularly for those who are still growing.
- Make developing aerobic capacity a high priority for all athletes, particularly those who participate in endurance or endurance-related sports.
- Progressively increase the volume and intensity of anaerobic training. In this stage, athletes are capable of coping with lactic acid accumulation.
- Improve and perfect the techniques of the sport. Select specific exercises that will ensure the athletes are performing the skills in a manner that is biomechanically correct and physiologically efficient. Athletes should perform difficult technical skills frequently during training sessions, incorporate them into specific tactical drills, and apply them in competitions.
- Improve individual and team tactics. Incorporate game-specific drills into tactical training sessions. Select drills that are interesting, challenging, and stimulating and that require quick decision making, fast action, prolonged concentration, and a high level of motivation from the athletes. Athletes should demonstrate initiative, self-control, competitive vigor, and ethics and fair play in competitive situations.
- Increase the number of competitions progressively so that by the end of this stage the athletes are competing as frequently as senior-level competitors. It is also important to set objectives for competitions that focus on developing specific skills, tactics, and motor abilities. Although winning becomes increasingly important, do not overemphasize it.
- Athletes should practice mental training. Incorporate drills and exercises that develop concentration, attention control, positive thinking, self-regulation, visualization, and motivation to enhance sport-specific performance.

As children approach adolescence, coordination does not develop at the same rate as it does during prepuberty. Children's ability to synchronize movements slightly improves after the growth spurts of puberty and culminates during postpuberty, when improvement in coordination is constant. Athletes fare much better than nonathletes, who often look awkward if they perform unfamiliar moves.

Despite the concentration on sport-specific training at this stage, postpubescent athletes should still practice a variety of skills, train for multilateral activities, and pay attention to continuing coordination development. To ignore this and focus only on specific training may stop the improvements in coordination that are crucial for perfecting the skills required for the selected sport. That's why, as discussed in chapter 1, it's important that multilateral training composes 20 percent of an athlete's program during the specialization phase.

Designing a Program

The main objectives of coordination training are to be able to perform increasingly complex skills and exercises and to improve skill acquisition. Parents and instructors should expose young athletes to the basic skills of sprinting, jumping, throwing, catching, balancing, climbing, gymnastics, and swimming. As athletes acquire these skills, they can improve coordination by extending the complexity of skills and exercises and by enhancing the difficulty of performing them. At the same time, instructors should teach the athletes new skills from the selected sport or other sports, progressively demanding higher quality performance. As mentioned earlier, coordination proficiency and learning ability may plateau if the athletes do not constantly challenge themselves but rather perform the same skills all the time.

The form of the training program for coordination is simpler than that of the other training programs in this book. Because improvements in coordination are difficult to measure, no specific training methods exist for measuring the load or number of sets and repetitions for coordination exercises.

Table 2.1 suggests a long-term, comprehensive periodization model for coordination, agility, balance, and skills. Exercises become more challenging as the athlete progresses

Table 2.1 Periodization Model for Motor Skills Training

Stage of development	Form of training	Exercises
Initiation	Preparatory exercises for skill acquisition	• Rolling • Kicking • Throwing • Dribbling • Catching
	Simple balance	• Walking on narrow lines • Jumping onto and off of low objects
	Simple rhythm and reaction time	• Catching
	Simple spatial orientation and sense of body and limb position	• Crawling and rolling • Front somersault • Throwing • Catching
	Simple hand–eye coordination	• Dribbling • Throwing • Catching
	Skill-enhancing exercises	• Ball exercises • Ball exercises with partner • Ball hits and throws • Catching skills • Rebounding ball catch • Dribbling • Relays
	Advanced balance exercises	• Scissors-kick handstand • Backward roll • Cartwheel • Cartwheel against the wall

Stage of development	Form of training	Exercises
Athletic formation	Advanced hand–eye coordination	• Ball throws and catches • Ball hits • Rebounding ball catches
	Limbs coordination	• Coordination for limbs • Skipping rope • Ball throws and catches
	Advanced spatial orientation	• Skipping rope • Backward roll • Scissors-kick handstand • Cartwheel
	Signal analysis and reaction to various stimuli	• Handstands • Ball exercises with partner • Games • Relays
	Advanced hand–eye coordination	• Jumps with turns and ball throws • Games • Relays
Specialization	Skill perfection	• Rolls and rotations • Ball throws and catch games • Relays
	Complex spatial orientation	• Jumps with turns • Games • Jumps over objects • Rolls and jumps
	Balance, body control, and body awareness	• Rolls and turns • Jumps over objects and turns • All variations of body balance • Games • Relays
	Anticipation improvement	• Rolls and turns • Throws and catches with partner • Balance exercises • Games
	Analysis and reorientation	• Rolls and turns of 180-360 degrees • Rolls, ball throws, and catches • Games • Relays

Note: Refer to exercises at the end of this chapter.

through each development stage. During the initiation and athletic formation stages, the coach tries to develop the main elements of coordination. This will eventually lead the athletes to a sport-specific form of training in later stages that includes complex, performance-oriented activities. The model does not pretend to exhaust all the possibilities. Rather, use it as a guideline that enriches your experience and expertise.

Table 2.2 Sample Workout for Prepuberty

Part	Scope	Forms of training	Duration (min)
1	Warm-up	• Jogging • Stretching	5
2	Coordination and balance	• Preparation for skill acquisition • Hand–eye coordination • Spatial orientation • Simple balance	10-15
3	Play, game	Skill acquisition from the chosen sport	20-30
4	Cool-down	• 2-3 relays • Easy stretching	5

Note: See table 2.1 for examples of exercises for each form of training.

Exposing children to coordination exercises in the early years (i.e., prepuberty) of athletic development is essential to skill acquisition. Good coordination will make a child learn a skill faster, which will translate into better performance in their late teens. This is why it is crucial during prepuberty and puberty to include exercises for developing coordination, balance, spatial orientation, and body awareness (e.g., those in table 2.2) in every physical activity. Because many of the suggested exercises are simple, coaches, teachers, or parents can incorporate them in any formal training session they organize in a backyard, basement, or playground.

All age groups should do 10 to 15 minutes of coordination, agility, and balance work at every workout. It should be done in the early part of a training session, such as immediately after the warm-up, because children learn best when they are fresh. Table 2.2 shows an example of a typical workout for the initiation phase. As children improve in coordination or grow older, increase the difficulty of the coordination and balance exercises.

Some exercises that we suggest for the initiation or athletic formation phases could be used during the specialization phase as well. Select exercises according to the individual's abilities and athletic potential. For the more difficult exercises such as a somersault, cartwheel, or jumps, children need assistance and support from a parent or instructor to avoid discomfort or injury. It is important to constantly follow a good progression. Simple exercises should lead to more complex ones (e.g., learn the target kick first and then the foot dribble), and familiar exercises should lead to unfamiliar ones (e.g., the athlete can progress from a cartwheel to a handstand).

Exercises and Skills

Although performance on the motor skills described throughout this chapter is largely genetically determined, the skills are highly trainable. We have designed the games and exercises in this chapter to help young athletes improve coordination, agility, and balance. Young athletes who repetitively perform these skills over time will show better accuracy, timing, and precision and an improvement in overall performance.

To make this book practical for all users, we suggest several exercises that each athlete should perform. Athletes can perform most of the exercises at home or outdoors, but some they must perform in a gym or fitness club. An adult should always supervise children during exercise. These exercises do not exhaust all that are available in the field; however, they will develop coordination in the basic skills of jumping, batting, dribbling, kicking a ball, and so on using a variety of equipment such as reaction balls (a basic rubber ball that children play with), baseballs, and medicine balls. Medicine balls are so named because they have been used in therapeutic medicine and rehabilitation for more than 100 years. The best medicine balls are made of rubber. Some medicine balls have one or two handles and can bounce. They are available in different sizes and weigh between 3 and 14 pounds (1.3 and 6 kg).

Front Somersault

Focus: coordination, agility, body awareness

1. Squat with the arms extended in front of the body.
2. Place the hands on the floor, tuck the head, bend the elbows, and slowly extend the knees for a forward front roll, keeping the back rounded.
3. When the roll is complete, bend the knees to end up in a squatting position.

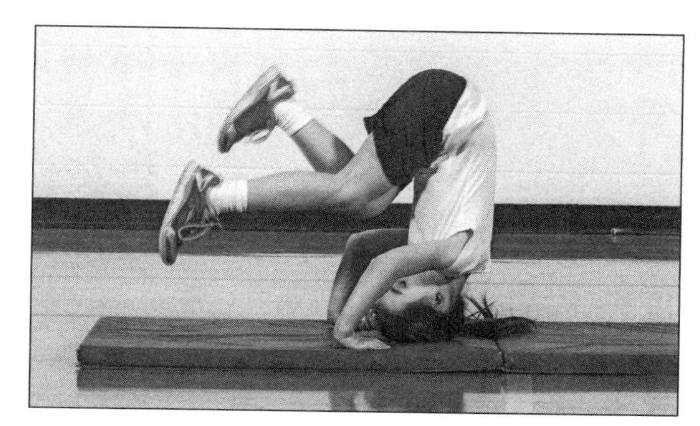

Basketball Dribbling

Focus: hand–eye coordination, timing

1. Begin in a standing, kneeling, or sitting position.
2. Perform two-hand dribbling and then one-hand dribbling.

Variation

Dribble the ball back and forth with a partner.

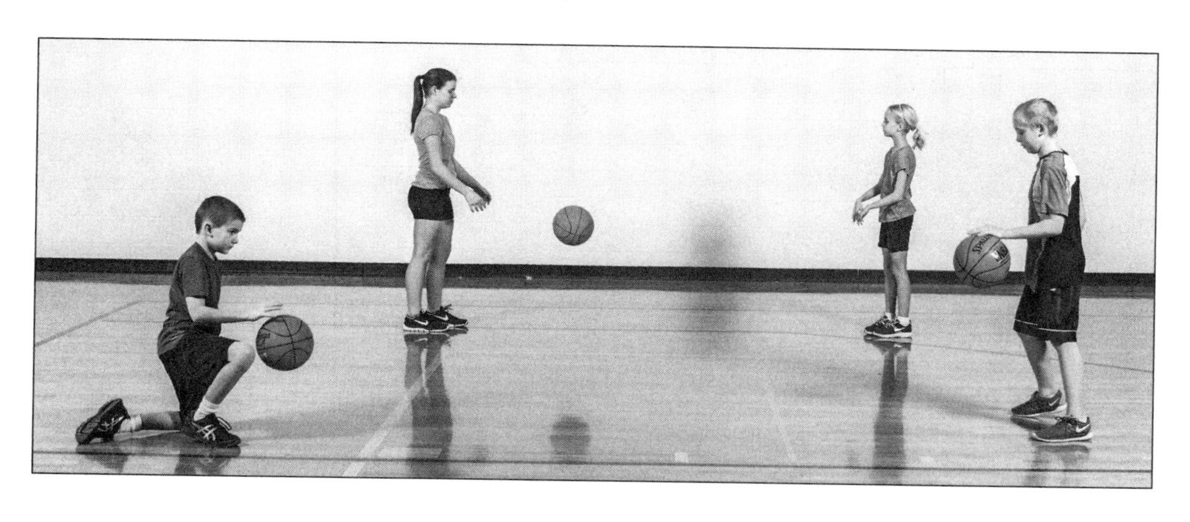

Target Kick

Focus: coordination, awareness (distance, direction), passing and kicking accuracy

1. Begin in a standing position.
2. Kick the ball, with each leg alternately, toward the target (e.g., another ball, a cone, and so on).

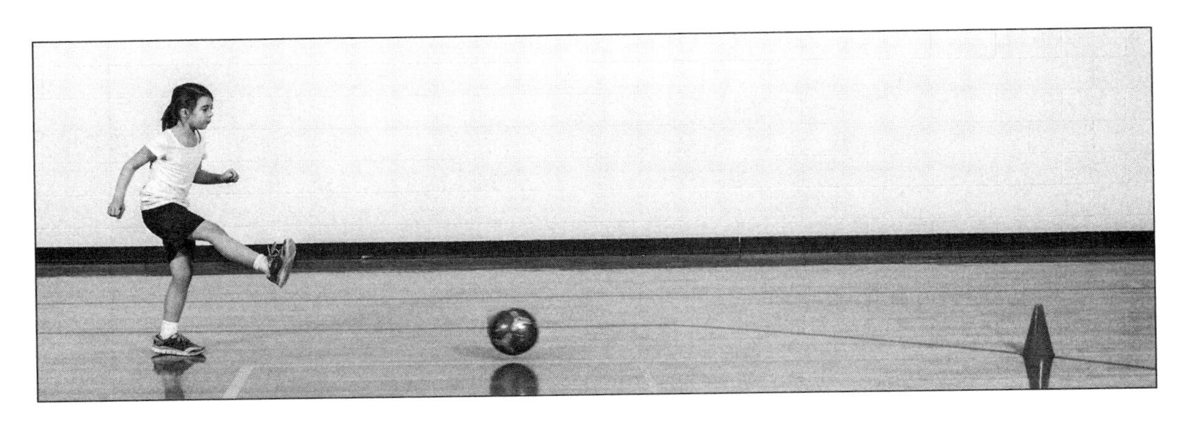

Foot Dribble

Focus: leg–eye coordination

1. Stand with the ball on the ground in front of one foot.
2. Dribble the ball forward, sideways, with both feet, and with both sides of the foot.

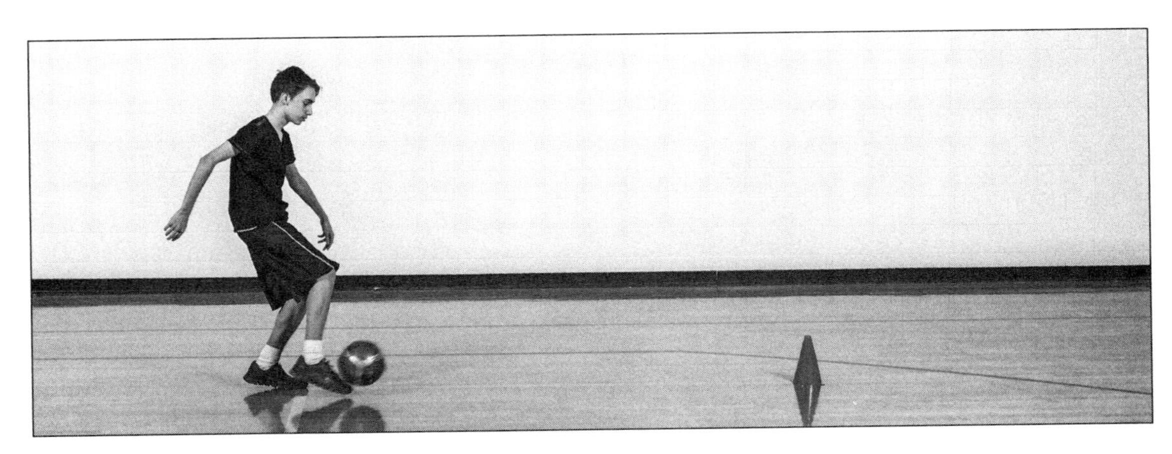

Coordination for Limbs

Focus: limb coordination

1. Stand with the arms at the sides.
2. Circle both arms forward (figure *a*).
3. Circle both arms backward.

Variations

- Circle one arm at a time in both directions.
- Circle the left arm forward while circling the right arm backward (figure *b*).

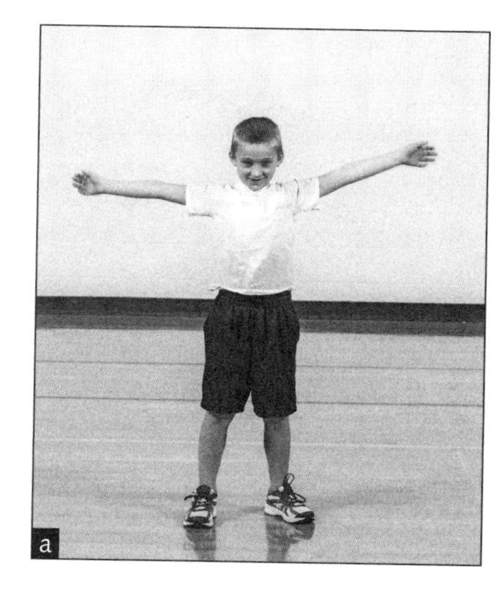

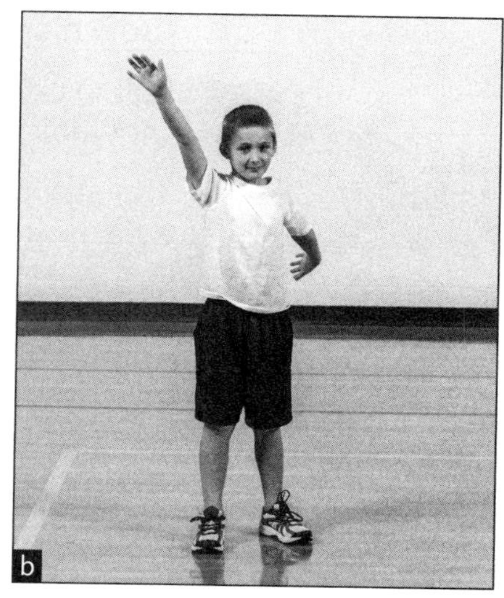

Skipping Rope

Focus: limb coordination

1. Stand holding one end of the rope in each hand.
2. Do continuous jumping. Keep arms close to the body and rotate arms in a forward circular position while performing small continuous jumps.

Variations

- High tuck jumps. Keep arms close to the body and rotate arms in a forward circular position while jumping higher and lifting knees high off the ground to jump over rope.
- Jump on one foot; repeat using the other foot. Perform small jumps on one foot and alternate to other leg.
- Straight jumps, crossing the arms. When skipping with arms close to body using small jumps, cross arms in front of body while rotating arms forward while continuing skipping motion.

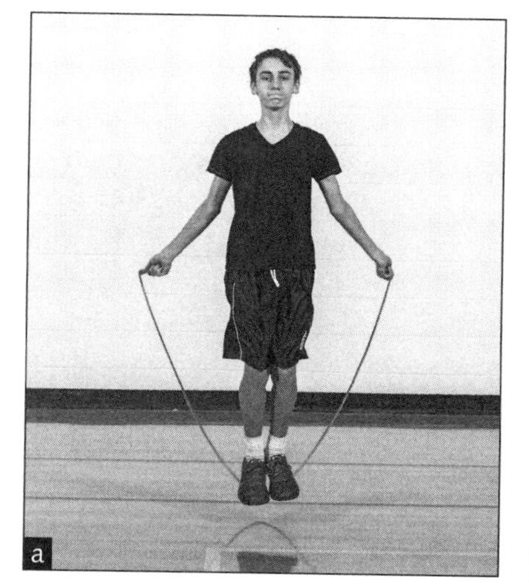

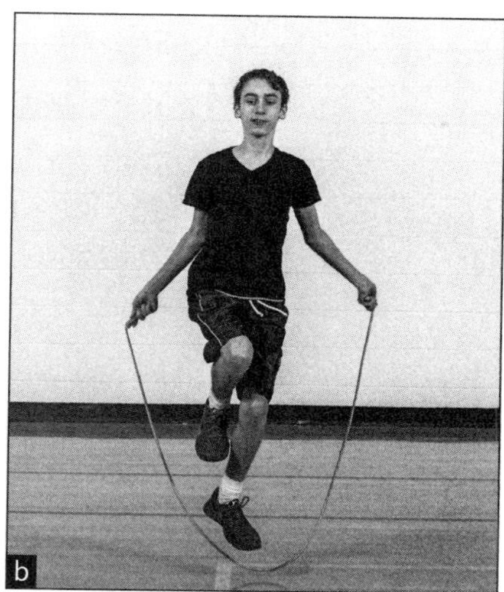

Backward Roll

Focus: limb coordination, spatial orientation

1. Crouch down and grab the knees with both hands.
2. Roll backward onto the back, palms ready to be placed on the floor below the shoulders.
3. Straighten the legs, touch the toes, and then push with the arms to complete a backward roll into a squat position.

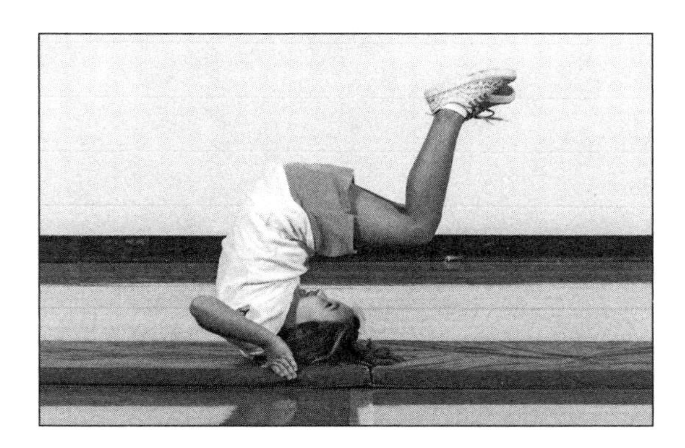

Scissors-Kick Handstand

Focus: balance, spatial orientation

1. Stand with arms above the head and one leg extended in front of the body.
2. Step forward, placing the hands on the floor. Keeping the arms straight, kick one leg up and then kick the other leg up. Bring the first leg down and then the second leg down and resume a standing position.

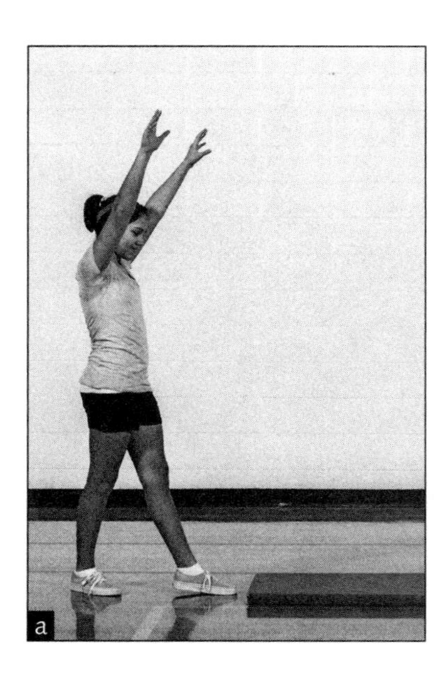
a

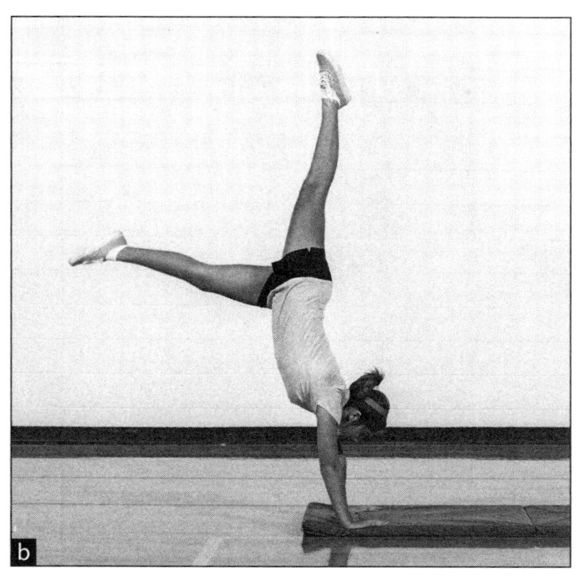
b

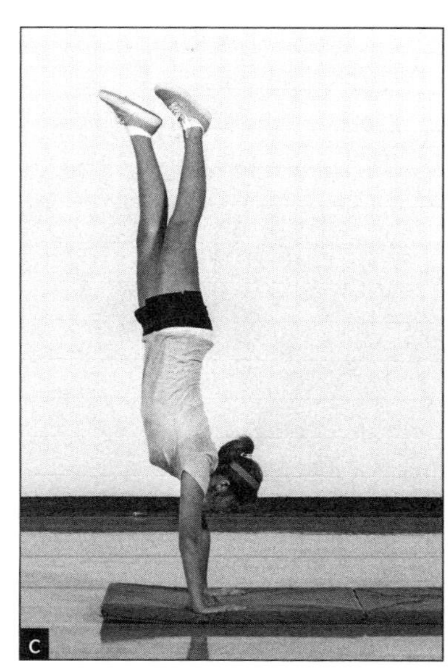
c

Cartwheel

Focus: balance, spatial orientation

1. Stand with the feet apart and arms extended above body.
2. Lower the hands to the floor and, keeping the arms straight, kick the legs up and over the hands.
3. Bring the first leg down and then the second leg. End in a standing position similar to how you started the movement with the legs apart, but facing the opposite direction.

Variation

Cartwheel against a wall and then cartwheel back down.

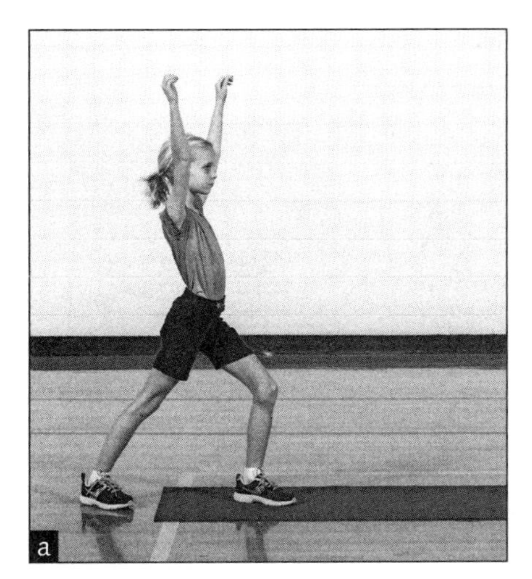
a

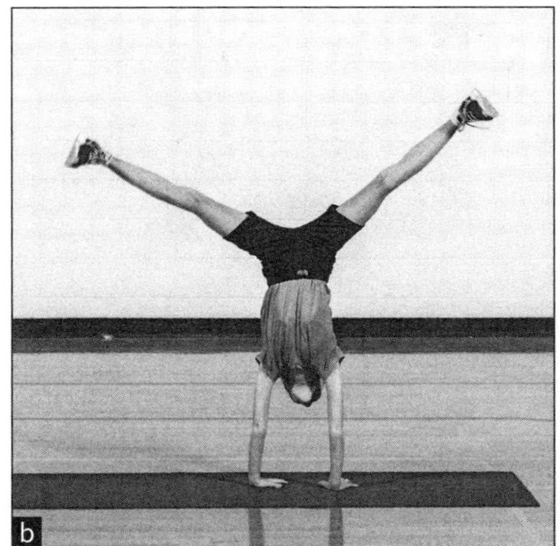
b

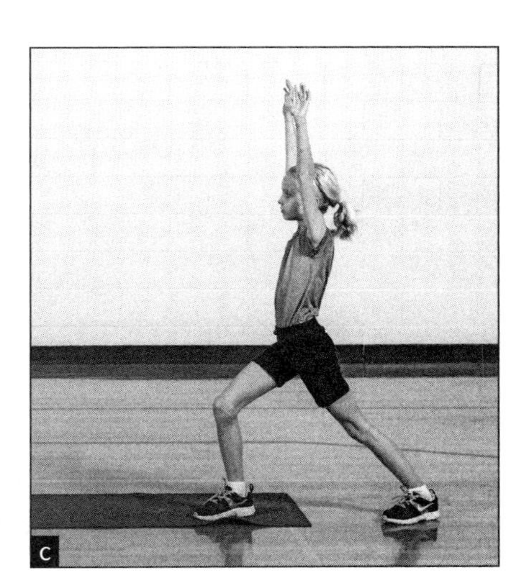
c

Behind Overhead Throw

Focus: skill, hand–eye coordination

1. Stand with the feet apart. Hold the ball behind the buttocks.
2. Bend the body forward at the hips and throw the ball up and forward.
3. Extend the body and catch the ball above the head.

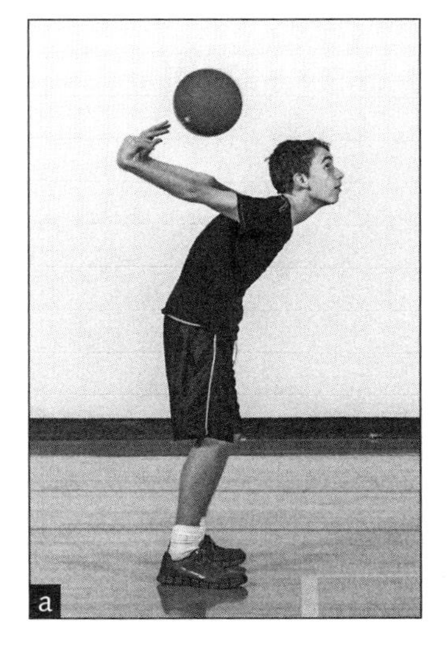
a

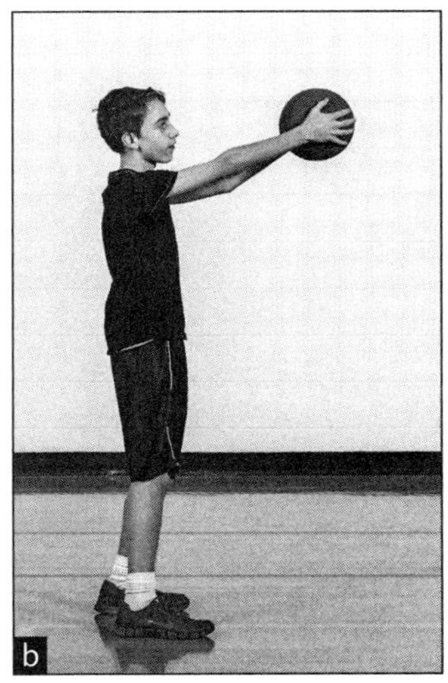
b

Between-Leg Throw

Focus: skill enhancement, hand–eye coordination

1. Partners stand facing each other about 10 feet (3 m) apart.
2. Partner A bounces the ball between the legs to partner B.
3. Partner B catches the ball and bounces the ball between the legs back to partner A.

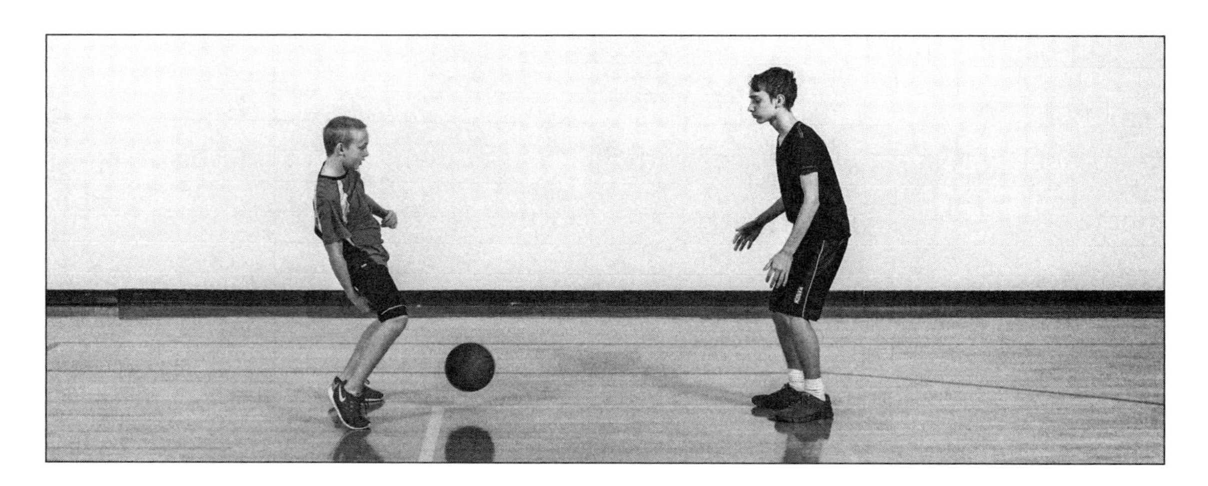

Overhand Simultaneous Throw

Focus: hand–eye coordination

1. Partners stand facing each other two to four feet (.6-1.2 m) apart. Each partner holds a ball in one hand.
2. Each partner simultaneously bounces the ball to the other partner.
3. Each partner catches the ball in the opposite hand.
4. Each partner then bounces the ball back to the other partner using the hand that caught the ball (i.e., the opposite hand).

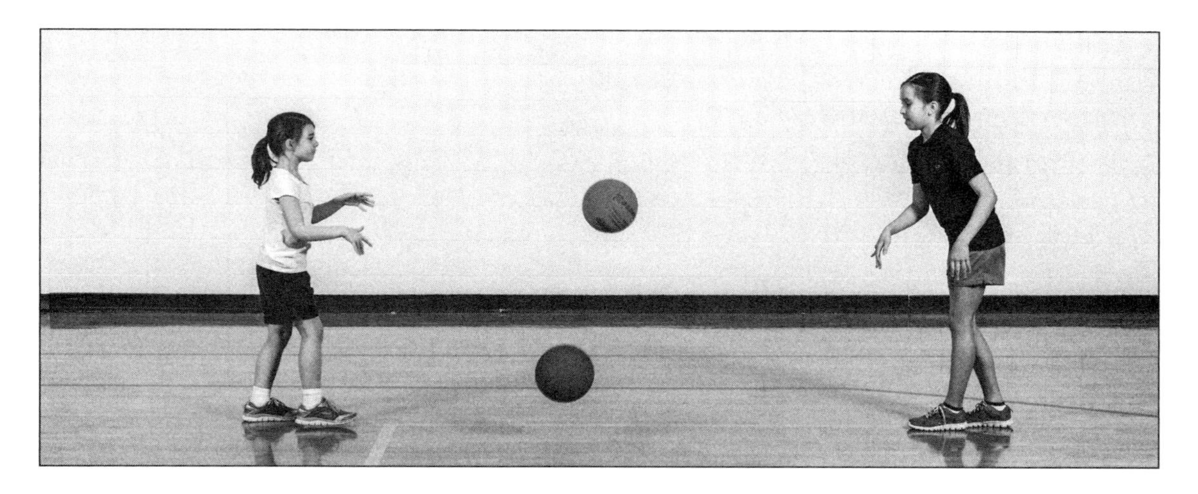

Rebounding Ball Catch

Focus: hand–eye coordination, throwing and catching accuracy

1. Stand in front of a wall or wooden fence.
2. Throw the ball against the wall, let it rebound off the ground, and catch it.

Variations

- Throw the ball against the ground, let it rebound off the wall, and catch it.
- Two players: Rebound toward the wall and then toward the player who catches it.
- Throw the ball against the wall and catch it without letting it rebound.
- Perform the rebound against wall and catch the ball with one hand.

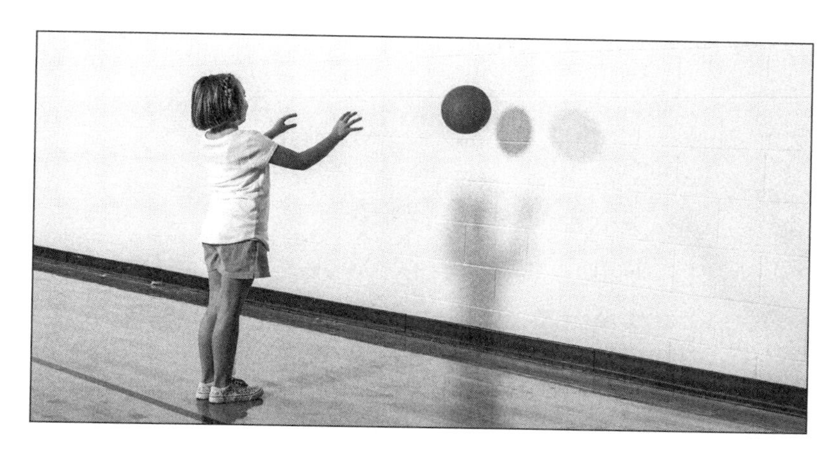

Two-Hand Chest and Overhead Pass

Focus: hand–eye coordination, passing and catching accuracy

1. Two rows of players stand facing each other 10 to 15 feet (3-4.5 m) apart. One partner holds a ball.
   - Two-hand chest pass: Stand with arms bent and hold ball at chest level. Extend arms and push the ball forward.
   - Overhead Pass: Stand with arms over head and bent with ball behind head. Extend arms forward and throw the ball forward.

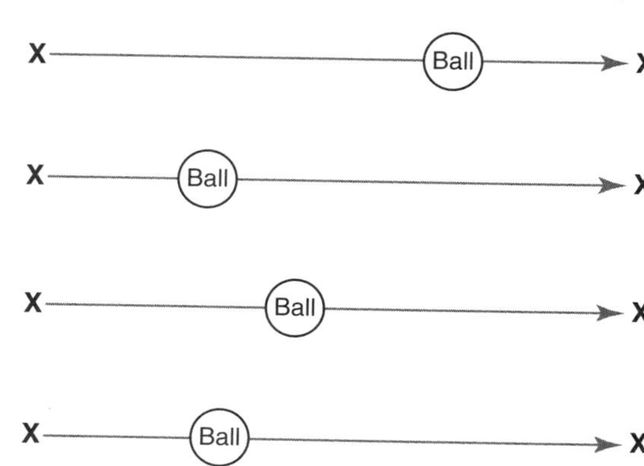

2. The player with the ball passes the ball toward a player in the opposite row. The player catches the ball and then passes it back to the player in the opposite row.

Variation

Do the same drill above but only use one hand. Alternate hands.

Overhand Zigzag and Target Throw

Focus: hand–eye coordination, throwing accuracy

1. Two rows of players stand facing each other 10 to 15 feet (3-4.5 m) apart. One player holds a ball (e.g., tennis ball, baseball, and so on).
2. Overhand throw toward a player or a target. If using a target, draw a box on an outside wall using chalk or create a target with tape on the wall and toss ball toward target. Retrieve ball and repeat with both hands.

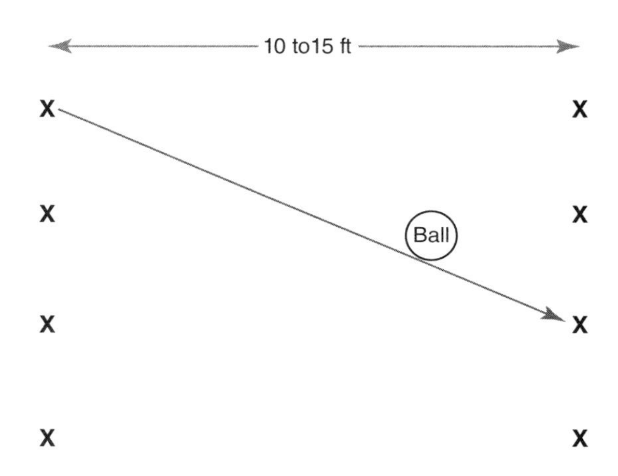

Overhand Throw Relay

Focus: hand–eye coordination, passing accuracy

1. Divide the group into two teams. Players in each group line up one behind the other. One team member from each group stands about 10 feet (3 m) opposite the team, holding a ball.
2. The team member standing opposite the group throws the ball to the first team member standing in line. That team member catches the ball, throws it back to the person who threw it, and sits down at the back of the line.
3. This continues until the whole team is seated. The team that finishes first is the winner.

Note: Make the teams as equally skilled as possible.

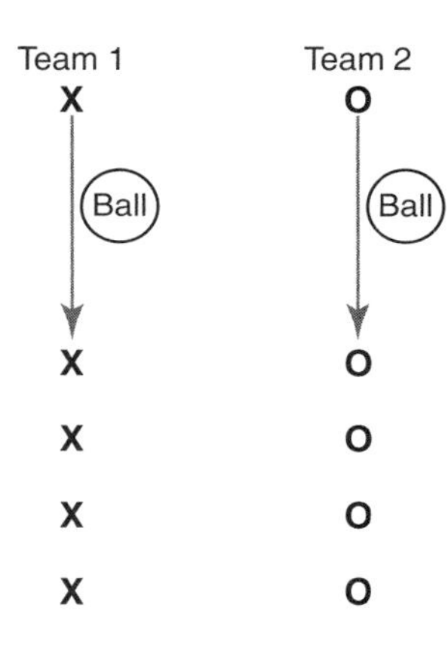

Handstand

Focus: balance, skill

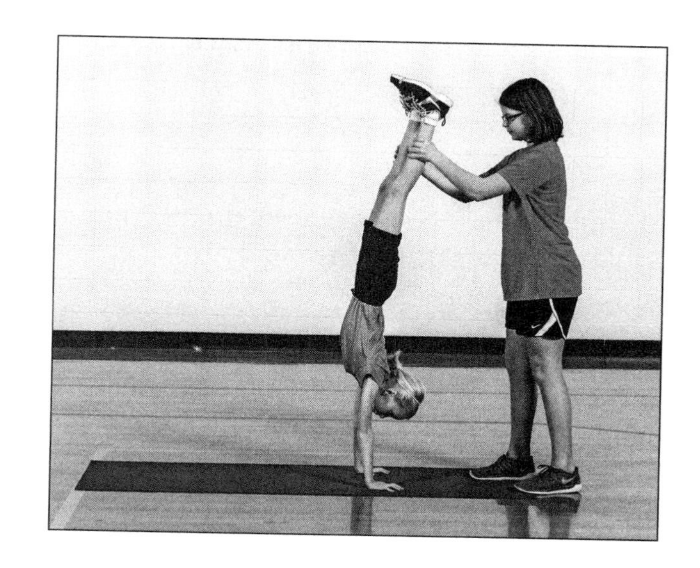

1. Stand facing the instructor.
2. Take a short step forward, extending the arms toward the ground.
3. Kick one leg upward toward the spotter. (The spotter catches the athlete by the shins.)
4. Bring the other leg forward into the handstand position.
5. Return to the starting position.

Rolls With Turns

Focus: balance, spatial orientation

1. From a standing position, perform a front roll to a standing position and jump up performing a half turn to the right side.
2. Stop, repeat front roll and jump to the left side.

Variations

- Perform a front roll, with a jump turn to the right or left side, followed immediately with a back roll with a jump turn to the right or left side. Continuously repeat the movement.
- Perform 3 to 4 forward rolls with jumps continuously in a row.
- Perform the movement with a 360-degree turn. This variation should only be performed when athlete has mastered the forward and back rolls with half turns.

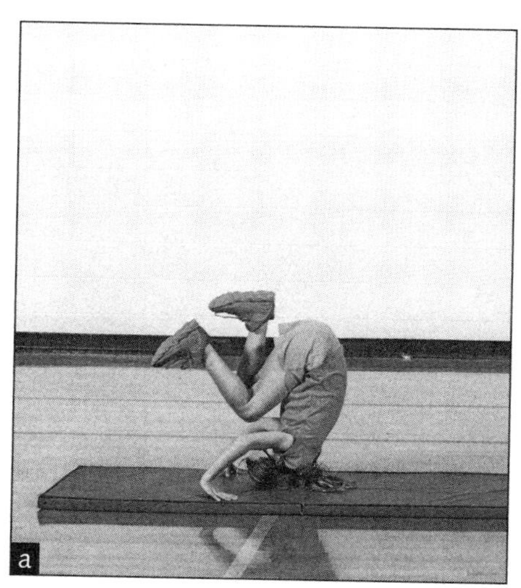
a

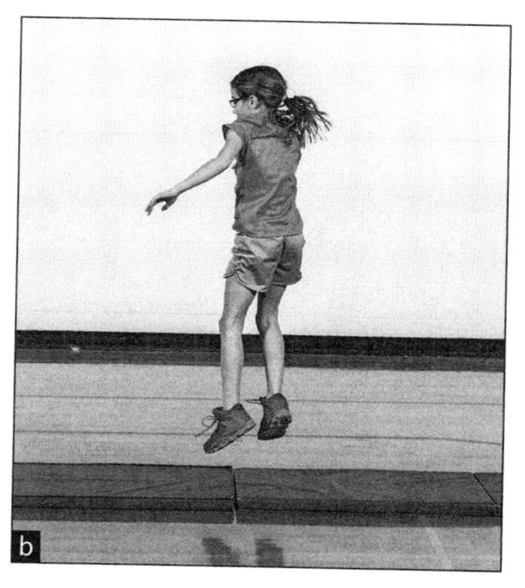
b

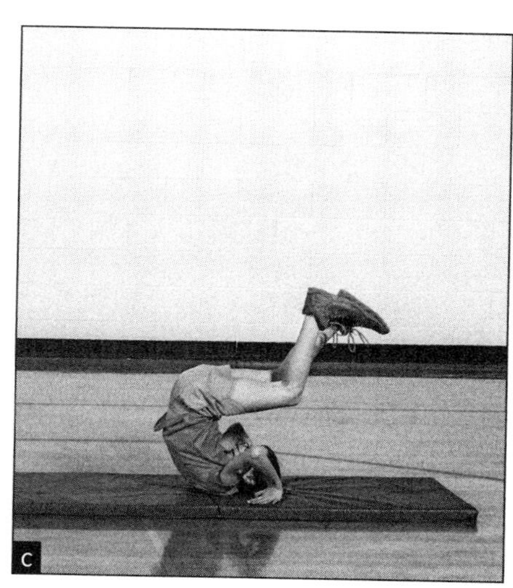
c

Jump and Roll With Turn

Focus: spatial orientation, body control

1. Stand on one side of a rope or ribbon that is suspended parallel to the ground. The height of the rope is dependent on the age and skill level of the athlete. Height can range from inches to a foot off the floor.
2. Jump over the rope. Upon landing, immediately perform a front roll followed by a half turn (180 degrees).
3. Turn around, jump back over the rope, again performing a front roll with a half turn upon landing.

Variation

- Continuously repeat the movement (i.e., jump over the rope, front roll, jump, half turn).

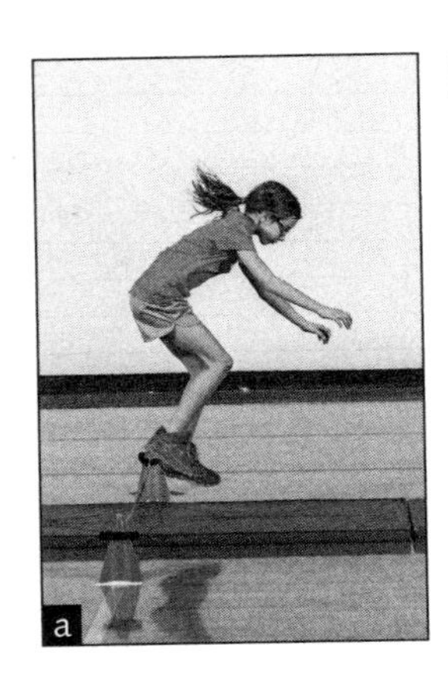
a

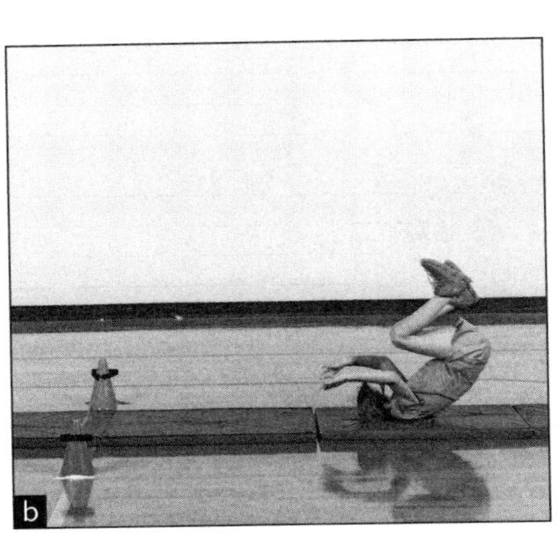
b

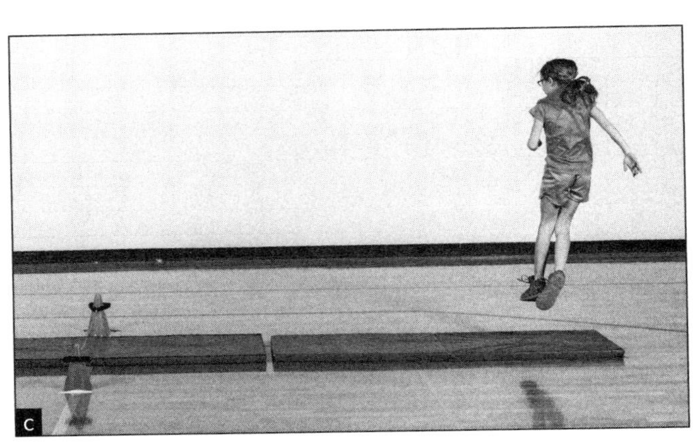
c

Throw, Roll, and Catch

Focus: spatial orientation, body awareness

1. Begin in a standing position, holding a ball.
2. Throw the ball up and forward.
3. Perform a front roll.
4. Catch the ball.

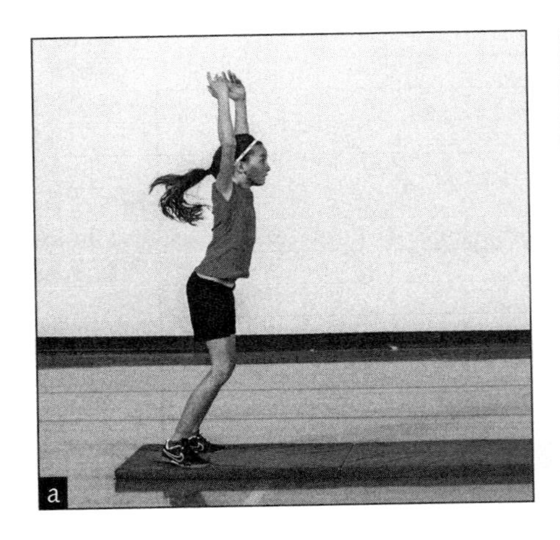
a

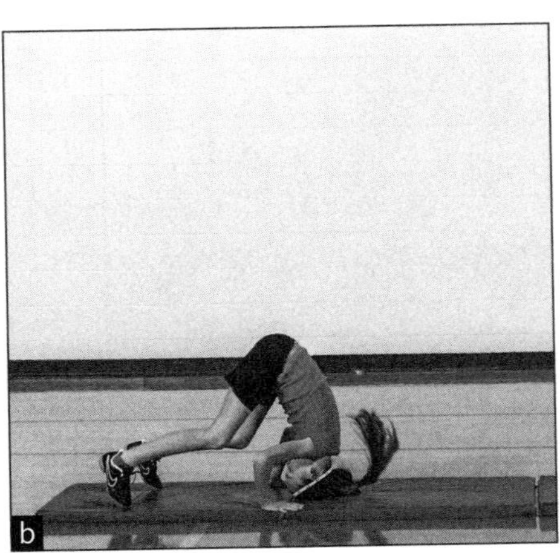
b

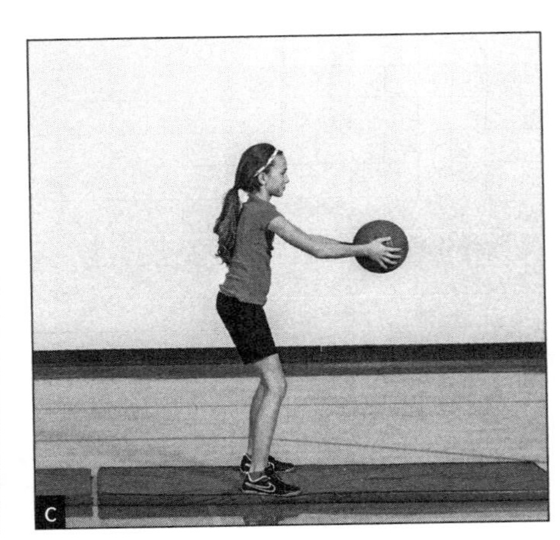
c

Rolling Target

Focus: hand–eye coordination, throwing accuracy

1. Divide the class into small teams. One at a time, each team throws rubber balls at a medicine ball that is rolled across the gym floor. The players must stand behind a designated line and should throw using both the left and right arms.
2. Record each team's score (i.e., number of hits).

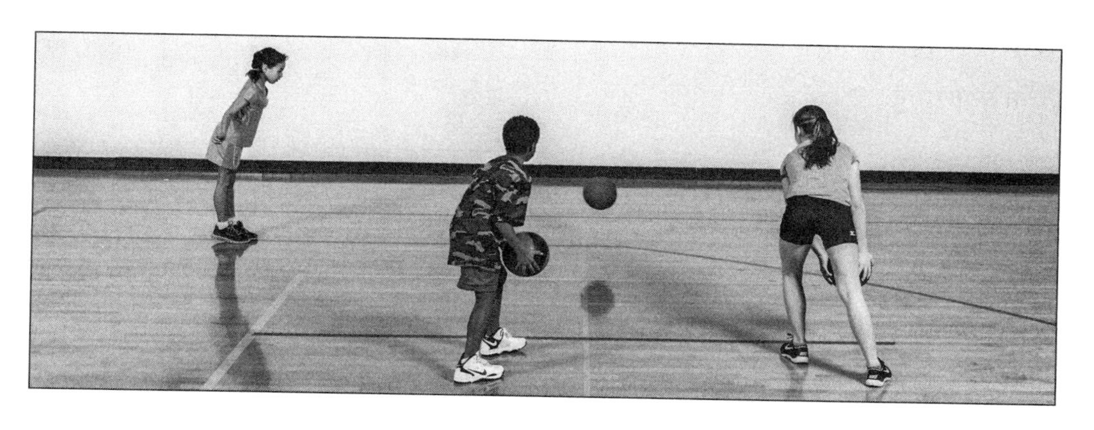

Dodge Game

Focus: hand–eye coordination, throwing accuracy

1. Divide the players into two teams. Each team starts at an opposite wall. Place three balls in the center of the gym.
2. At the start the players dash for the balls. The players who get them first throw from their side of the gym to hit members of the other team. Hit only below the waist.
3. If hit, a player is considered captured and must go stand along the wall on the opponents' side of the gym.
4. If an errant ball comes within reach of a player who has been captured, he may use it to hit an opposing player.
5. The game ends when one entire team has been captured.

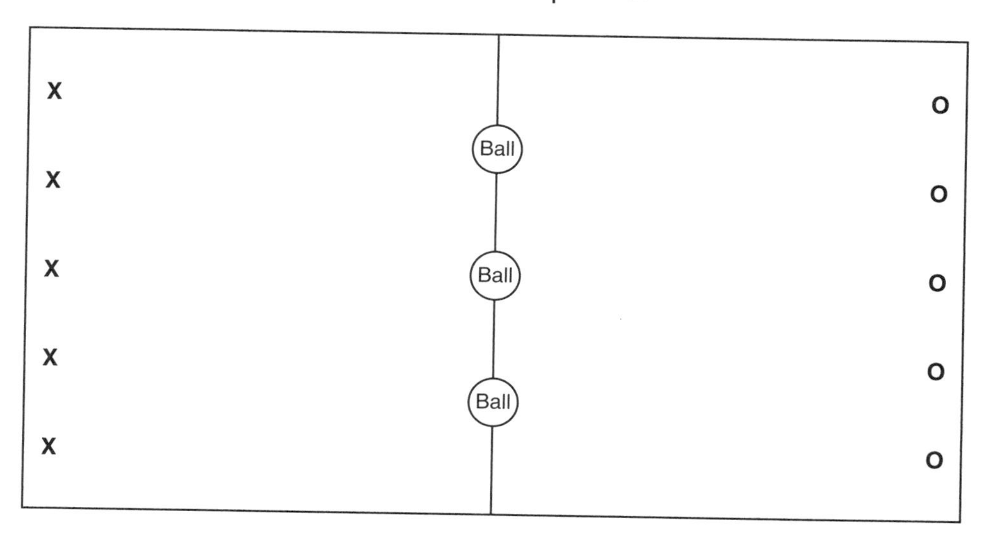

V-Sit Balance

Focus: balance

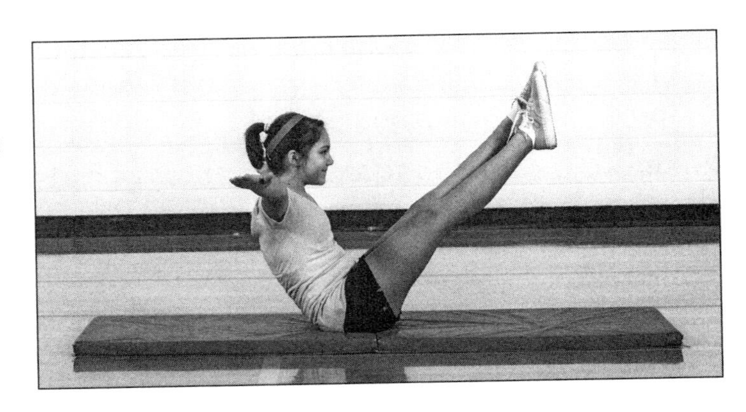

1. Sit with the palms on the floor at each side of the body.
2. Raise the arms to horizontal and extend the legs up in front of the body.
3. Maintain balance in this position.
4. Return to the starting position.

Walk the Plank

Focus: balance, body control

1. Stand at the end of a two-by-four plank.
2. Walk forward, sideways, and backward without falling off the plank (figure *a*).

Variations

- Walk the plank while performing circles, forward and backward, with the arms.
- Do crossover steps in both directions.
- Standing on the plank, raise a bent or straight leg with the arms out to the sides (figure *b*).
- Walk forward and backward over several utility balls placed two feet (.6 m) apart.
- Hold a balancing move (e.g., bent or straight leg with arm to the side) for three to six seconds.
- Walk across the plank on the toes.
- Turn 180 degrees on the toes.
- Turn 360 degrees on the toes.
- Walk forward and leap slightly at the end of the plank.

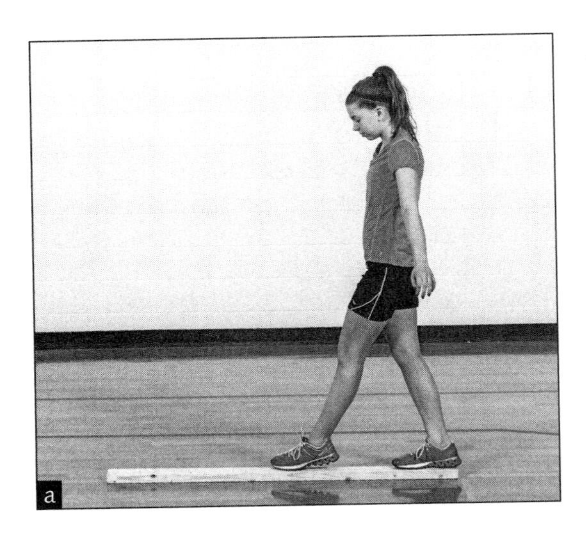

a

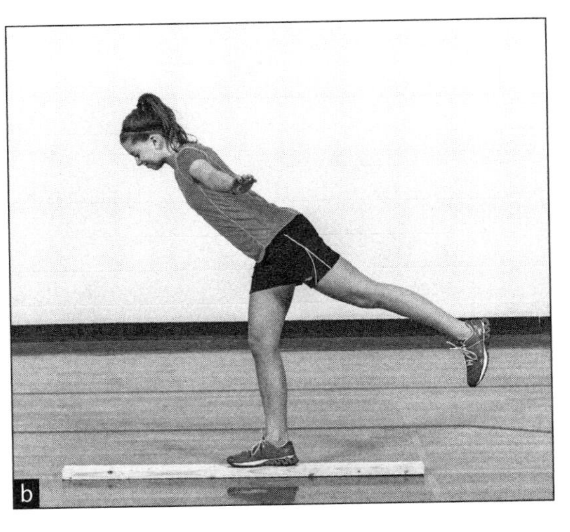

b

Reaction Ball Forward Drop

Focus: agility, hand–eye coordination

1. Stand in a quarter-squat position knees slightly bent and with the upper body leaning forward with the right arm extended in front of the body, holding a reaction ball.
2. Drop the reaction ball and attempt to catch it after one bounce.
3. Repeat 8 to 10 times.

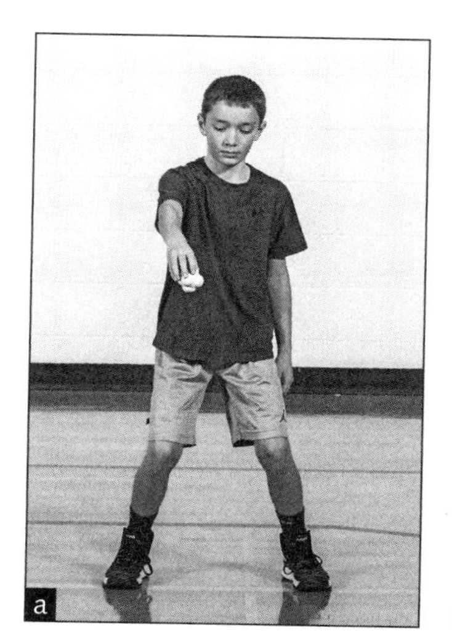

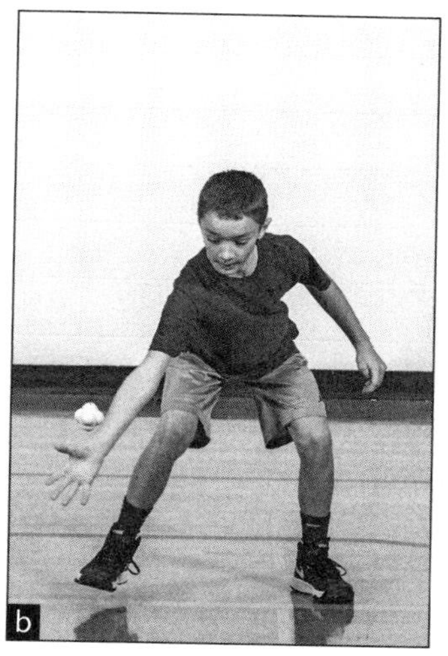

Reaction Ball Toss Against Wall

Focus: agility, coordination

1. Stand in a quarter-squat position with knees slightly bent and body leaning forward approximately six to eight feet (1.8-2.4 m) away from a wall.
2. Using an underhand throw, lightly toss the ball against the wall. Catch the ball as quickly as possible after the first bounce. Continue performing the drill until the ball is caught.

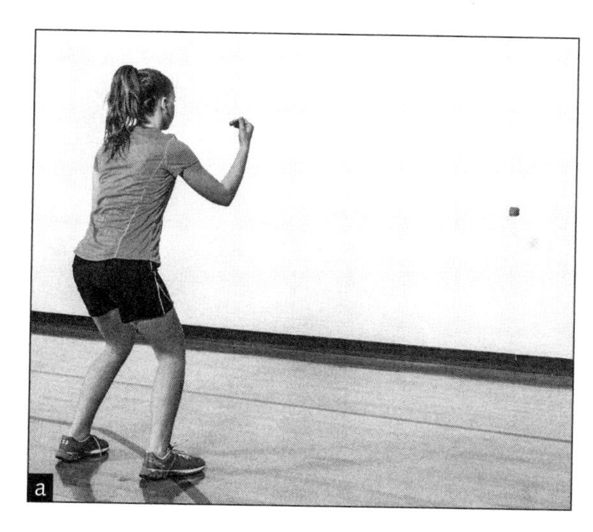

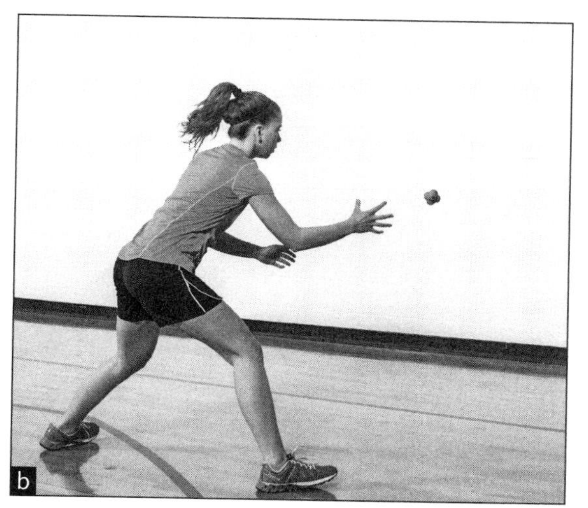

Reaction Ball Team Drill

Focus: agility, coordination

1. Divide the players into two teams. The teams stand in single file lines facing each other approximately 10 to 15 feet (3-4.5 m) apart.
2. Using an overhead throw, the first player on team A tosses the ball onto the floor and toward team B. The players on team B attempt to quickly react and catch the ball. The player on team B who caught the thrown ball then tosses the ball back to team A with an overhead or underhand throw.
3. Repeat the drill until each player has caught the ball five to eight times.

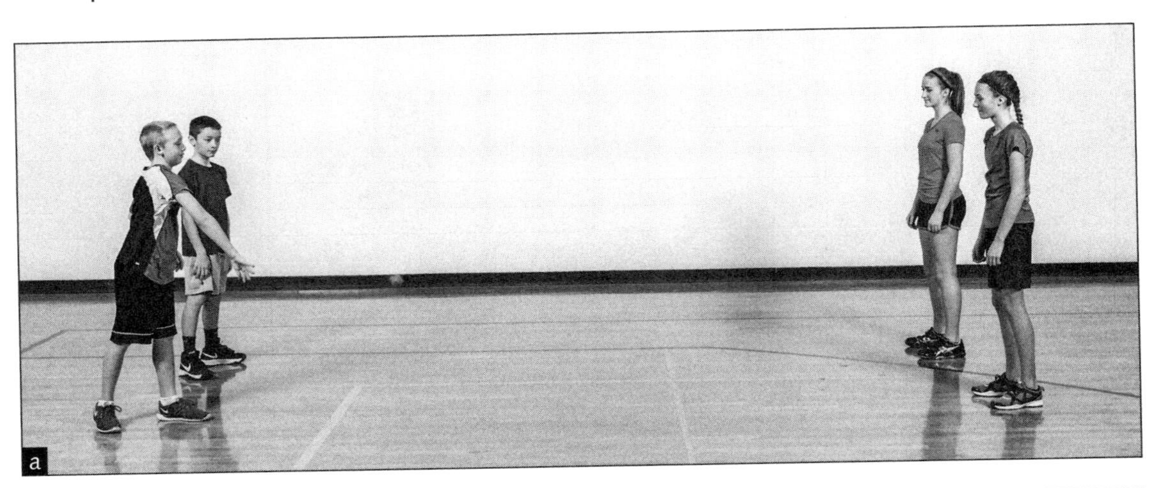

a

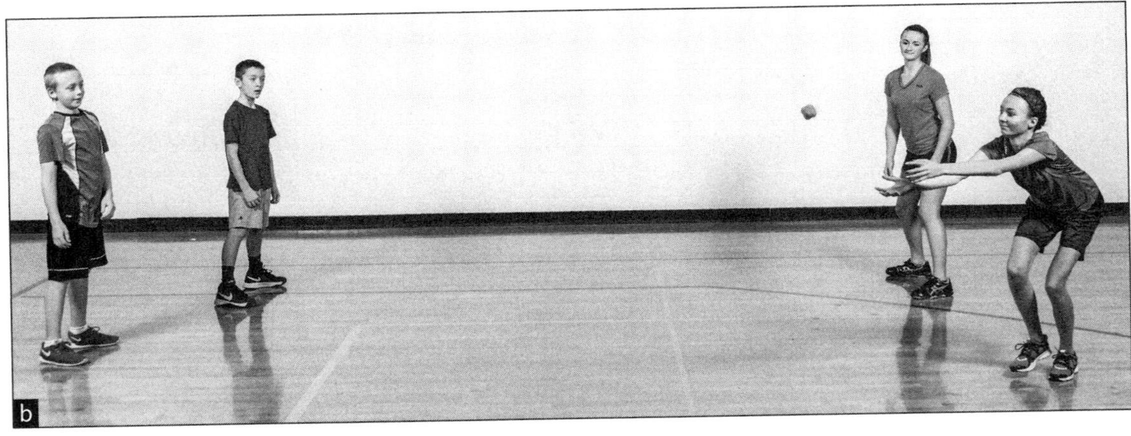

b

High Performance—19 Years of Age and Over

A well-designed training plan based on sound principles of long-term development will lead to high performance. Exceptional performance results that athletes achieved during the initiation, athletic formation, or specialization stages do not correlate with high performance results as a senior competitor. As table 2.3 demonstrates, the majority of athletes are most successful after they have reached athletic maturation.

This book is concerned only with the first three stages of development. For further information on training for high performance, consider the following books:

- Bompa, T., and Haff, G. 2009. *Periodization: Theory and methodology of training.* 5th ed. Champaign, IL: Human Kinetics.
- Bompa, T., and Buzzichelli, C. 2015. *Periodization training for sports.* 3rd ed. Champaign, IL: Human Kinetics.

The coming chapters discuss methods and specific programs for developing flexibility, speed, strength, and endurance. For each, we progress the difficulty of the training and suggest exercises that can be incorporated into a long-term training program. Consider our suggestions discretely and apply them according to your training environment and the characteristics of your individual athletes.

Table 2.3 Average Age of Participants at the Olympic Games Between 1968 and 1992

Sport	Average age (yr)
Athletics	24.1
Basketball	24.7
Boxing	22.7
Canoeing	24.2
Cycling	23.4
Equestrian	31.2
Fencing	24.1
Field hockey (men)	25.4
Gymnastics (women)	17.2
Gymnastics (men)	22.6
Judo	24.0
Rowing	24.2
Sailing	30.3
Shooting	33.2
Soccer	24.1
Swimming (women)	18.9
Swimming (men)	21.6
Volleyball (men)	25.2
Water polo (men)	25.3
Wrestling	24.8

chapter 3

Assessing the Young Athlete

Children's participation in competitions requires ongoing assessment, including medical supervision by a physician and monitoring by parents and coaches. To properly assess athletes' improvements and reactions to training, every coach and parent should, as scientifically as possible, monitor techniques. Some coaches and clubs have access (and financial means) to laboratories that can administer physiological, psychological, and biomechanical testing to evaluate athletes' improvements, performance, efficiency, technical effectiveness, and mental power. Others do not have such opportunities. Irrespective of the testing opportunities available, the simple and practical monitoring charts included in this chapter are useful for each athlete because tests are administered just a few times a year. The tests in this section are simple for parents and instructors to organize. By keeping records of each test, you will be able to monitor the improvements of your young athlete.

Throughout a training program, a coach must have feedback about the young athlete's physiological and psychological responses to the load or weight used in training. Such feedback helps the coach monitor improvements and effectively plan for strength-training progressions. You can record this feedback daily on the charts included in this chapter. The heart rate chart allows parents and coaches to monitor the physiological effects of training. The psychological traits and appetite chart tracks psychological reactions to training, including quality and quantity of sleep, level of fatigue, appetite, and willingness to both train and compete.

Two versions of each chart are provided. The first version is an example of an athlete's chart, and the second is a blank chart that you can photocopy and use for your young athlete. At the top of each chart is space to write the name of the athlete and the month of the year. Each chart is designed for 31 days. Every athlete should fill in the charts daily. The charts can be kept at home, preferably in a log book, for parents to see, and the athlete can take them to training sessions to show the instructor.

It is essential that the coach look at the charts of each athlete before a training session in order to modify the training program according to each athlete's psychological state and fatigue level. For instance, if the heart rate chart indicates a high level of fatigue, or if the psychological traits and appetite chart shows that the athlete got just four hours of restless sleep, then the daily program must be easy with no high-intensity work, which normally increases fatigue.

Heart Rate Chart

Heart rate is useful for monitoring the athlete's reaction to the previous day's training program. Before using the heart rate chart, the athlete must know his or her base heart rate (BHR), which is the heart rate taken in the morning before stepping out of bed. To determine the BHR, count the number of pulse beats for 10 seconds, then multiply this number by 6.

On the first day of each month, take a blank heart rate chart and, in the number 1 column, place a dot in the row of the number that corresponds to your heart rate (e.g., 49 on the sample chart). Record your heart rate in the same manner on each subsequent day. At the end of the month, connect the dots to view the variability of your heart rate over this period. Continue to take your BHR daily, entering a dot in the appropriate line of the next column and joining it to the previous dot to form a curve.

The BHR also reacts to the intensity of the previous day's training. When the BHR increases by six to eight beats per minute over the standard curve in one day, it could mean that the previous day's training program was not well tolerated or that the athlete did not observe a normal athletic lifestyle. For example, the athlete may be fatigued from illness or from staying up too late the previous night. The coach should talk with the athlete to learn the cause of the increased BHR and change the planned training program so it does not add to an already high level of fatigue. When the BHR decreases to its standard levels, the normal program can resume.

The BHR illustrates the athlete's physiological state and reaction to training. Under normal conditions, the curve does not have many deviations. The dynamics of the curve could change, however, according to the training phase and the state of the athlete's adaptation to the training program. As an athlete adapts to training, the BHR curve drops progressively: The better the adaptation, the lower the curve. Certainly, the shape of the curve depends on the chosen sport. For example, athletes from endurance-dominant sports usually have lower BHR levels and thus the shape of the curve is lower than anaerobic dominant sports.

Psychological Traits and Appetite Chart

The athlete should also complete each element of the psychological traits and appetite chart daily. This chart has a high correlation with the heart rate chart. As an athlete's level of fatigue or overtraining increases, sleeping patterns are disturbed and appetite decreases, as does the athlete's willingness to train and compete.

The sample chart represents a real-life situation of an athlete training to compete in the Olympic Games. By adequately changing the training program and improving the diet, which included supplements, the athlete recuperated and competed in the Games as expected (and placed fourth).

These simple and practical charts for monitoring training are extremely useful for the serious athlete. Many undesirable situations, such as overtraining, can be prevented when the athlete spends a minute a day filling in the charts and has the coach examine them before every training session.

Sample Heart Rate Chart

Name ____________________ Month ____________________

Heart rate	1	2	3	4	5	6	7	8	9	10	11	12	13	14	15	16	17	18	19	20	21	22	23	24	25	26	27	28	29	30	31
72																															
71																															
70																															
69																															
68																															
67																															
66																															
65																															
64																															
63																															
62																															
61																															
60																															
59																															
58																															
57																															
56																															
55																															
54																															
53																															
52																															
51																															
50																															
49																															
48																															
47																															
46																															
45																															
44																															
43																															

Heart Rate Chart

Name ________________________ Month ________________________________

Heart rate	1	2	3	4	5	6	7	8	9	10	11	12	13	14	15	16	17	18	19	20	21	22	23	24	25	26	27	28	29	30	31
72																															
71																															
70																															
69																															
68																															
67																															
66																															
65																															
64																															
63																															
62																															
61																															
60																															
59																															
58																															
57																															
56																															
55																															
54																															
53																															
52																															
51																															
50																															
49																															
48																															
47																															
46																															
45																															
44																															
43																															

From T. Bompa and M. Carrera, 2015, *Conditioning young athletes* (Champaign, IL: Human Kinetics).

Sample Psychological Traits and Appetite Chart

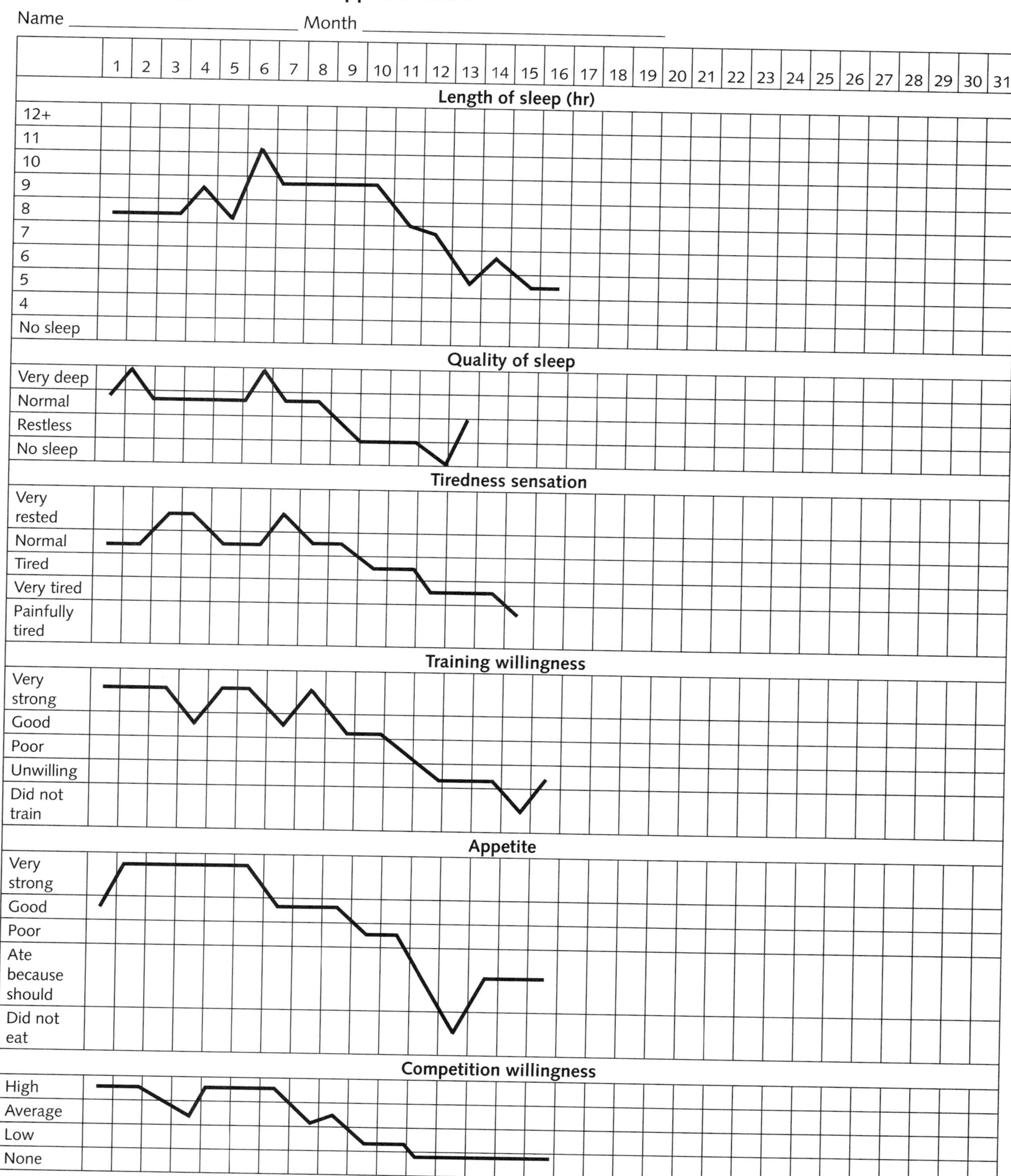

From T. Bompa and M. Carrera, 2015, *Conditioning young athletes* (Champaign, IL: Human Kinetics).

Psychological Traits and Appetite Chart

Name ____________________ Month ____________________

	1	2	3	4	5	6	7	8	9	10	11	12	13	14	15	16	17	18	19	20	21	22	23	24	25	26	27	28	29	30	31
Length of sleep (hr)																															
12+																															
11																															
10																															
9																															
8																															
7																															
6																															
5																															
4																															
No sleep																															
Quality of sleep																															
Very deep																															
Normal																															
Restless																															
No sleep																															
Tiredness sensation																															
Very rested																															
Normal																															
Tired																															
Very tired																															
Painfully tired																															
Training willingness																															
Very strong																															
Good																															
Poor																															
Unwilling																															
Did not train																															
Appetite																															
Very strong																															
Good																															
Poor																															
Ate because should																															
Did not eat																															
Competition willingness																															
High																															
Average																															
Low																															
None																															

From T. Bompa and M. Carrera, 2015, *Conditioning young athletes* (Champaign, IL: Human Kinetics).

Assessment Tests for the Young Athlete

Both parents and coaches can use simple tools and tests to monitor improvements in strength, power, speed, and aerobic endurance. As previously mentioned, few teams have access to a battery of scientific laboratory tests and computer software that can track an athlete's progress in various strength and power parameters along with changes in body composition throughout the season and year to year. Most coaches have little time and resources for planning a significant strength-training program, let alone a budget for a laboratory testing protocol.

As we state often throughout this book, to be successful in sport you don't have to do what is new but what is necessary. The same applies to testing. Coaches and parents want the best for the athletes, including the opportunity to follow a training program that improves fitness and sport performance. Improvements in sport and fitness can be gauged on the field, in the water, or on the ice. Is the athlete able to last longer before fatigue is evident? Is the athlete hitting the ball harder or farther? Has the athlete improved his 100-yard sprint time? Is the athlete able to physically defend in the corner? These are questions that coaches and parents ask themselves each time an athlete competes. The goal is always to push the athlete to run faster, jump higher, hit harder, or last longer. This is the purpose of strength, power, speed, and aerobic training in sport—to provide tools off the field that will make the athlete better on the field.

Tracking improvements in load, repetitions performed, and rest between sets is good for tracking improvements in strength. In addition, a few universal tests that can be performed two or three times a year can be used as benchmarks for assessing an athlete's level of strength and fitness development. These tests can be used as general, nonsport-specific measurements in most sports and can provide parameters for setting individual goals for improvement. To the young athlete, a simple test such as the push-up test can inspire a renewed commitment to training, especially if the athlete is competing against teammates. During the 2014 National Hockey League (NHL) draft, one player in particular made headlines for being the top pick—and for his inability to complete even one pull-up. Although his lack of upper-body strength may not have affected his draft ranking, in one article he claimed to be disappointed in his results and wanted to improve his pull-up score (Gillis, 2014). The skill of a hockey player is not determined by his pull-up score, but given the physicality of the game, upper-body strength is a must. Improving such strength doesn't require fancy equipment or expensive computer testing—just a bar and a body. If it's good enough for the NHL draft, we think coaches and athletes should start pulling up!

Most of the tests in this chapter require very little equipment and can be performed in a gym or open field with the use of a stopwatch, measuring tape, and marking cones. We recommend that the coach or parent keep a file that lists each date of testing, the athlete's score, and any comments that the athlete, coach, or parent have regarding the testing protocol. For example, how did the athlete feel on that day? How long since the last fitness test? Did the athlete have any injuries or muscle soreness? What was the weather like? Some detailed information regarding the testing day can help put the results into context. Also, coaches may find it useful to collect all data from the tests, both to use in pre- and posttest comparisons with current athletes and to help establish testing norms for athletes they work with in the future.

In chapter 2 we discussed four stages of athletic development:

- Initiation stage (6-10 years of age)
- Athletic formation stage (11-14 years of age)
- Specialization stage (15-18 years of age)
- High-performance stage (19+ years of age)

Both general and sport-specific testing is useful in all stages of athletic development. In the later stages—in particular, the late athletic formation stage and the specialization stage—fitness testing is especially important, both for monitoring improvements in overall strength, power, speed, and endurance and for collecting data that will help the coaches and trainers better devise a detailed training plan that meets the needs of the athlete and challenges further development. Thankfully, improvements in sport-specific strength, power, speed, and endurance are transferred to improvements in valuable fitness indices such as maximum push-ups, maximum pull-ups, and sprint time. Even with the sophisticated equipment and resources available, too many professional and semiprofessional sport teams, trainers, and coaches rely on standard measures of strength such as total pull-ups, total push-ups, and short sprints when evaluating athletic progress. As athletes progress in age and specialization, laboratory tests such as anaerobic power tests or maximal oxygen consumption tests, along with body fat percentages, become much more important measures of fitness and sport-specific specialization.

The following eight tests are useful for all stages of development, with some modifications for the initiation stage of development. The initiation stage of development is just that—an initiation to many basic patterns of running and jumping that are part of overall athletic development. One cannot judge fitness during this stage of development by push-up, pull-up, or sprint scores. For kids in this stage of development, fitness is best gauged and trained on the playground. Especially in the early part of the initiation phase, young athletes should be encouraged to climb the rock wall, swing on the monkey bars, balance on risers, and slide down poles. As kids mature both physically and emotionally they can participate in more direct fitness tests in both physical education class and sport.

Young athletes in the athletic formation stage, regardless of the sport, will benefit from completing the assessment tests in this chapter. Push-ups and pull-ups are a foundation of upper-body strength and can help a young athlete improve strength as her body matures. Although female athletes will not be able to complete as many repetitions as males in either test, they should be nonetheless encouraged to practice both exercises as a way of developing muscle strength and the central nervous system in preparation for following a thorough strength-training program.

Athletes in most team sports, including hockey, baseball, football, volleyball, and soccer, will benefit from utilizing these tests. The goal is not to compare the athlete's score with relative norms of other athletes but rather to help them visualize their level of fitness and thus set goals for future improvement. Sometimes it isn't enough for an athlete to feel like he has improved. Results from a number of assessment tools such as the ones listed here can help athletes better understand what is expected from them as they progress. We have been involved in many community-based programs in which the main purpose of competition is fun and play. We have coached both winning teams and losing teams. We start each season by conducting a fitness test that includes exercises similar to the ones listed here. At the end of the short season we conduct a retest and—regardless of whether we are coaching a winning team or a losing team—the kids are always amazed at how much they improved in most, if not all, measures. By simply playing the game and not necessarily following a strength-training protocol, athletes improve in most variables. The more time you put into play, the greater the fitness results. Not all athletes will become professional athletes, but young athletes who are given an opportunity to challenge themselves and see the results of their labor will likely make goal setting and fitness challenges an important part of their lifestyle. It all starts when they are young.

Athletes in the specialization and high-performance stages can also benefit from these fitness tests. At these levels of play, more sport-specific tests—tests that assess an athlete's ability to compete in a particular sport or position—would be administered. As we see in the National Football League, push-ups, pull-ups, the standing long jump (also known as the broad jump), the vertical jump, and the 40-yard dash are foundational exercises used in testing, along with many sport-specific tests, anatomical assessments, blood work, and body composition tests.

Important Points Before Testing

Administering a battery of tests to a group of 20 to 25 athletes can be time consuming and seem unproductive. Although you may want to get through the testing as quickly as possible, it is important that athletes are given enough time to rest between sets or attempts at a particular test. Take at least three minutes of rest between strength and power tests, especially sprinting, push-ups, and pull-ups tests. For power tests, allow for at least three attempts and record the best result.

Begin by recording the athlete's body weight and height. We don't recommend calculating body mass index (BMI) because the interpretation of BMI is different for children than for adults and because children go through growth spurts, which can quickly change the BMI value. We would rather focus attention on testing, training, and proper nutrition to give the young athletes the tools for bettering themselves physically and mentally. A BMI value that potentially indicates the need for weight loss can discourage a kid from participating in sport, especially if their BMI value increases due to a growth spurt. Although BMI interpretations for children are different than those for adults, take into consideration differences in body fat between boys and girls, and use sex-specific percentiles (Mei et al., 2002), we prefer not to include BMI in our data collection. Nonetheless, if coaches are interested in BMI, it can be calculated using the height and weight of the young athlete. Measuring body weight and height provides a full snapshot of the athlete's physicality at the time of the test.

The following eight fitness tests can be used to test young athletes in most sports. We include recommendations for staging and tips for better positioning, and variations for each test.

Test 1: Push-Up Test

Measurement

- Tests upper-body strength and endurance.
- Record the total number of repetitions.

Stage

Appropriate for late initiation stage (10-year-olds can attempt the push-up technique) and all other stages of development.

Position

- Start in the push-up position, with legs extended, toes on the floor, and the back straight. Keeping the arms straight, place the hands on the floor approximately shoulder-width apart.

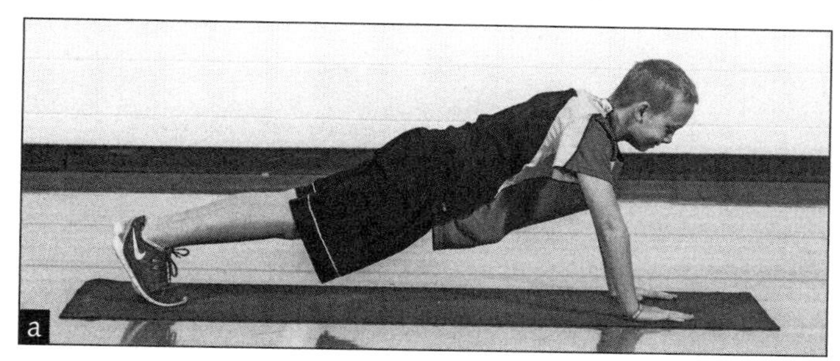
a

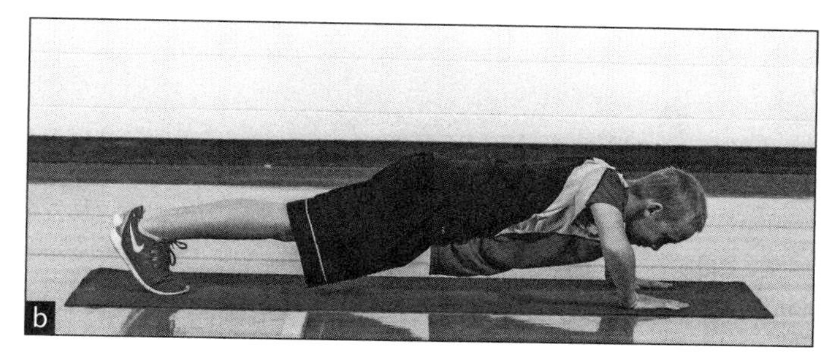
b

- While keeping back and abdominals tight and the body straight, bend the elbows until the arms are at a 90-degree angle. Return to the starting position. Perform as many repetitions as possible while maintaining form.
- Coaches can choose to use the failure rule (i.e., athletes perform as many repetitions as possible without a pause at the top of the movement until they can do no more) or the one-stop rule (i.e., athletes are allowed to pause at the top of the movement for three seconds before performing a few more repetitions to failure).

Tips

- To improve an athlete's technique, a teammate can place his fist on the floor directly below the athlete's chest. The athlete extends his arms once he makes contact with the fist.
- To better challenge athletes, coaches can administer a weighted push-up test. The athlete performs the push-ups as described previously, but the coach places a 5- or 10-pound (2.3 or 4.5 kg) weight plate on the athlete's upper back. (Another athlete can hold the plate in place, if needed.) Test and retest with the same weight each time.

Variations

Although coaches should keep the push-ups as standard as possible for testing, push-up variations can be used in training. Incline push-ups, decline push-ups, and wide-grip push-ups are all great variations for challenging the athlete and improving upper-body and core strength.

Test 2: Pull-Up and Bent-Arm Hang Tests

Measurement

- Tests upper-body strength and endurance.
- Record the total number of repetitions for pull-ups and the total time for the bent-arm hang.

Stage

- Athletes in the early athletic formation stage can attempt the bent-arm hang test.
- Athletes in the late athletic formation, specialization, and high-performance stages can complete the pull-up test.

Position for the Pull-Up Test

- Grab an overhead bar with an underhand grip (palms facing the body; see figure *a*).
- Extend the arms and place the hands approximately shoulder-width apart.
- Pull the body up until the chin clears the bar, and slowly return to the starting position. The feet should not touch the floor between repetitions.
- The test is stopped when the athlete can no longer perform the test with proper technique.
- The movement should be smooth and controlled—no jerking or swinging is allowed.

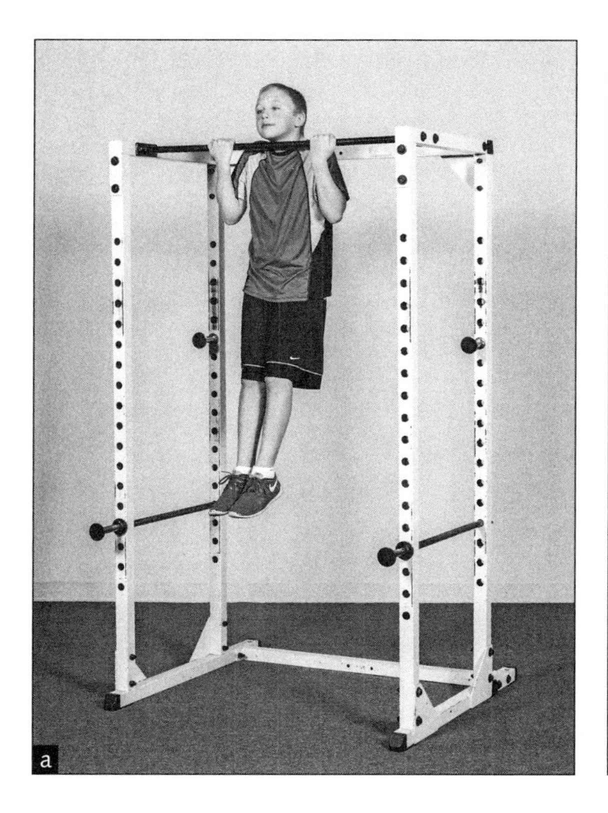

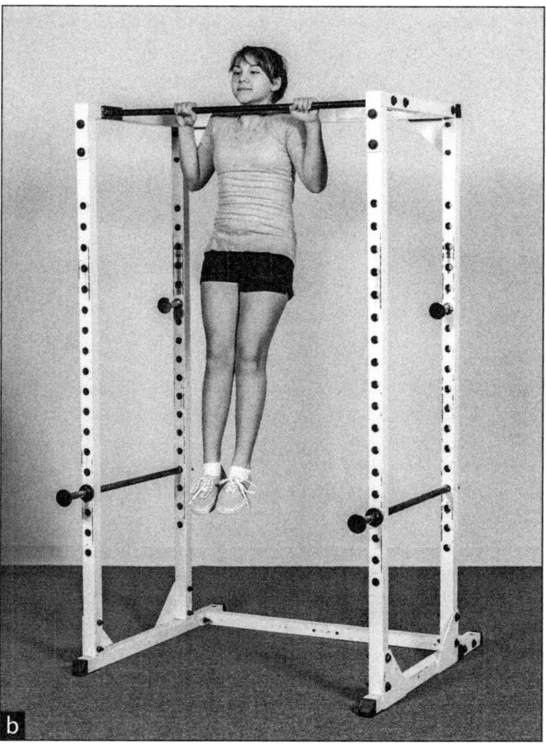

- Resting is allowed in both the up and down phases as long as the legs do not touch the floor and the athlete does not rest the chin on the bar.

Position for the Bent-Arm Hang Test

- Instead of the standard pull-up test, female athletes can perform the bent-arm hang test (see figure *b*).
- Pull up, jump up, or step up to the pull-up bar until the chin is at the level of the bar. Use a reverse or forward grip. Make sure to use same grip for retest.
- Hang and maintain this position for as long as possible. Stop the test when athlete can no longer maintain the chin at the level of the bar.
- Male athletes can also perform this test to complement the pull-up test.

Variations

- Some coaches use the horizontal bar of an in-ground goalpost to conduct the pull-up test. Although this is possible, keep in mind that the standard goalpost bar is thicker than the pull-up bar and can negatively affect the total number of repetitions performed because the thicker bar will fatigue the forearm muscles faster. If coaches conclude that the goalpost option is safe, then the same goalpost should be used for retesting until a new approach is formulated.
- Coaches can also purchase a portable pull-up or chin-up bar that can be attached to a door frame. These bars are relatively inexpensive, are easy to use, and can be used for both indoor testing and training.

Tip

Use various grips (e.g., wide grip, short grip, reverse grip) for training variety.

Test 3: Standing Long Jump and Three-Step Jump Tests

Measurement

- Tests power performance.
- Measure the length of the jump using a measuring tape.

Stage

Great for all stages of athletic formation, including the initiation stage.

Position

- Stand with the feet shoulder-width apart and the toes placed on a start line (marked with a cone, tape, or chalk; see figure *a*).
- Perform a countermovement jump by rapidly bending the knees and swinging the arms alongside the body (figure *b*).
- Propel the body forward as far as possible and stick the landing by bending the knees and holding the landing positon.
- Measure the distance from the start line to the heel of the foot that is farthest back upon landing.
- Repeat the movement three times and take the best score.
- For the three-step jump (figure *c*), the athlete's position is the same as that for the standing long jump. This time, instead of stopping after the first jump, the athlete quickly jumps again two more times for a total of three consecutive jumps.
- Measure the distance from the start line to the heel of the foot that is farthest back upon landing. Repeat the test three times and take the best score.

Tip

- Both the standing long jump and three-step jump are good measures of lower-body power.
- It is useful to perform these tests on the competition surface used in the particular sport. Thus, soccer players can perform the tests on grass, and basketball and tennis players can perform them on the court. For hockey, these tests can be performed on a regular gym floor, grass, or concrete. Note that the surface must be the same for both the test and retest in order to accurately assess changes and improvements.
- To guarantee accurate results, athletes should be properly warmed up and given an opportunity to practice the tests.

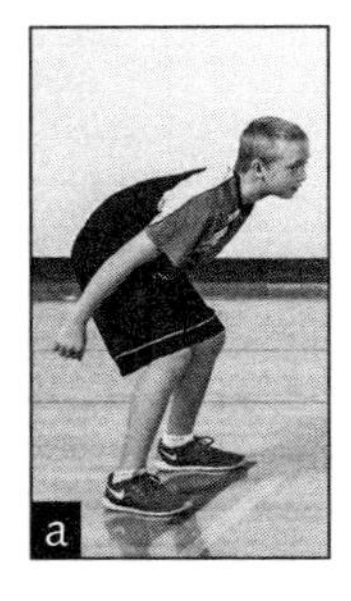
a

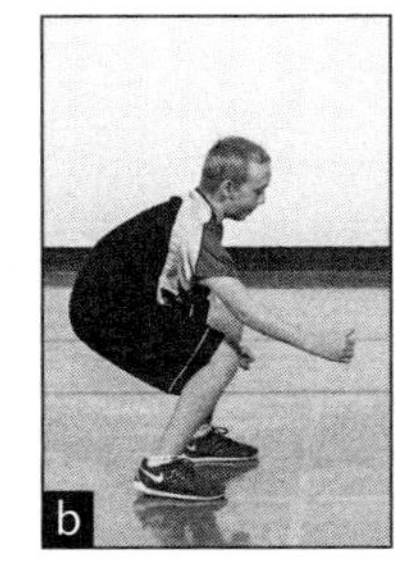
b

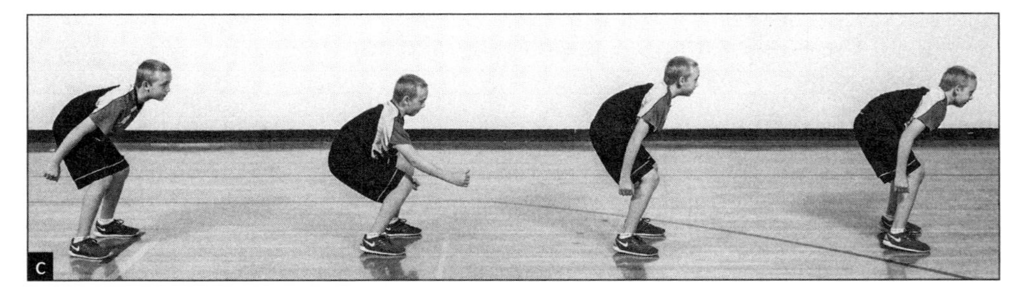
c

Test 4: 30-Meter and 60-Meter Sprints

Measurement

- Tests speed and power.
- Use a stopwatch to record the fastest time.

Stage

Use short distances, such as 15 to 20 meters, for athletes in the initiation stage and increase to 30 meters for athletes in the in late initiation stage. Use the 30- and 60-meter sprints for athletes in other stages.

Position

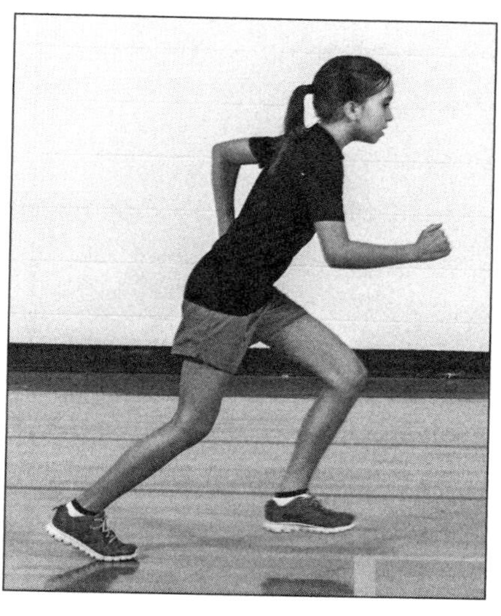

- The coach marks both a 30-meter distance and a 60-meter distance using a measuring tape and cones.
- Maintain a standing sprint stance at the start line, and run the prescribed distance as fast as possible.
- Allow for proper recovery between sets, and perform two or three sets of each sprint. Take the best time.

Variations

- Coaches can use the 30-meter sprint test, 60-meter sprint test, or both. Both tests are a good measure of speed and power.
- Athletes in team sports such as basketball, volleyball, and hockey can perform these sprints outdoors on a field or track. Coaches in these sports may also choose to administer a sprinting test on the court or ice to complement these two sprint tests.

Test 5: Vertical Jump

Measurement

- Tests lower-body power.
- Use chalk or sticky tape and a measuring tape to measure.

Stage

This test is great for all stages of development, regardless of sport. It is especially beneficial for athletes in the initiation and athletic formation stages because the vertical jump is an important indicator of leg strength and power; it can provide insight into possible weaknesses and help customize an athlete's programming. In later stages of development, the vertical jump is used to assess power in sports or events that have a vertical component—for instance, basketball, volleyball, and the high jump.

Position

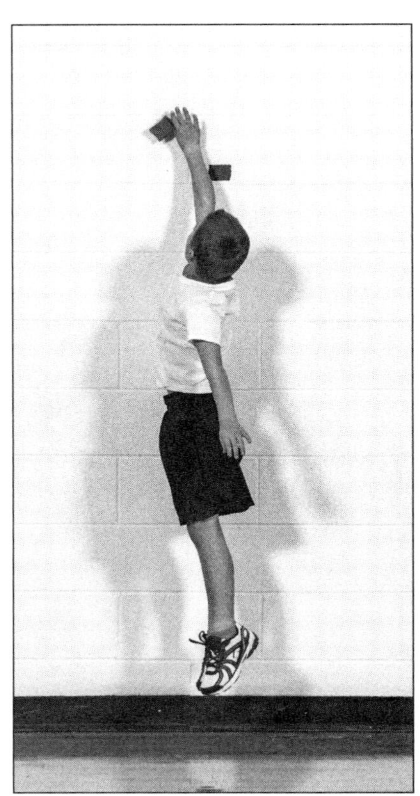

- Stand sideways against an indoor wall, holding a piece of tape in the right or left hand up against the wall.
- Keeping the body close to the wall, extend the arm overhead and mark the starting position with tape.
- Hold another piece of tape in the hand with the hand close to the wall. Rapidly bend the knees and perform a quick countermovement jump. Jump up as far as possible, extending the arm up and sticking the tape to the wall.
- Measure the difference (in centimeters) between the starting position and the jump height tapes.

Variations

If performed outdoors, mark the starting position (with one arm extended) and the jump height with a piece of chalk rather than with sticky tape.

Test 6: Plank and Modified Plank Tests

Measurement

- Tests core strength (abdominals and lower back) and upper-body endurance.
- Use a stopwatch to record the total length of time.

Stage

Athletes in the initiation stage can practice the modified plank test as a way to improve balance and coordination. Athletes in the early athletic formation stage can use the modified plank test. Athletes in the late athletic formation and other stages of development can use the standard plank test of core strength.

Position

- Start in the push-up position, with the toes on the floor and the back straight. Keeping the arms straight, place the hands on the floor approximately shoulder-width apart.
- Bend both elbows and support the upper body on the elbows while maintaining balance on the toes and holding the body in a straight line (figure *a*).
- Hold the position as long as possible, or until the hips begin to lower.
- Record the total time to failure in seconds.

Variation

A variation of the traditional plank test is the modified plank test (see figure *b*). This test is more appropriate for younger kids, especially those in the initiation stage who are beginning to practice balancing movements. For this group, use time to failure to indicate when to stop the test, as hip sway may be prevalent throughout the entire test. With the modified plank test, start in the push-up position, with the hands and toes on the floor and the back straight. Stop the test when the hips begin to drop or the body begins to sway.

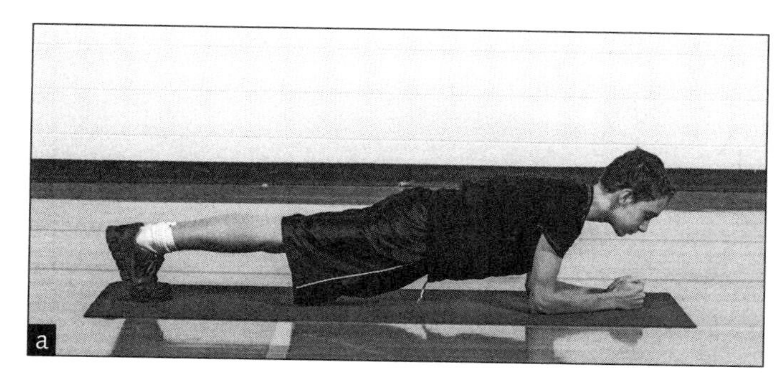
a

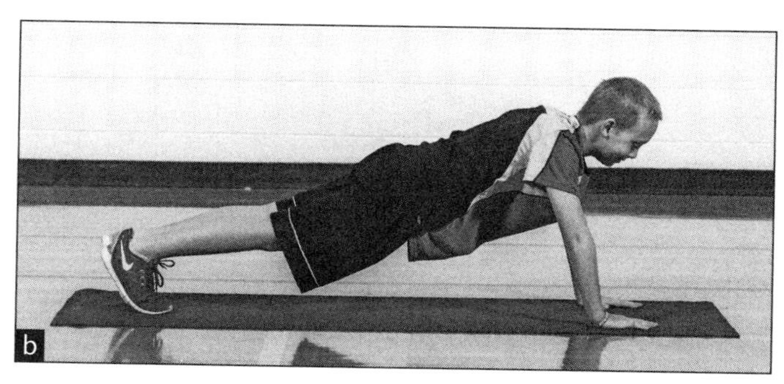
b

Test 7: One-Mile (1500m) Aerobic Test

Measurement

- Tests cardiovascular fitness.
- Use a stopwatch to measure time to completion.

Stage

One mile is too great a distance for athletes in the initiation stage of development; one-quarter or one-third of a mile are more appropriate distances for this age group. For athletes in other stages, the one-mile test is appropriate.

Position

- The coach marks a one-mile distance on the field or in the surrounding neighborhood.
- Walk and run one mile. Time how long it takes to complete the distance.

Variation

The one-mile test is a good indicator of the aerobic fitness level of an athlete. Coaches are encouraged to create their own aerobic tests that can be performed on a field or in a gym. For instance, one soccer coach we spoke to uses the length of the soccer field as a test marker. Although it is time consuming, the coach has each athlete run the test alone and measures how long it takes the athlete to run four full lengths; he also records how long it takes the athlete to complete each of the four lengths. This helps the coach determine each athlete's average fatigue rate and whether each athlete is trying his best.

Tips

- Encourage the athletes to give their all. Some coaches set up a reward program, but from our experience—especially with athletes in the athletic formation and specialization stages—acknowledgement of a job well done is usually enough to spark the interest of the athlete and motivate future effort and performance.
- Use some form of the one-mile test. Improvements in cardiovascular fitness and time to complete the test occur quickly, and thus can serve to motivate the athlete and inspire greater work effort.

Test 8: Four-Cone Agility Test

Measurement

- Tests starting speed and speed in changing directions.
- Use five cones, a measuring tape, and a stopwatch.

Stage

This is a fun agility test for athletes in all stages of development. It is easy to remember, and the cone touches challenge the athlete to master her footwork in order to regain control and accelerate. Athletes in the athletic formation, specialization, and high-performance stages can use agility tests of greater difficulty.

Position

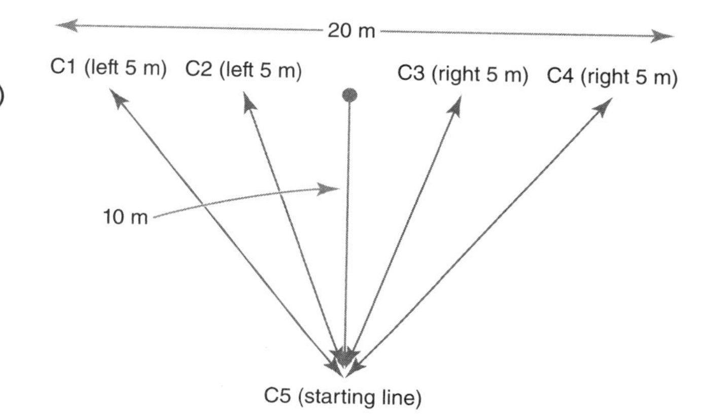

- The coach puts four cones in a straight line, placing cone 1 (C1) and cone 4 (C4) 20 meters apart. The coach then places cone 5 (C5) 10 meters from the line and between cone 2 (C2) and cone 3 (C3). C5 is the starting point.
- Start at C5. Sprint to C4 and touch the base of the cone with the right hand. Turn and return to C5 and touch the base of the cone with the right hand.
- Continue to C3 and touch the base of the cone with the right hand. Turn and return to C5 and touch the base of the cone with the right hand.
- Continue to C2 and touch the base of the cone with the left hand. Turn and return to C5 and touch the base of the cone with the left hand.
- Continue to C1 and touch the base of the cone with the left hand. Turn and finish by sprinting to C5 and touching the base of the cone with the left hand.
- The coach times the entire trial.

Variations

- Coaches can use many variations of agility tests to test their players. Whatever test they choose should also be used for retesting. The goal of each agility test is to test an athlete's speed as well as her ability to change direction.
- As a variation, athletes can sprint to the cone and then shuffle back to the starting cone (C5) before sprinting to the next cone. After completing the last cone (C1), the athlete should sprint (rather than shuffle) back to C5 to end the test.

Tip

Encourage the athletes to run as fast as possible, and use the test as a training measure to help athletes improve agility in competition.

To ensure that athletes are improving in both skill and fitness, it is important to evaluate progress both in competition and outside of competition. Conducting a proper fitness test that tracks strength, power, speed, and aerobic endurance is an easy way to monitor progress in training and thus assess whether the training program is achieving its expected goal. Fitness testing does not need to be completed in an expensive laboratory or research center. Data can be collected by simply using some standard tests that require little equipment but offer valuable insight into the athlete's level of fitness. Regardless of the stage of development, all athletes can benefit from some, if not all, of the fitness tests in this chapter. Tracking the data over the years will help coaches and parents evaluate progress and fine-tune an athlete's programming.

One does not have to become a professional athlete to be successful in sport. Success can be achieved by carrying the qualities of good sportsmanship and a healthy and fit lifestyle into adulthood. Success does not require fancy equipment or Olympic training centers. The only requirements are the desire to work hard and the ability to sometimes skip over what is new and focus on what is necessary.

chapter 4

Flexibility Training

Flexibility refers to the range of motion around a joint. Improving flexibility is a fundamental element of a young athlete's training program because good flexibility enables the athlete to perform various movements and skills easily and helps prevent injury.

The ability to successfully perform many movements and skills depends on the range of motion, which has to be greater than the skills of the sport require. For instance, to hit a high ball during a soccer game, players have to lift their leg to chest level, so they must be flexible enough to go beyond that level. If they don't have that flexibility, they won't be able to learn and perfect the various movements required for the sport. Flexibility is not improved in one or two stretching sessions but rather with an ongoing emphasis on statically and dynamically engaging the various muscles and joints with a variety of stretching exercises. Regular stretching can improve force, speed, and jump height (Shrier, 2004). Because flexibility is more difficult to improve in adulthood, it is best to start young and make both warming up and stretching an important part of the training program.

Flexibility training is also an injury-prevention strategy. Most sports involve repetitive movement, often through a limited range of motion, such as running. This can lead to muscle tightness and possibly muscle strains and tears. A careful and progressively increased flexibility program will stretch the muscles, thus relieving muscle tightness and helping prevent injury.

Furthermore, while inflexibility can lead to injury, so can a low level of fitness. The groin and adductor muscles don't appear to be directly engaged in running and sprinting, yet soccer players need a tremendous amount of hip and groin flexibility when sliding and tackling. Thus, it is important that flexibility, like all other sporting attributes, be given an opportunity to allow the muscles to adapt and enhance the quality and effort of play (Herbert and Gabriel, 2002; Ingraham, 2003). Flexibility needs to be multifaceted and include more than basic static stretching before a practice or game—it must be an ongoing training factor that provides more than the necessary range of motion required for the activity. For instance, soccer players may spend time stretching their quadriceps muscles and hamstrings but neglect their groin and adductor muscles.

The best time to perform stretching exercises is at the end of a general warm-up (i.e., jogging and calisthenics), during the rest interval between exercises, and at the end of the training session.

Developing Flexibility

Young children are flexible, but flexibility performance often decreases with age after puberty—especially in boys, presumably because of gains in muscle size, stature, and muscle strength. Flexibility therefore requires training throughout all stages of a young athlete's development. Because athletes can more easily develop flexibility at a young age, it must be part of the training program for each young athlete irrespective of sport specialization. Once an athlete achieves the desired degree of flexibility, the objective of the flexibility-training program is to maintain that level. Year-round maintenance is important because athletes quickly lose flexibility with inactivity, and reduced flexibility can make them prone to injury.

The initiation stage is therefore the ideal time to start a program for developing flexibility. Emphasizing overall flexibility that involves all the joints of the body will result in good basic development. This is important because specialization does not occur until later stages of athletic development, and no one knows which muscles will require the most flexibility as a result of training for a specific sport.

Flexibility exercises can involve static stretches, low-intensity dynamic stretches, and calisthenics such as arm swings, toe touches, and jumping jacks. Although generally used as part of the warm-up, these three exercises help stretch joints—especially the shoulder, hip, and ankle joints. During the initiation stage, children enjoy playing at playgrounds that offer a number of activities, including monkey bars, climbing walls, and slides. These activities, to name a few, are fun and challenging and help improve strength, agility, balance, and flexibility. We know a community-league soccer coach who works with children in the initiation stage of development. He takes the time to practice kicking, cone drills, and other skills, but always ends his practices by sending the kids to a nearby playground, where they are happy to jump, climb, and swing. The coach knows the value of playground activities, and the parents are more than happy to tire out their kids!

As boys start to build stronger muscles and grow in size, they begin to show some decline in flexibility, reaching the lowest level in the second part of pubescence. At the same time, girls continue to perform well. Puberty is the development stage when sex differences in flexibility are the largest. During postpuberty, the trend of sex differences continues. Girls still show better flexibility than boys, although the difference is not as large as during puberty. As girls approach adolescence, however, they seem to reach a plateau (Alaranta et al., 1994; Kohl and Cook, 2013), which might maintain or even decrease during maturity. This is why overall flexibility training should be a constant concern for everyone involved in athletics.

Methods of Stretching

The best way to improve flexibility is to perform stretching exercises. Stretching exercises can be performed statically, dynamically, and using proprioceptive neuromuscular facilitation (PNF). Before briefly exploring each method, it is important to mention that some contradiction exists regarding which method is most efficient. Many coaches and athletes prefer the static method, fearing that the ballistic method may lead to muscle pulls. Although the application of PNF has some limitations, it is often the preferred method.

Static stretching involves stretching to the limit of motion without forcing the stretch and then holding the position without movement for a given time. Throughout the performance of static flexibility exercises, the athlete should attempt to relax the muscles to achieve the maximum range of motion.

For both the static and PNF methods, the athlete tries to position the joints to enhance the sought flexibility. Then the athlete statically maintains the position for a number of seconds for each set. The time spent stretching should progressively increase over a long period. Static stretching involves pressure applied solely by the athlete's own force, whereas PNF involves pressure applied by a partner.

Dynamic stretching involves bobbing or active movements that reach the limits of motion. The athlete does not hold the final position. For instance, take a standing position with the arms above the head and the feet apart. Lower the trunk dynamically toward the knees to reach maximum range of motion. Repeat this several times, in each repetition attempting to reach the most acute angle. Stop upon feeling any discomfort or pain.

PNF involves stretching to the limits of motion and then doing a static contraction for a few seconds against the resistance of a partner. The athlete then lifts the limb voluntarily to a more acute angle beyond previous limits. After lifting the limb voluntarily, the athlete then again performs a static isometric contraction against the resistance of a partner.

Getting Practical

Every game and practice should begin with a progressive warm-up. Increased blood flow and temperature prepare the muscles for activity and aid in force and power development. Every warm-up should begin with 10 to 15 minutes of cardiovascular activity and include a number of static and dynamic stretches. Coaches may also choose to split athletes into groups of two to practice PNF stretching, especially for the muscles of the lower body. As a general rule, coaches can begin each warm-up with a 10- to 15-minute jog followed by 5 to 10 minutes of static or PNF stretching and can end the warm-up with 5 to 10 minutes of dynamic stretches and activities that incorporate medicine balls or explosive body movements (e.g., squat jumps, burpees, rhythmic arm swings, and knee lifts).

A recent study (Faigenbaum et al., 2005) looked at three warm-up protocols and their immediate effects on children's performance on the vertical jump, shuttle run, long jump, and V-sit. Group 1 performed a 5-minute walk followed by 5 minutes of static-stretching exercises, group 2 performed 10 minutes of dynamic exercise, and group 3 performed 10 minutes of dynamic exercise plus three drop jumps from a 15-centimeter (6 in.) box. The groups that performed dynamic exercise (groups 2 and 3) showed improved performance in the vertical jump and shuttle run. Only the group that performed dynamic exercise plus drop jumps (group 3) showed improved long jump performance. The group that completed the 5-minute walk plus static stretching (group 1) showed no improvements in any measure. None of the three warm-ups produced significant improvements in V-sit flexibility.

Static stretching is needed in all training environments, and we recommend performing static stretches in a cluster of exercises as part of the warm-up. More important, athletes should also perform static-stretching exercises outside of the competitive environment as part of a healthy and active lifestyle—where the benefits of stretching are best attained.

Designing a Program

As noted earlier, the best time to start developing flexibility is during the initiation stage because the early stages of anatomical development in children involves general low-intensity play which emphasizes all muscles and joints, and thus provides a solid base on which to improve flexibility in the absence of muscle soreness and other joint restrictions that can occur as a result of intense activity. During this stage, training programs should focus on developing all joints, especially the hips, shoulders, and ankles. Ankle flexibility is crucial for any skills requiring running and jumping, and athletes must use flexion and extension to bring the toes toward or away from the calf. We suggest using the static method, whereby attention is given not to overstretch the muscle beyond the point of discomfort. Don't overdo it!

Flexibility training should also be emphasized throughout the formation stage. This allows the child to continue developing strong joints while addressing the anatomical problems (e.g., the legs growing disproportionately to other parts of the body and a change in leverage between the legs and the trunk) that may occur during puberty. The more time an athlete dedicates to developing flexibility during prepubescence and pubescence, the fewer problems that appear in the later stages of athletic development.

A flexibility session should not be boring! You can combine it with play and games; however, do not create a competitive environment because this can result in overstretching and eventual harm.

During prepubescence, athletes develop general flexibility; the flexibility they develop from pubescence on is sport specific. As such, parents, instructors, and coaches should pay attention to the flexibility of joints required in a given sport, particularly ankle and hip flexibility, because these areas have been underemphasized in the past. This does not mean that other joints should be neglected. Athletes need a maintenance program in place during puberty and throughout their athletic careers for the nonspecific joints.

In the specialization stage the athlete should work on maximizing specific flexibility. Because athletes perform certain sport movements dynamically, the athletes have to train to perform moves dynamically and with the highest amplitude. It is the lack of such training—not the dynamic exercises themselves—that results in injuries. If an athlete does not have adequate flexibility, even dynamic stretching might not help. Develop good flexibility to protect athletes from injury and remember that greater flexibility will produce greater development of power and force.

Athletes must strive to gain most of their flexibility during the off-season. Regard the competitive season as a maintenance period, when athletes will direct their energy and the strain they place on muscle groups toward specific training. Regardless of whether athletes are working on gaining flexibility or maintaining it, flexibility training has to be part of everyday training year round. Athletes should incorporate flexibility exercises into the end of the warm-up part of a training session and should increase the range of motion of an exercise progressively and carefully. At first, athletes may perform exercises with an amplitude, magnitude, and extension that does not challenge them; in this case they should increase progressively up to their limits. From this point on, each repetition should aim at reaching this maximum and slowly and carefully progressing the stretch but never pushing beyond the point of major discomfort.

View the following exercises as guidelines only. Parents and instructors can incorporate many other exercises into training as long as the athletes perform them in a progressive manner. All the exercises in this chapter are appropriate for all stages of athletic development. Some of the exercises have dynamic and PNF options that may be used with athletes in the specialized stage of training. Refer to tables 4.1 and 4.2 for examples of an appropriate progression.

Table 4.1 Periodization Model for Flexibility Training

Stage of development	Training method	Exercises
Initiation	Static Low-level dynamic exercise (playground activities)	• Trunk and hip flexion • Large body circles • Flex to opposite leg • Ankle double touch • Seated toe touch • Straddle stretch • Opposite toe touch
Athletic formation	Static PNF Introduction of dynamic stretching	• Hamstring stretch • Bow shoulder stretch • Ankle stretch • Diagonal ankle press • Double kick • Exercises (on the floor and standing) with a partner to enhance flexibility using the static and PNF methods
Specialization	Static PNF Dynamic	• Perform stretching exercises with and without a partner using static and PNF methods. • You can use most partner exercises for dynamic flexibility. For dynamic stretching, be careful at the extreme points of the stretch (point of discomfort).

Note: Refer to the exercises in this chapter.

Table 4.2 Periodization of Flexibility in an Annual Plan for Puberty and Postpuberty

Phase	Scope of flexibility training	Training methods
Preparatory		
General	Improve general and specific flexibility	Static PNF
Specific	Maximize specific flexibility	All methods
Competitive	Maintain general flexibility	All methods
Transition	Improve general flexibility	Static PNF

Note: Even during the annual plan there is a progression from static to PNF and then to all methods, including ballistic.

Trunk and Hip Flexion

Areas stretched: hips and side of the trunk

1. Stand with the feet shoulder-width apart and arms reaching out at the sides, palms facing up.
2. Bend the body to the left, swinging the right arm over the head until the palms are touching. Keep the elbows straight. Hold for four to six seconds.
3. Repeat to the right side.

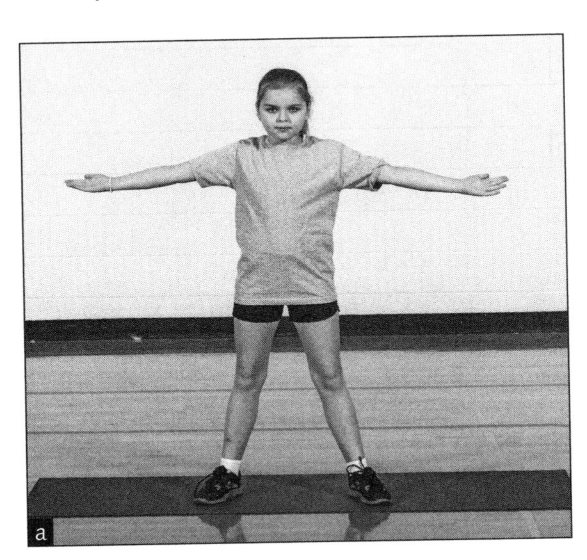
a

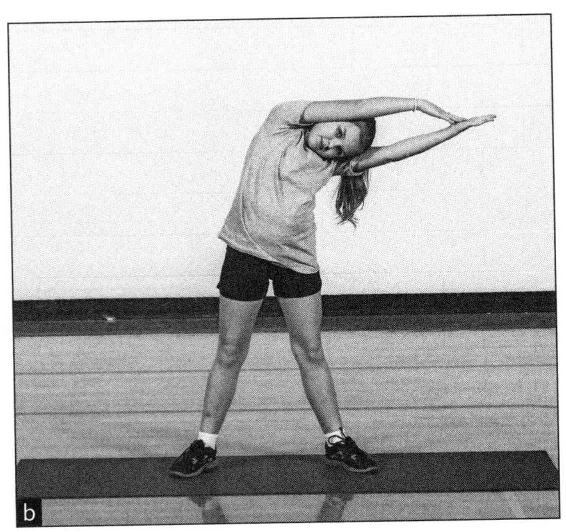
b

Large Body Circles

Areas stretched: trunk, hips, and hamstrings

1. Stand with the feet shoulder-width apart and the arms above the head, palms together.
2. Make four large rotations with the arms and body, traveling down the left side to the floor and up the right side to above the head.
3. Perform four rotations in the opposite direction.

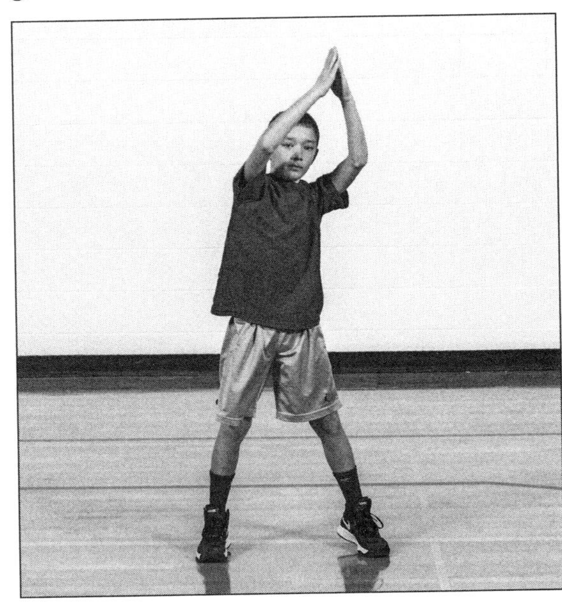

Flex to Opposite Leg

Areas stretched: hips, trunk, and hamstrings

1. Stand with the feet wider than shoulder-width apart and the arms above the head.
2. Flex the hips and drive the right arm toward the left foot, leaving the left arm up. Hold for four to six seconds.
3. Return to the starting position.
4. Repeat the movement with the left arm toward the right foot, leaving the right arm up. Hold for four to six seconds.
5. Return to the starting position.

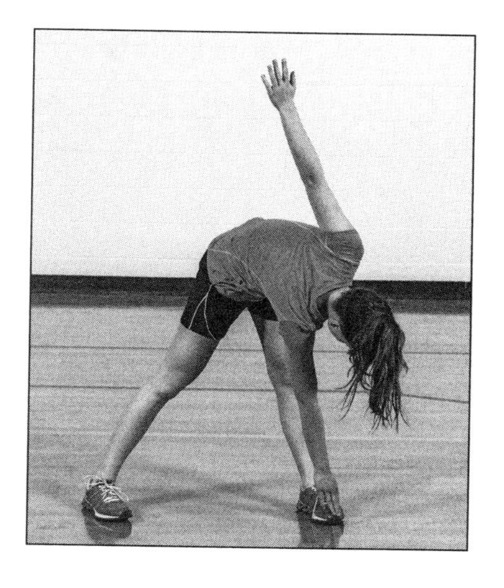

Ankle Double Touch

Areas stretched: hips, chest, shoulders, and hamstrings

1. Stand with the feet apart and the arms reaching out to the sides.
2. Flex the upper body, touching the opposite leg with each hand by crossing the arms. Hold for four to eight seconds.
3. Bring the upper body to the horizontal, swinging the arms to the side and up.
4. Return to the starting position.

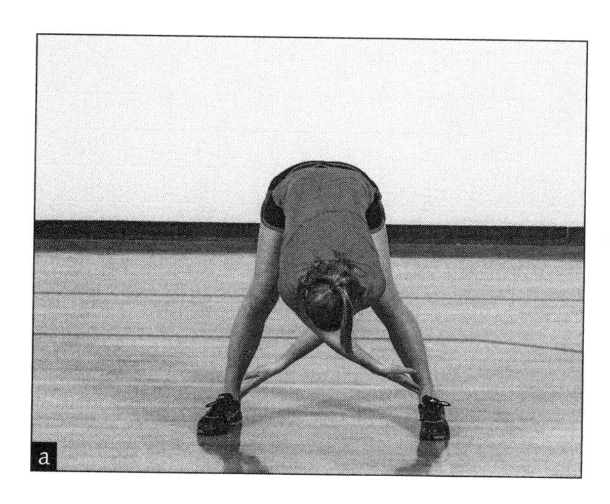
a

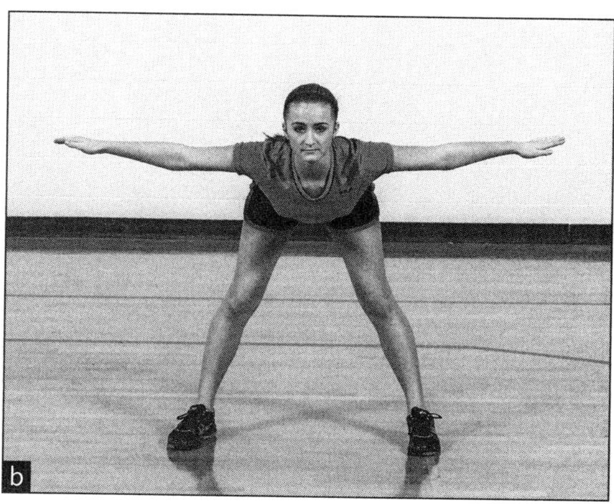
b

Seated Toe Touch

Areas stretched: hips, hamstrings, and calves

1. Sit with the legs straight and the arms extended above the head.
2. Flex the upper body forward while exhaling and extend the arms as far as possible toward the toes. Hold for four to six seconds.
3. Return to the starting position.

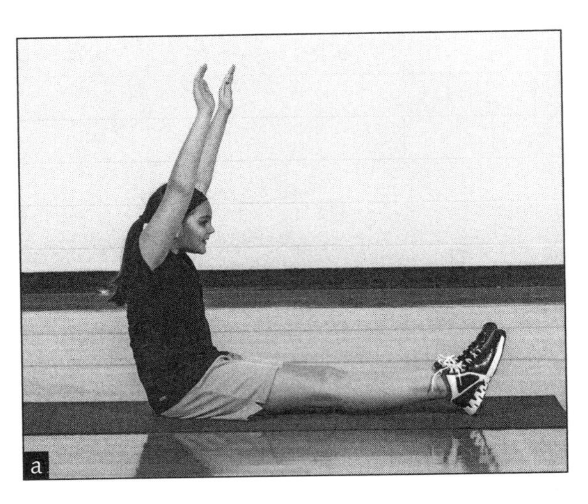

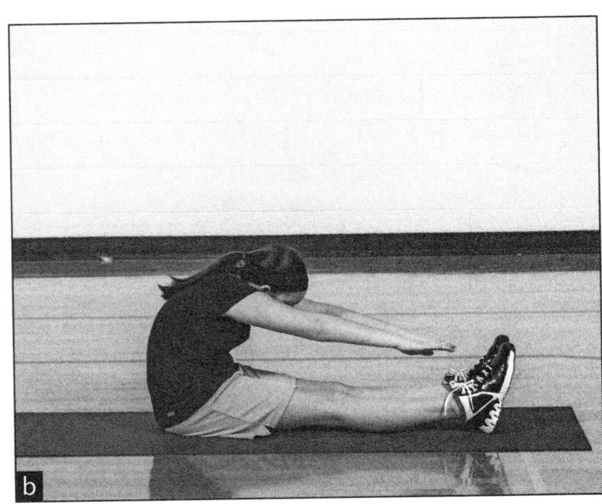

Straddle Stretch

Areas stretched: hips, shoulders, and calves

1. Lie on the back with the arms stretched overhead and the toes flexed.
2. Raise the upper body and flex it over the legs, attempting to touch the hands to the toes. Hold for four to six seconds.
3. Return to the starting position.

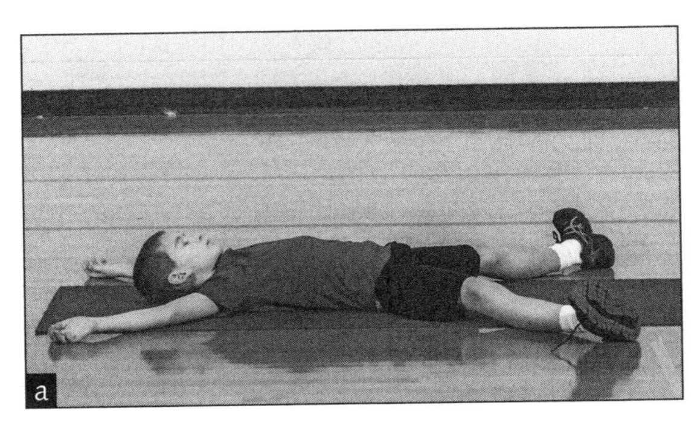

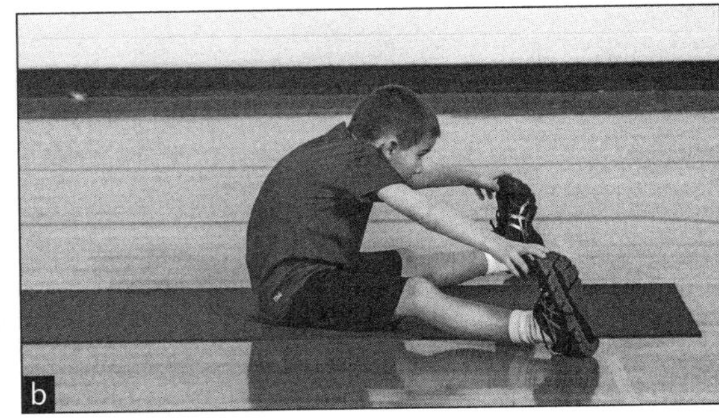

Opposite Toe Touch

Areas stretched: hips, hamstrings, and shoulders

1. Kneel on the right leg with the left leg extended forward. Raise the arms to shoulder level.
2. Twist the trunk to the left while touching the right hand to the left toes. Hold this position for three to six seconds. Extend the upper body and bring the right leg back to the starting position.
3. Repeat by kneeling on the left leg with the right leg extended forward.
4. Repeat with the opposite leg.

Variation

Perform this exercise by extending the leg diagonally rather than forward.

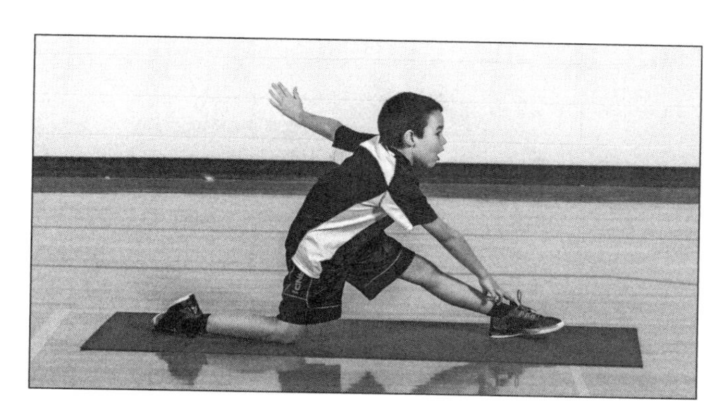

Hamstring Stretch

Areas stretched: hamstrings and hips

1. Flex the knees and hips, and place the hands on the floor.
2. Extend the knees, keeping the hands on the floor. Hold for three to five seconds.
3. Return to the starting position.

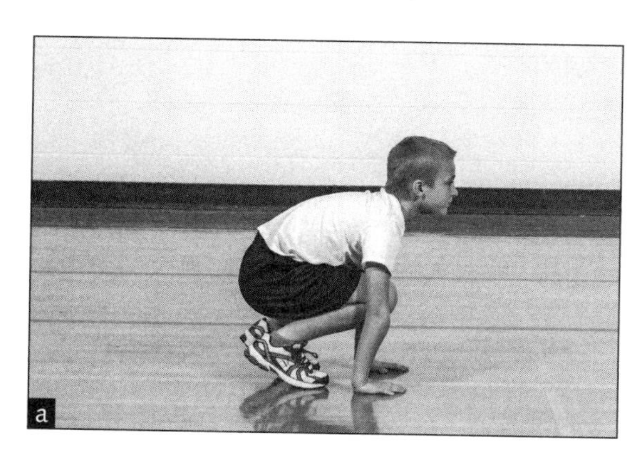
a

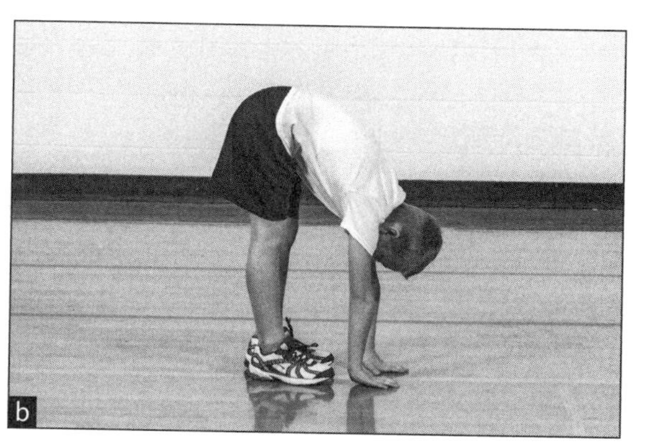
b

Medicine Ball Straddle Rotations

Areas stretched: shoulders, groin, hips, and hamstrings

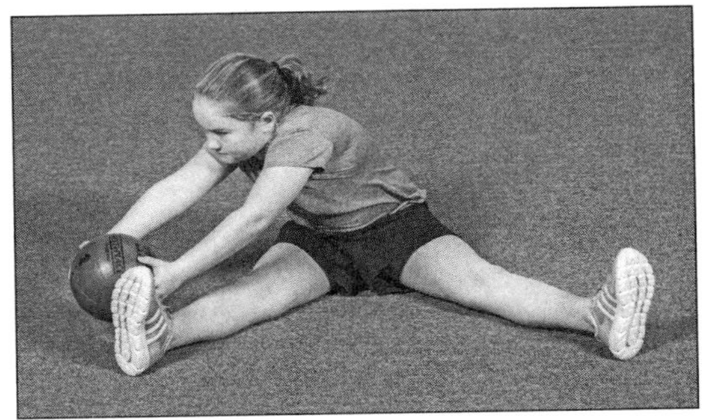

1. Sit with the legs far apart, holding a medicine ball in front of the chest.
2. Perform a complete, large rotation to the right extending the arms toward the right toes and towards the left toes. Return to starting position.
3. Repeat by extending arms to the left toes and rotate to the right.

Bow Shoulder Stretch

Areas stretched: shoulders and chest

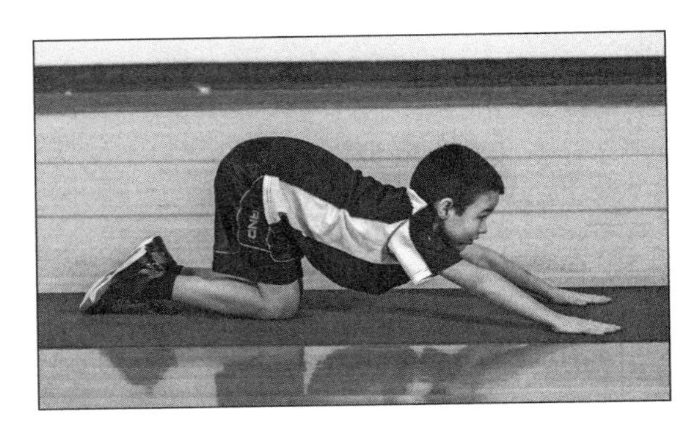

1. Kneel on both legs, with the hips flexed and the arms on the floor above the head.
2. Press the chest toward the floor. Hold for four to six seconds.
3. Return to the starting position. Repeat three to six times.

Ankle Stretch

Area stretched: calf muscles

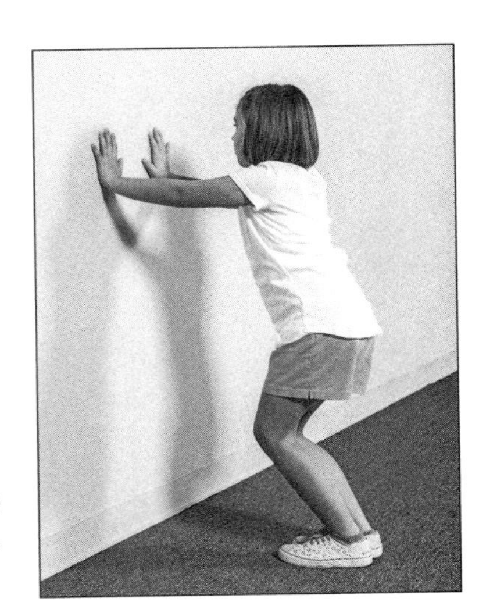

1. Stand in front of a wall with the feet together. Stand far enough away from the wall that the knees don't touch the wall when the legs are bent. Place the hands on the wall at chest level.
2. Bend the ankles and knees toward the wall without lifting the heels off the floor. The pressure should be mainly on the ankles. Hold for six to eight seconds.
3. Return to the starting position.

Note: To perform this exercise ballistically, the athlete should bend the knees and quickly return to the starting position six to eight times.

Diagonal Ankle Press

Areas stretched: calf muscles

1. Stand in front of a wall with the feet together. Place the hands on the wall at chest level. Move the feet as far away from the wall as possible.
2. Bend the knees slightly, forcing the ankles to bend as much as possible without lifting the heels off the floor. Hold for 6 to 10 seconds.
3. Return to the starting position.

Note: For a ballistic stretch, raise the heels off the floor and back down quickly and dynamically.

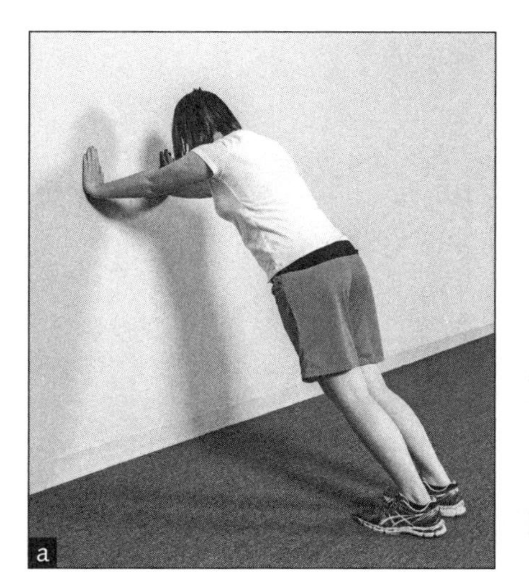

a

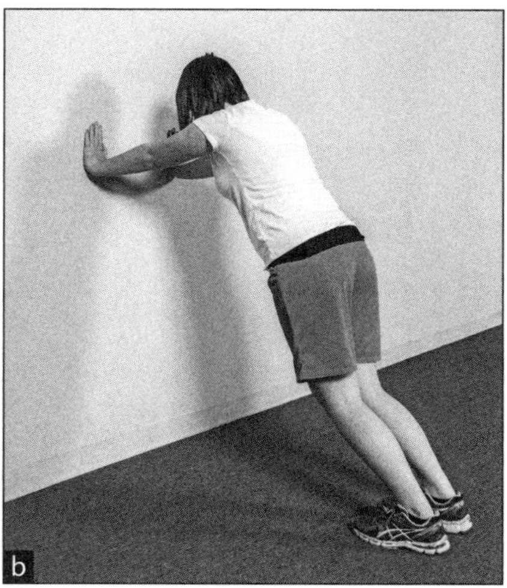

b

Sea Lion Stretch

Areas stretched: trunk and groin

1. Lie on the stomach, flexing the arms and placing the hands on the ground at shoulder level.
2. Extend the arms, arching the upper body while keeping the hips on the ground. Hold this position for two to four seconds.
3. Flex the arms and lower the upper body to the starting position.

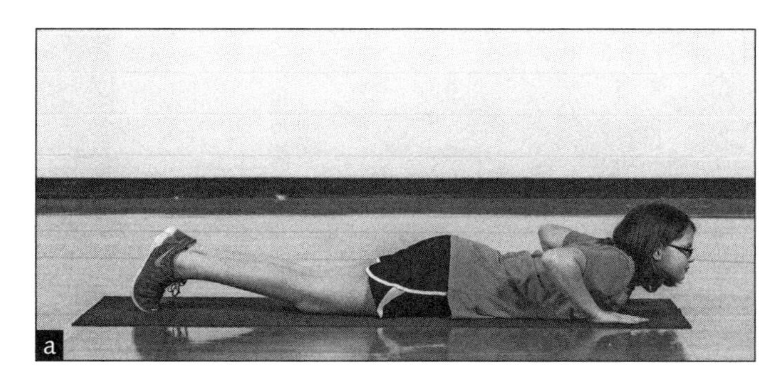

a

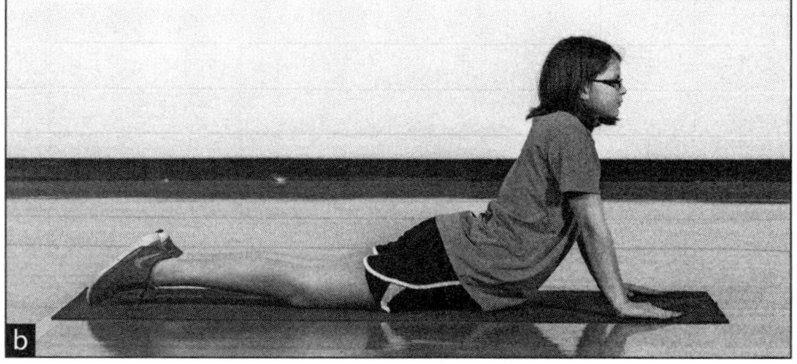

b

Double Kick

Areas stretched: shoulders, back, and groin

1. Kneel with the hands on the floor.
2. Dynamically swing the right leg and left arm upward, arching the back.
3. Return to the starting position.
4. Repeat the movement with the opposite limbs.
5. Return to the starting position.

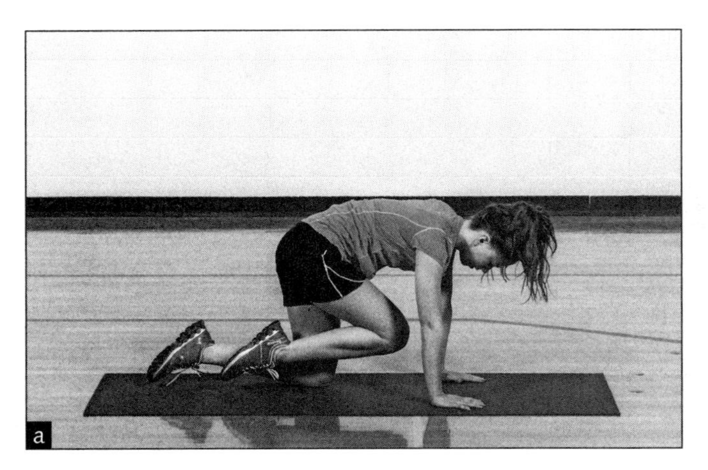

a

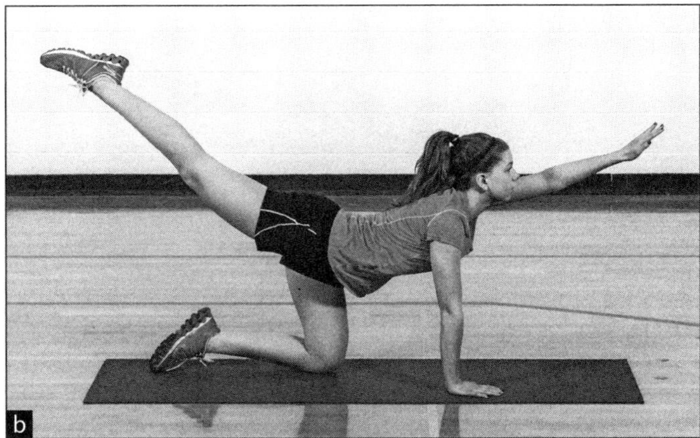

b

Seated Hip Flexion

Areas stretched: hips and hamstring muscles

1. Partner A sits on the floor with the arms extended. Partner B stands behind A and places the hands on A's back.
2. B presses A's upper body forward and down. They both hold the position for four to six seconds.
3. They both relax and return to the starting position.

Note: To perform the stretch ballistically, B presses A's trunk dynamically six to eight times.

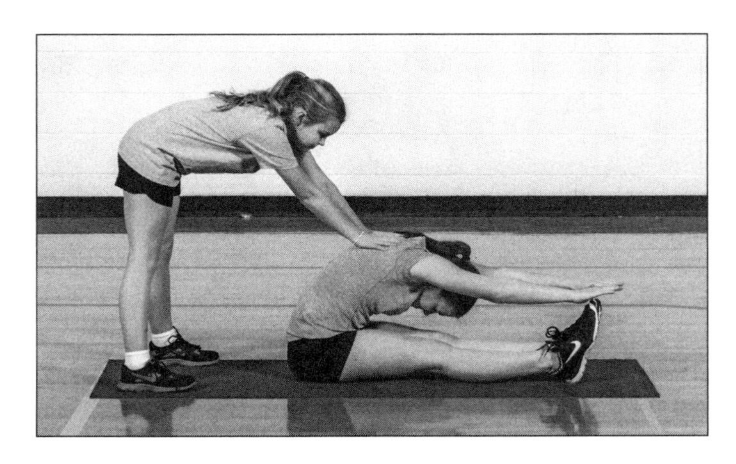

Standing Shoulder Stretch

Areas stretched: chest and shoulder muscles

1. Partner A stands with the arms above the head. Partner B stands behind A, placing the right hand below shoulder level on A's back and grasping A's hands with the left hand.
2. B presses A's upper back forward and pulls A's arms to extend them backward. They both hold the position for four to six seconds.
3. They both relax and return to the starting position. Alternate roles continuously.

Note: To perform the stretch ballistically, B pulls A's arm backward dynamically four to eight times.

Partner Shoulder Stretch

Areas stretched: chest, shoulders, groin, and abdominal muscles

1. Partner A lies on the stomach with the arms above the head. Partner B stands with the legs straddling A's upper body and grasps A's hands.
2. B slowly raises A's arms and holds the position for four seconds.
3. They return to the starting position.
4. Repeat with partners changing roles.

Scale Stretch

Areas stretched: groin, quadriceps, and trunk

1. Partner A stands three feet (1 m) in front of partner B.
2. A raises the left leg back and up, keeping the upper body vertical. B catches A's ankle with both hands.
3. B slowly presses A's leg upward and holds this position for two to six seconds.
4. B lowers A's leg and returns to the starting position. Alternate leg action and partners' roles.

Note: For a ballistic stretch, B bobs A's leg upward three to six times.

Variation

While in the hold position, A flexes and extends the knee of the supporting leg.

Partner Hamstring Stretch

Areas stretched: hamstrings, hip muscles

1. Partner A lies on the back with the arms above the head. Partner B stands at A's left side.
2. A raises the right leg. B catches A's ankle with both hands.
3. B applies a constant pressure downward against A's leg.
4. A returns the leg to the starting position.
5. Alternate legs and then partners' roles.

Note: For a ballistic stretch, bob the leg downward four to eight times.

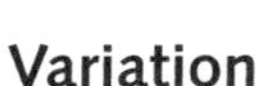

Variation

A pulls the leg above the head while B holds A's opposite leg against the ground.

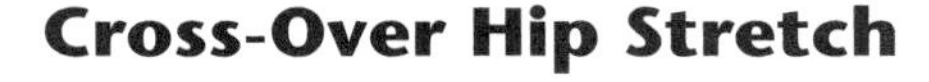

Cross-Over Hip Stretch

Areas stretched: hips, glutes, and lower back

1. Lie flat on the back with the left knee bent.
2. Place the right hand on the left leg and rotate the thigh to the right as close to the floor as possible. Keep the left shoulder flat on the floor while performing the stretch.
3. Perform the stretch on both sides of the body.

Variation

Perform this stretch with a partner. Partner A places one hand on partner B's rotated leg (around knee area) and the other hand on B's shoulder to help anchor B's body to the floor. Perform the stretch on both sides of the body.

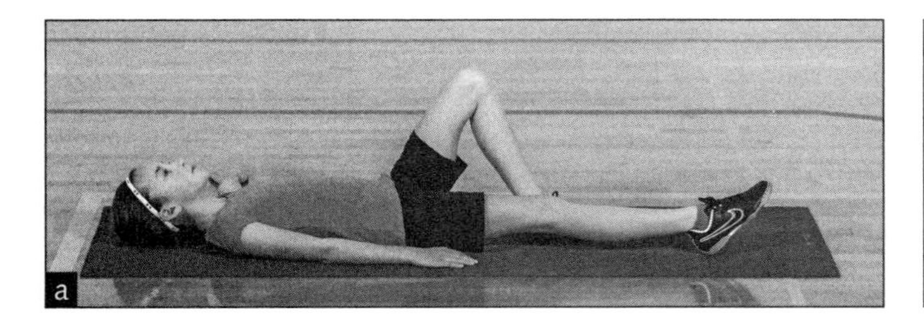

a

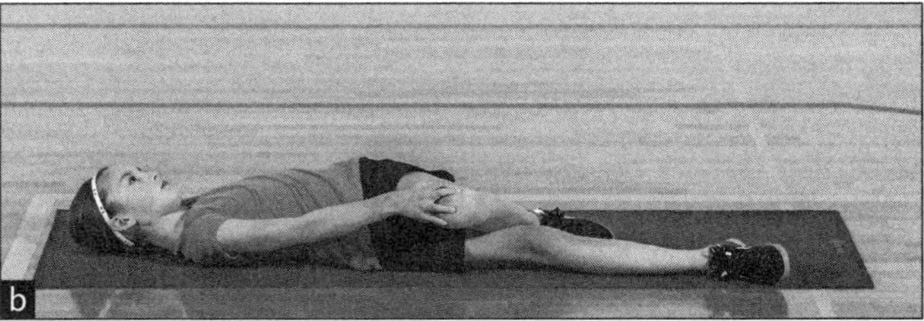

b

Quad and Hip Flexor Stretch

Areas stretched: quadriceps, hip flexors, and groin muscles

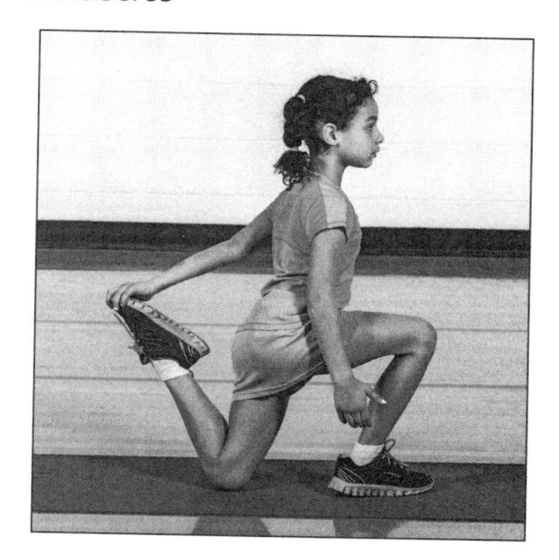

1. Place the left knee bent on a mat and the right leg forward, with the right foot flat on the mat and the leg bent approximately 90 degrees.
2. Keeping the upper body straight, lean forward at the hips to stretch the front of the left thigh. Hold for 10 to 15 seconds. Then, grasp the left foot with the left hand and slowly pull the foot to the glutes, further emphasizing the stretch in the quadriceps.
3. Repeat with the right side of the body.

Medicine Ball Swing

Areas stretched: hips, thighs, lower back, and shoulders

1. Stand with the feet shoulder-width apart and the knees slightly bent. Hold a light medicine ball in front of the body.
2. Bend the knees and drive the hips back. With the arms extended, lower the medicine ball between the legs (keeping the back straight) and slowly swing the ball up and over the head.
3. Repeat ballistically 8 to 10 times.

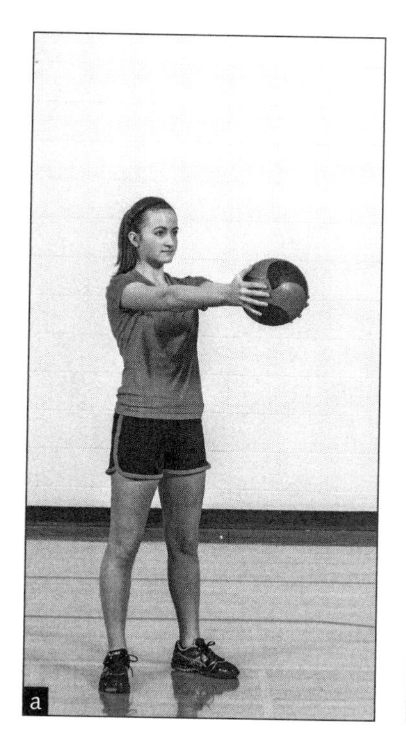
a

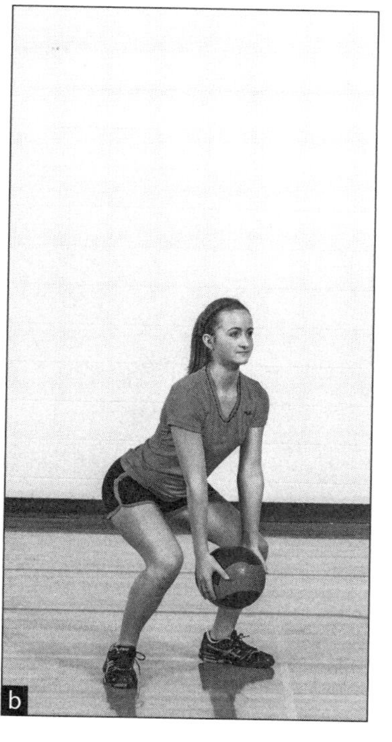
b

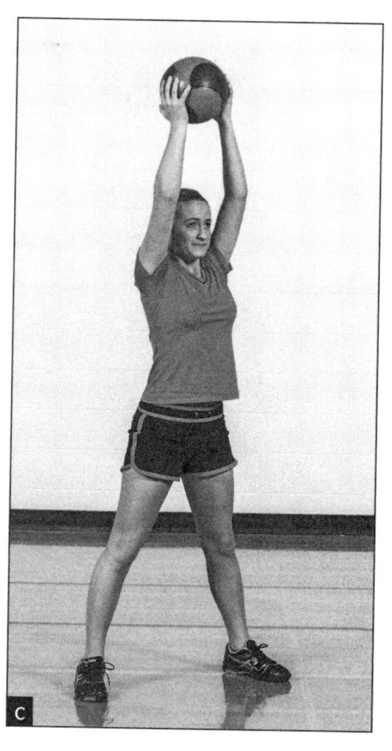
c

chapter 5

Speed Training

Speed is one of the most important qualities necessary to excel in sports such as track and field and team sports performed on large fields (e.g., football, rugby, baseball). In a few other team sports, such as basketball, handball, and lacrosse, athletes must run and move, react, or change direction quickly. In this case athletes must both be fast and have a high level of agility. To have speed and agility, one needs to develop strength and power—an athlete can't be fast or agile if she is not strong and powerful. The term *speed* incorporates three elements: reaction time (the motor reaction to a signal), movement time (the ability to move a limb quickly, as in martial arts, batting, or passing a ball), and speed of running (including the frequency of arm and leg movement).

In team sports an athlete rarely performs action in a straight line, such as sprinting in track and field. Players who can quickly change directions to receive a pass or deceive an opponent are highly regarded. In this case, elements of speed—reaction time and speed of running in different directions—are combined. Another example of speed is the quick arm or leg action required in martial arts when an athlete is either delivering a fast blow to an opponent or quickly blocking or avoiding a fast blow from an opponent. Such an athlete has to be fast or have a fast movement time. This is why it is important to understand and train the different elements of speed.

Each sport has a specific type of speed and quickness training. However, parents and coaches can help their young athletes by incorporating additional speed work into the athlete's training program. The exercises at the end of this chapter will assist in your quest for gains in speed.

Many sport specialists believe that sprinters are born, not made, because speed depends on the athlete's muscle-type composition. Speed depends on the following:

1. *Genetics.* The higher the proportion of fast-twitch to slow-twitch muscle fibers, the faster the reaction and more powerful the muscle contraction.
2. *Strength and power level of the athlete.* Children cannot be expected to display a high level of speed before getting stronger.

Irrespective of genetic qualities, athletes can develop speed through training. Even athletes who do not have a natural talent in speed-related activities can significantly improve their speed. It is important for young athletes to emphasize speed training during childhood. Running speed, reaction time, and quick footwork improve continuously from five years of age to maturity.

Speed improvement also depends on the ability of muscles to contract forcefully so that the body or a limb moves fast. Therefore, a forceful contraction in any type of quickness or speed relates to strength training. Because children's strength is visible mainly from puberty on, they achieve most gains in speed during puberty and postpuberty. However, speed improvements are also visible during prepuberty as a result of neural adaptation, meaning that as children perform quickness and speed activities, the muscles learn to work together and become more effective. Therefore, speed gains during prepuberty are not the result of powerful muscle contractions but rather the outcome of neuromuscular adaptation.

Regardless of the physiological adaptation responsible for improving speed during prepuberty, children are encouraged to run, skip, and jump in many directions and at various levels of intensity. The scientific literature shows that children who do not participate in activities that challenge the neuromuscular system and the development of motor skills early in life may not be able to approach activities in sport in the later years with vigor, determination, and physiological proficiency (Faigenbaum et al., 2013). Even in the absence of traditional strength training, children are encouraged to play hard and give 100 percent effort in play. While strength training with dumbbells and barbells and choosing exercises should consider the age of the athlete, children are encouraged to work hard and intensely when performing running, jumping, skipping, and other bodyweight activities. Doing so will help develop muscle mass and improve body composition, bone health, and motor skills (Barbieri and Zaccagni, 2013).

Speed-Training Model for Initiation

The ability of prepubescent children to perform quick motions increases progressively in this early stage; both boys and girls develop speed in the later stage of athletic formation. Most speed gains come from learning sprinting skills and from developing better muscle coordination.

Some children, especially those who do not experience multilateral development, may have poor arm and leg coordination. Because arm drive directly influences leg frequency, a low level of coordinating arm and shoulder force impedes children's ability to run fast. The main reason for this is that boys start gaining strength during puberty due to an increase in hormones such as testosterone, whereas girls have very low, and therefore modest, gains. The coordination of the arms and legs can be improved by repeating short distances (20-30 meters) with medium speed. In such an exercise, learning limb coordination—not running fast—should be the objective.

Sex differences in running speed are not visible during early prepubescence. These differences start to show as children approach puberty; the trend is that boys perform speed-related activities better than girls. This is seen in all running phases, with marked differences in speed development after the age of 15 years (Papaiakovou et al., 2009). Other forms of speed and agility display the same trend (Bailey et al., 1985; Hebbelinck, 1989). Furthermore, regardless of sex, the chronological age of the athlete will determine running speed. An 18-year-old boy will run faster in a 30-meter sprint than a 15-year-old boy will. Similar results are found in female athletes (Papaiakovou et al., 2009). Variations in speed development should be taken into consideration when developing programs for male and female athletes.

Scope of Speed Training

One main goal of prepubescent sport activities is to develop play-specific speed. Through exposure to play, games, and relays, children will learn how to coordinate their arms and legs, make them move faster, and run on the balls of the feet. Children's movement time will improve as a result of such motor experiences. They will learn how quickly to start moving parts of the body at a signal or in a play situation.

Prepubescent speed development is mainly the result of nervous system adaptation that children achieve through play and games. As a result of this motor experience, the nervous system learns how to coordinate the actions of the arms and legs most effectively. Consequently, a child will progressively cover a certain distance, change directions, and react more quickly. One way to challenge motor coordination and neural patterns of movement is to perform activities on difference surfaces. Because most school yards are paved in asphalt, which can be stressful on the joints, children are also encouraged to play on softer surfaces such as grass. Doing so will lessen the impact on the joints, improve balance, force the muscles to contract more fully by dampening ground reaction forces, and provide variety in training.

Children enjoy knowing that they are fast. They have fun and like performing physical tasks in which speed is important, during both play and relays. Variety in speed exercises is important because it improves motor experience. At the same time, children should not neglect the upper body. Simple throws using baseballs, tennis balls, or light medicine balls are useful for developing upper-body movement time. Also, relays and exercises using medicine balls for throwing and carrying will benefit upper-body strength, which will positively influence movement time later. For these exercises, see chapter 7.

Children can progressively participate in simple speed drills as their limb coordination improves, especially as they approach puberty. Similarly, for those involved in organized training such as team sports, the instructor can perform specific drills for speed, in most cases using a ball. The instructor can organize sport-specific drills as part of training, and children can perform other types of speed training in addition to the technical work.

Unless children participate in sex-specific teams, most games, plays, and relays—especially in the school curriculum—should be coed because no visible differences between boys and girls exist at this developmental stage (Bailey et al., 1985; Laemmle and Martin, 2013).

Program Design

When playing outdoors or recreationally with friends, children should be encouraged to play at their own pace. The guidelines in this section are for predetermined training programs or play that is performed under the umbrella of "training." Casual play with other boys and girls should be fun, and intensity should be unrestricted. We have all seen children who appear to have endless energy when playing. They transition from 10 minutes of jumping on the trampoline to 20 minutes of playing tag before finishing with a 30-minute bike ride or basketball game. Playing different activities and pushing each other in play helps improve children's self-esteem and skill and gives them the opportunity to determine their own level of intensity. Some children will push harder to catch up with those who are superior in fitness, and others will use their skills to be smarter in play. In either approach, children will benefit both mentally and physically by participating in fun, leisurely activities with family and friends.

You should view any speed-training program for prepubescence as an opportunity to utilize exercises that initiate an early nervous system adaptation to a variety of movements. As the coordination of muscle nerves improves, so will the children's capacity to be faster.

The duration of a drill or the distance to run should not be long. Children should not experience discomfort at this age. They should not run fast and continuously for longer than four to six seconds because longer distances require specific training. If they pause for two or three minutes, then they can repeat the same action with enjoyment. Children do not have fun when they experience discomfort and pain.

Instructors should plan training programs for speed, like anything else, over several years. The instructor should use a variety of exercises that involve the whole body and stimulate running speed and movement time for both the arms and the legs. Play, games, and relays should be the major elements of a training program for improving speed in prepubertal children.

Young athletes, especially children who are approaching puberty, should increase distance progressively over years, from 20 meters or yards to 40 to 50 meters or yards. Children should perform primary running exercises in a straight line. As children approach puberty and become stronger, you can incorporate running in zigzag, stop-and-go, and slalom patterns and running with quick turns in training. Stop and Go is a speed drill in which the athletes run as fast as possible for 5 to 15 meters or yards and then, at the signal *stop*, stop running as quickly as possible. At the signal *go*, they then run as fast as possible in another direction, which the instructor points out, for 5 to 15 meters or yards.

In team-sport training or during games, the instructor can combine speed tasks with skill performance (e.g., throwing and kicking a ball). Such drills are typical combinations for developing running speed and movement time. Prepubescent children have good trainability for speed, especially as they approach puberty; however, you should carefully plan and progressively implement everything including running, kicking, and throwing drills.

Table 5.1 presents several elements of speed training that are useful in most sports. The "form of training" column lists the types of activities children can perform, and the "duration or distance of activity" column suggests how many minutes, meters, or yards to run. The next column suggests how many times to repeat an activity. Between repetitions, children need to rest, relax, and avoid undesirable stress; the final column lists appropriate rest intervals.

For prepubertal children, the duration of a game does not have to be longer than 20 or 30 minutes. In hockey or soccer, children can play the game for two periods. We do not recommend that prepubescent children play a game for the same duration as adult athletes because children at this age do not have the conditioning potential to play a 90-minute soccer game or three 20-minute hockey games. An exhausted child hardly thinks about the next game, whereas one who has been tired but enjoyed it eagerly waits for the next game. Many soccer leagues in Canada and the United States have compressed each soccer game for prepubesecent children to 60 minutes; the first 30 minutes are devoted to practice and the remaining 30 minutes are devoted to a game. This model helps the children properly warm up and mentally prepare for the game and encourages a quick transfer of the skills and techniques used in practice to the game. Technical skills are rarely learned in a game because ball touch is minimal, but athletes can touch the ball 100 to 300 times during practice, depending on the length. This

Table 5.1 Periodization Model for Speed Training for Prepuberty

Form of training	Duration or distance of activity	Reps	Rest interval (min)
Games	20-30 min	1-2	—
Relays	10-15 m/10-55 yd	3-5	2-3
Speed training	10-50 m/10-55 yd	4-6	3-4
Speed training with turns, changes of direction, and stop and go	5-15 m/10-55 yd	4-8	2-3

Table 5.2 Sample Speed-Training Session

Part	Objective	Exercises	Duration or reps
1	Warm up	Same as table 2.1	10 min
2	Improve speed		6 × 25 sec
	Improve game-specific speed	Short and fast technical or tactical drills with quick direction changes	8 × 15 sec
		Game or scrimmage with technical or tactical goals	20-30 min
3	Cool down, relaxation, enjoyment	Relays	3 reps
		Relaxed, easy jogging	3 min

quick transition from practice to play results in greater confidence and application of skills in the game.

Children can easily repeat relays performed over 10 to 15 meters or yards three to five times, especially if they use different relays. However, irrespective of how eager children may be to repeat a relay, make sure they have a rest interval between relays.

For team sports, speed training has to take the form of running with turns, direction changes, and stop and go. Because the distance for this type of work is not long, children can perform more repetitions (four to eight) with a two- or three-minute rest interval between them. Table 5.2 shows the structure of a sample workout for speed training.

Exercises that improve reaction time need not be complicated or require the use of sophisticated equipment. A simple game of soccer or tag will suffice. Both activities require sudden bursts of speed and changes in direction, which improve power and agility. One study looked at the upper-body and whole-body reaction times of boys and girls between the ages of four and six years. The study compared children who liked dynamic activities, such as skipping or tag, with those who preferred static play, such as playing house, reading, or building blocks. Children who preferred static activities measured slower reaction times, whereas children who liked to play soccer or tag showed faster whole-body and upper-limb reaction times (Miyaguchi et al., 2013). This is not meant to discourage static play, which offers numerous mental benefits, including improvements in creativity and focus, but rather to encourage a multidisciplinary approach that offers a combination of active play and static activities.

Speed-Training Model for Athletic Formation

Speed development increases during puberty. Most children—both boys and girls—experience an acceleration in speed development during this stage. Such improvement may relate to increases in body and muscle size.

Strength gains positively influence speed development. From puberty on, the testosterone level in boys starts to increase dramatically, as does the ability to increase strength. The direct result of strength gains is improvement in both running speed and movement time.

Although boys show clear improvements from the later stages of pubescence, girls seem to plateau in their rate of speed development. Some speed gains can result from improved nervous system coordination of the muscles involved in quick actions, but most are the consequence of strength development and the ability of the muscles to contract more powerfully. As a result, the arms can drive more forcefully and the legs can push against the ground with more power.

Gains in upper-body power, especially the arms, improve movement time, reflecting the ability to throw the ball farther or bat more powerfully. On the other hand, improved leg strength translates into kicking the ball with more power. For most team sports in which running speed is important, the ability to quickly change directions is also significant. This skill is the result of improved nervous system coordination and strength gains of the muscles involved.

Scope of Speed Training

To improve speed to higher levels, speed training during puberty has to be specific. However, it should still be a part of multilateral athletic development, and children should do it in connection with developing other abilities.

During puberty, quickness and acceleration training lead to better nervous system adaptation, which results in enhanced coordination of the muscles performing the arm and leg actions. As strength starts to improve, especially for boys, movement time improves, which influences upper-body quickness and running speed. Similarly, as leg strength improves, children start to push more forcefully against the ground and are able to drive their bodies forward much faster.

Although coed speed training may occur during prepubescence, we advise that you separate the sexes starting at pubescence. Boys become stronger from puberty on, which positively influences the rate of limb movement and speed. As a result of these differences, it is better for girls and boys to train in separate groups.

Teaching Correct Running Technique

To improve running efficiency, athletes should work on running form. A crucial component in achieving running efficiency is good arm drive. The arms are driven back, forward, and up to the face level. Leg frequency increases as the rate of arm drive increases because the rate of leg movement is led and coordinated by arm drive and frequency. The thigh of the driving leg (for our example, this is the right leg) should reach a horizontal line; from this point on the foot of the same leg is projected forward and down. The back of the foot lands on the ground through a brushing action. As the body moves forward, the other (left) leg is driven forward. The right leg is now pushing against the ground, projecting the body forward. These actions are repeated for as long as the sprints last.

As children perform these exercises, the coach or teacher should constantly observe them for good form—keeping the shoulders down and relaxed, driving the arms simultaneously, and bringing the knees high. The position of the body should be vertical, and the eyes should be focused ahead. The foot should strike the ground quickly, coming underneath the body as it moves forward. The running step has the following phases:

1. The propulsion phase, in which the foot pushes against the ground with power to drive the body quickly forward.
2. The drive phase, in which the opposite leg drives forward with the thigh horizontal. The opposite arm also drives along the body, with the hand at shoulder height (arms are bent 90 degrees). It is essential to keep the ankle locked until the landing phase.
3. The landing phase, in which the foot strikes the ground and quickly comes underneath the body.
4. The recovery phase, in which the heel of the propelling leg quickly drives toward the buttock while the opposite arm quickly moves forward.

Program Design

As children approach postpubescence, they can increase the total amount of speed training. Whether using play, games, relays, or even sprinting routines, they can progressively increase the distance run with high velocity from 20 to 50 or 60 meters or yards.

Speed training can be fun for children and instructors alike. Children can perform a variety of exercises involving play, games, and especially relays. Instructors can organize relays in ways that use many exercises, such as sprints, sprints with turns, runs around cones with direction changes, carrying or throwing medicine balls, or jumps over safe equipment at a low height.

Instructors should also organize special exercises that improve reaction time. The objective is to decrease the time it takes for the child to move a limb—for instance, the arms and legs in running or the arms in throwing a ball. Such a goal can be achieved in two simple phases:

1. During the early part of improving movement time, the instructor positions herself in front of the children, facing them. At her signal—visual (clap) or sound (whistle)—the children perform the task. Because children can see the instructor, they can start the action faster.
2. As children improve their reaction time, after a few months or one to two years, the instructor selects a position behind the children so she can see the children but they cannot see her. Now the children will rely on sound only. The purpose of this exercise is the same: At the signal the children perform the task as quickly as possible.

Parallel with speed and movement time exercises, children should participate in simple exercises for power improvement. For the upper body, they can use a variety of medicine ball throws. Tennis and baseball throws for distance, alternating the arms for balanced development, are fun and beneficial for developing power in the upper body. Children can develop leg power by performing simple jumps on, off, and over low and safe equipment. (Refer to chapter 7.)

As postpubescence approaches, children can progressively increase to the maximum intensity (speed) and power of exercises to improve neuromuscular coordination. As children show better adaptation to training they can also increase the number of repetitions, depending on their work tolerance.

A critical element in speed training is the duration of the rest interval between repetitions. Because the ability to repeat high-quality exercises depends on the freshness of the neuromuscular system, the rest interval between repetitions must be as long as necessary to almost fully recover and restore the fuel needed to produce energy.

As table 5.3 illustrates, instructors can use relays for developing speed in pubescent children, and these relays can be of longer distance than those used for prepubertal children: 10 to 30 meters or yards, repeated four to six times, with a rest interval of two or three minutes. Children can repeat speed training in a straight line of 20 to 50 meters or yards five to eight times with a longer rest interval (four or five minutes) between each repetition. During the rest, the children should stretch the muscles for better relaxation. For team sports, children can perform speed training with changes of direction, turns, and stop and go for 5 to 25 meters or yards, repeated 5 to 10 times, with a rest of two or three minutes. Performing game-specific skills fast also develops specific speed.

If in a training session children repeat just speed training or speed with turns and direction changes, the number of repetitions can be much higher. After such training the coach will do either technical and tactical drills, play games, or scrimmage.

Table 5.3 Periodization Model for Speed Training for Puberty

Form of training	Distance of activity (m/yd)	Reps	Rest interval (min)
Relays	10-30	4-6	2-3
Speed training (including starts)	20-50	5-8	4-5
Speed training with turns, changes of direction, and stop and go	5-25	5-10	2-3

The structure of a training session for pubescent children can be the same as that shown in table 5.2. However, for each form of training the instructor should use the distance and number of repetitions shown in table 5.3.

Speed-Training Model for Specialization

Speed improvement comes with age. As children enter the postpuberty stage, gains in speed and movement time are more visible, especially for boys. Girls show the highest speed gains during late puberty and early postpuberty. From this point on, they seem to reach a plateau that may last throughout postpuberty unless they implement a speed-training program.

Boys maintain speed development throughout postpuberty. As they become stronger, they also become faster. The biggest difference between boys and girls is probably in the area of upper-body strength because from puberty on the upper-body strength of boys is constantly increasing.

For children involved in sport, speed gains may also relate to improved muscle coordination. As a result of multilateral training, they learn how to use their muscles and how to coordinate them for the best efficiency. As such, speed improvement also comes from better muscle and limb coordination. In addition, the nervous system learns to be more selective in choosing how fast and in what manner to react to an athletic situation. As a result of processing the signal or a game situation, the nervous system selects the action and stimulates the necessary muscles to contract and perform the quick movement.

Scope of Speed Training

Speed training during postpubescence should become specific and relate to the needs of the selected sport. Instructors should reduce the amount of time allotted to play games in order to leave time for sport-specific speed training.

For any athlete who intends to climb the ladder of high performance, postpubescence is the key rung. On one hand, athletes can still correct anything they missed during the first two stages of development. On the other hand, failing to address the sport-specific needs of speed training during prepubescence can drastically impair athletes' chances of reaching high performance. Although speed training becomes progressively more sport specific, athletes should not totally dismiss fun and elements of multilateral training.

Most speed training has to be dynamic and performed with high intensity to constantly stimulate the neuromuscular system. This type of training will result in running with higher leg frequency and velocity.

A constant concern in speed training is for the athlete to learn to relax the antagonistic muscles as the agonistic muscles contract to perform the movements. Allot special time for training lessons in which athletes learn how to relax and perform smooth, easy, flowing, and well-coordinated skills or movements. This is possible by first performing repetitions of speed work with lower velocity so the athlete can concentrate on relaxing the antagonistic muscles. As they achieve this, they can progressively increase the velocity until they can do the same repetition with maximum velocity. However, athletes will not achieve this training goal in a day, a week, or even a month. Sometimes it may take one or two years. Considering the benefits of learning to run smoothly, relax, and perform flowing actions, it is worth the time. If athletes do not do this at this development stage, they will run rigidly. Rigidity means higher energy expenditure and unnecessary muscle contraction that lowers velocity.

From the later stages of postpubescence, the coach has to apply annual periodization and planning. From this point on, the coach must organize a training program to meet the needs of training for a well-defined competitive season. The coach will have a preparatory (preseason) training phase for maintaining multilateral training and addressing compensation work for certain muscle groups. Training is specific from the late preparatory phase throughout the preparatory phase; during this time the coach or teacher uses mostly exercises and drills that will directly improve performance. Finally, in the transition or off-season phase of the annual plan, training is once again multilateral, informal, and relaxing. This is the time for removing fatigue, relaxing mentally, and maintaining some physical activity, play, and fun.

Program Design

Postpubescent speed training is more complex than what we suggest for the other two developmental phases. In addition to speed training, athletes must train the following elements to develop speed and movement time:

- *Speed.* High-velocity, high-frequency training at the highest intensity should be an important part, approximately 60 to 70%, of the total time dedicated to speed training.
- *Movement time.* Movement time is the time elapsed between the first overt movement of a response and the completion of that movement (Anshel et al., 1991). Movement time is not only a muscular reflex to a stimulus but also the ability of the muscles to contract quickly and powerfully. Training both speed and power will greatly improve the athlete's ability to move a limb quickly.
- *Ability to overcome external resistance.* In most sports, power—the force of a muscle contraction—is a determining factor in performing fast movements. During training and athletic competitions, external resistance to the athlete's quick movements exists in the form of gravity, the equipment, the environment (e.g., water, snow, wind), and the opponent. To defeat such opposing forces, athletes have to improve their power. By increasing the force of muscular contraction, they can increase the acceleration of movements and the speed to complete a skill. As part of training to overcome external resistance, athletes must improve the explosiveness of their kicking, hitting, throwing, and batting.
- *Technique.* The speed and frequency of a movement and of movement time are often a function of technique. Acquiring an effective form facilitates performing a skill quickly, correctly, and efficiently. Athletes must also place importance on consciously relaxing the antagonistic muscles in order to perform a skill with ease and coordination.
- *Concentration and willpower.* Rapid movements are facilitated by a high degree of power. Consequently, the quickness with which the central nervous system processes

the athletic information coming to it, the frequency of the nervous impulses, and the athlete's maximum concentration determine the speed of a movement. The athlete's willpower and maximum concentration are important factors for achieving high speed.

- *Muscle elasticity*. Muscle elasticity and the ability to relax the agonistic and antagonistic muscles alternately are important factors in achieving high frequency of movement and correct technique. In addition, joint flexibility is an important ingredient for performing movements with high amplitude (i.e., long strides), which is paramount in any sport requiring fast running. Consequently, including daily flexibility training—especially for calf and thigh muscles—is imperative.

Table 5.4 presents a periodization model for speed training for postpuberty. Although the table refers to many training forms, you may select only those required in your sport of interest.

High starts are important for all team sports in which players are constantly performing quick accelerations: soccer, football, baseball, hockey, lacrosse, and basketball. The athlete performs high starts standing, feet apart, in a ready position. At the signal, the athlete accelerates as quickly as possible for 10 to 30 meters or yards, repeating the same action 6 to 10 times. The instructor should give the athletes a three- or four-minute rest interval; relaxation and easy stretching maintain muscle elasticity. High starts can be performed separately from technical or tactical training in order to improve a fast start or as part of a specific drill.

Acceleration training is a form of training that increases maximum acceleration to increase maximum speed for both sprinting and team sports. Athletes can perform acceleration training over 20 to 60 meters or yards four to eight times, with a rest interval of three or four minutes. Speed endurance, on the other hand, is a form of training in which the scope is to maintain maximum velocity over a longer distance (60-120 meters or yards). Because this type of training is taxing physically and mentally, it is repeated three to six times but with a longer rest interval of four or five minutes. This form of training is important for wide receivers in football, baseball players, and track athletes.

Table 5.4 Periodization Model for Speed Training for Postpuberty

Form of training	Distance of activity (m/yd)	Reps and sets	Rest interval (min)	Speed sessions/wk
High starts	10-30	6-10	3-4	1-2
Maximum speed	20-60	4-8	3-4	2
Speed endurance	60-120	3-6	4-5	1-2
Sport-specific speed				
Accelerations	10-30	4-6	2	2-3
Decelerations	10-20	4-6	2	2
Stop and go	10-20	4-8	2	2-3
Accelerations with direction changes	10-30	4-8	2	2-3
Dynamic training (throwing, kicking, jumping)	—	2-4 sets, 5-10 reps	1-2	2-4

Note: Because these workouts are taxing, plan two to four forms of training per session, depending on the athlete's potential. Spend the balance of the sessions on technical or tactical work. Tables 5.5 and 5.6 provide examples of what types of training to perform on different days of the week.

Athletes must do sport-specific forms of speed training, such as using a ball in most team sports. For team sports, deceleration, or a quick stop from fast running, is as important as the ability to accelerate maximally. Because in team sports athletes rarely accelerate in a straight line, they must perform many sport-specific forms of training with turns, direction changes, and stop and go. The distance does not have to be long—10 to 30 meters or yards—repeated four to eight times. The rest interval is short (two minutes) to train the athlete to be able to accelerate and decelerate not only when rested but also in conditions of fatigue. Refer to chapter 6 for more agility drills.

In ballistic or dynamic training, athletes must perform dynamic, powerful throws, passes, kicks, hits, and jumps; for example, 5 to 10 repetitions, in two to four sets, with a one- or two-minute rest interval. Most team sports require these skills, for which athletes often train under the condition of fatigue.

We must also mention two important training considerations. First, athletes do not have to perform all forms of training in the same session. Sprinters in track and field may perform starts and maximum speed in the same workout. However, because of its difficulty, speed endurance is trained in its own session, separate from any other type of training. Wide receivers in football and baseball players would train high starts, acceleration speed, and accelerations with changes of directions in the same workout; in the case of baseball, changes of direction mean running around the diamond. Speed endurance, on the other hand, is performed on separate days and involves sport-specific form (e.g., changes of directions).

For most other team-sport athletes, the forms of training can be combined in the following way:

- One to two days per week: high start sprints, maximum speed training, and acceleration with changes of direction
- Two days per week: acceleration, deceleration, and stop-and-go sprints

The examples in tables 5.5 and 5.6 further clarify this. The second training consideration is that strength and power training, as suggested in chapter 7, will help the athletes improve maximum speed and movement time.

Table 5.5 Sample Training for Maximum Acceleration: Individual Sport

Monday	Tuesday	Wednesday	Thursday	Friday	Saturday	Sunday
Warm-up	Warm-up	Warm-up	Off	Warm-up	Warm-up	Off
Starts: 6-10 × 10-30 m/yd RI = 4 min	Maximum acceleration: 6 × 30 m/yd 4 × 50 m/yd 3 × 60 m/yd 4 × 30 m/yd RI = 4 min	Speed endurance: 4 × 60 m/yd 2 × 80 m/yd 2 × 120 m/yd 2 × 40 m/yd RI = 5 min		Starts: 4 × 10 m/yd 2 × 20 m/yd 2 × 30 m/yd	Speed endurance: 2 × 80 m/yd 2 × 120 m/yd 4 × 60 m/yd RI = 5 min	
Power training		Power training		Maximum speed: 3 × 40 m/yd 3 × 60 m/yd RI = 4 min	Power training	

Note: For power training, refer to chapter 7. Power training may be performed in the morning separate from speed training.

RI = rest interval. Light stretching during RI.

Table 5.6 Sample Training for Maximum Acceleration: Team Sport

Monday	Tuesday	Wednesday	Thursday	Friday	Saturday	Sunday
Warm-up	Warm-up	Warm-up	Off	Warm-up	Warm-up	Off
T drills acceleration–deceleration: 10 × 30 m/yd	TA drills direction changes, stop and go: 16 × 3 min	T drills maximum acceleration: 6 × 15 m/yd 6 × 30 m/yd RI = 4 min		T and TA drills for speed and agility: 12 × 30 m/yd RI = 4 min	Accelerations with turns: 6 × 30 m/yd	
T drills with turns and direction changes: 12 × 30 m/yd	Scrimmage RI = 2 min	TA drills: 12-14 × 1 min RI = 2 min		T and TA drills with turns, stop and go: 8-10 × 1 min	Acceleration–deceleration: 8 × 30 m/yd	
Scrimmage RI = 2 min	Ballistic or dynamic training	Ballistic or dynamic training		Scrimmage Ballistic or dynamic training	Stop and go: 10 × 30 m\yd RI = 2 min	

Note: On Saturday the program is performed individually (i.e., outside of the gym or ice arena). Add power training on Monday, Wednesday, and Friday per examples in chapter 7. You may organize power training on Monday, Wednesday, and Saturday mornings separate from specific training.

T = technical; TA = tactical; RI = rest interval.

As mentioned previously, from postpuberty on, the coach or instructor can start using annual periodization models. At this stage, athletes start to participate in more formal competitions, and training must follow a structured program. Instructors must base such a program on the concept of periodization, as in figures 5.1 through 5.3.

Figures 5.1 and 5.2 show that the progression for speed training starts from short-distance repetitions, in which the athlete seeks best form and maximum velocity for that development stage. When athletes reach their maximum velocity and best form for their particular stage of development, they should progressively increase distance up to that required in the chosen sport or in a dash race.

In team sports, the longest distance that athletes must run with maximum velocity depends on the position they play on the team. For instance, wide receivers or baseball players run with maximum velocity up to 80 meters or yards. In soccer, distance decreases to 40 to 60 meters or yards, whereas in basketball the distance is not longer than 15 to 20 meters or 16 to 22 yards, unless the athlete returns to his own basket with the same velocity. Irrespective of how far the athlete runs with maximum velocity, the instructor should organize special sessions for speed training that follow the concept of periodization and incorporate elements of maximum speed, speed power, and speed endurance. These types of training programs will make an athlete a fast runner who has good acceleration.

For team sports, the ability to accelerate quickly is not sufficient. The players have to be able to change direction and decelerate quickly so they can turn around and immediately accelerate in another direction. The stronger the legs, the faster an athlete can accomplish this. Therefore, an athlete should participate in strength training simultaneously with speed training.

In a 100-meter standard dash, an athlete does not achieve maximum velocity at once, and the running velocity is not the same throughout the race or run. From the start it takes an athlete four to five seconds to build up to the highest speed, which depends on leg power. Analysis of a 100-meter dash illustrates that athletes reach peak velocity at the 50- to 60-meter mark and maintain it up to 80 meters. From that point on, athletes tend to decrease velocity.

Figure 5.1 Periodization Model for Speed Training for Postpuberty

Month	Oct	Nov	Dec	Jan	Feb	Mar	Apr	May	Jun	Jul	Aug	Sep
Training phase	Preparatory						Competitive				Transition	
Types of speed training, distance, and percentage of max. velocity	Long tempo 8-12 times 400-200 m/yd at 50%	Short tempo 8-12 times 200-100 m/yd at 60-70%		Reps 20-40 m/yd at 95-100%	Reps 40-60 m/yd at 95-100% Low starts of 10-15 m at 80-100%		Reps 60-80 m/yd at 90-100% Starts of 20-40 m at 90-100%	40 m/yd to full distance, or over-distance without or with starts			Other physical activities Play/games	
Speed training	Anaerobic endurance			Maximum speed			Maximum speed, maximum acceleration, speed endurance				————	
Power training	Power endurance			Starting power			Starting power, power endurance				AA	

Note: Annual plan for speed training for a postpubescent sprinter, where peak performance must be reached in June and July. AA = Anatomical adaptation

Figure 5.2 Periodization Model for Speed Training for Late Postpuberty

Month	Oct	Nov	Dec	Jan	Feb	Mar	Apr	May	Jun	Jul	Aug	Sep
Training phase	Preparatory			Competitive		T	Preparatory		Competitive		Transition	
Types of speed training, distance, and percentage of max. velocity	Long tempo 400-200 m/yd at 50-60%	Short tempo 200-100 m/yd	Reps 20-40 m/yd at 95-100%		Reps 40-60 m/yd at 95-100%		Short tempo 200 m/yd at 75%	Reps 40-60 m/yd at 95-100%	Reps 60-80 m/yd at 95-100%	40 m/yd to full distance, or over distance without or with starts	Other physical activities Play/games	
Speed training	Anaerobic endurance		Maximum speed Maximum acceleration			/	Anaerobic endurance	Maximum speed Maximum acceleration		Maximum acceleration Maximum speed Speed endurance		
Power training	Power endurance		Starting power			/	Power endurance	Starting power		Starting power Power endurance	AA	

Notes: Annual plan for speed training for a late postpubescent child.

T = Transition phase

AA = Anatomical adaptation

Figure 5.3 Periodization Model for Speed Training for Postpuberty for a Team Sport

Month	May	June	July	August	Sept	Oct	Nov	Dec	Jan	Feb	March	April
Training phase	Preparatory					Competitive					Transition	
Types of speed training, distance, and percentage of maximum velocity	Long tempo 600 m at 50% 400 m at 60%	Short tempo 100 m-200 at 65%		Short reps 20-30 m/yd at 90-100% Specific drills 20-90 sec at 95-100%		Maintain maximum speed and acceleration					Other physical activities play/games, outdoor activities	
Speed training	Anaerobic endurance			Maximum speed: turns, stop and go, direction changes			Maintain maximum speed using specific drills/ scrimmages				————	
Power training	Power endurance			Power: acceleration and deceleration			Maintain power: acceleration and deceleration				AA	

Note: The league games are planned for October-February (i.e., basketball, volleyball, hockey, etc.).

In the early part of the race, high acceleration depends on power and speed power, whereas from 70 to 80 meters on, speed endurance is required to maintain the velocity. This brief analysis of sprinting speed shows that speed training is slightly more complicated than it may look. The instructor must know the three segments that compose a race, what is required for athletes to perform well in each segment, and which elements of speed (acceleration, maximum speed, and speed endurance) athletes must train to become fast runners.

Figure 5.1 illustrates a periodization model of an annual plan for speed training for a postpubescent athlete. In this example, the athlete must reach peak performance in June and July. At the top of figure 5.1 are the months of the year and the structure of the training phases. Below that are the types of speed training, distance, and percentage for a given segment of the plan. The program starts with long tempo, or a type of training in which the athlete does repetitions of 400 meters at the beginning and 200 meters at the end, repeating this 8 to 12 times at 50 percent of maximum velocity. The scope of this type of training is developing an aerobic–anaerobic base. The same training scope is planned in the next segment of the preparatory phase (late November to mid-January), but the velocity is higher: 8 to 19 repetitions at 60 to 70 percent of maximum velocity.

On the base created between October and mid-January, athletes progressively increase speed training to peak for the months of June and July. Maximum velocity should be developed by starting at short distances in late January and February and progressively increasing to full distance as competitions approach.

The distance that athletes repeat to increase maximum velocity depends on the form of running. In fact, running form dictates the distance and the number of repetitions the athlete performs. In the early part of the sprinting phase, athletes repeat distances of 15 to 20 meters, which requires them to keep a relaxed and correct form. When the athletes cannot maintain form, they are fatigued and lose the power of fast running.

When athletes can maintain form for 30 to 40 meters, the coach can plan repetitions of longer distances (40-60 meters)—in our example, from early March to mid-April. At the same time, the coach can plan low starts of short distance (10-15 meters) with 80 to 100 percent of maximum power and speed. Always demand good form.

After three months of speed training with short and medium distances, athletes can start to perform repetitions of 60 to 80 meters or yards. The coach can extend the distance when athletes are able to maintain maximum velocity with good form. From this point on, throughout the competitive phase, the athletes perform full distance or distances longer than the racing distance (i.e., overdistance) to develop maximum velocity and speed endurance.

From April through July, the number of repetitions depends on how much work the athlete can tolerate and the fatigue level she experiences. As competitions approach, it is better to undertrain than to overtrain the athlete. Maximum velocity is possible only when the athlete is rested, fresh, and unstrained.

The lowest two rows of figure 5.1 show the types of speed and power training the athlete must develop throughout the year if she expects to perform well in June and July. You do not have to rigidly apply the plan suggested in figure 5.1. Climatic conditions and athletes' training potential may necessitate some changes. However, irrespective of changes in the plan, do follow the suggested progression and type of training.

The difference between figure 5.1 and figure 5.2 is that the plan in figure 5.2 includes two competitive phases: indoor competitions from January to early March and outdoor races from late May to the end of July. Between these two phases are two weeks of transition in mid-March. The progression for each peak is similar to that in figure 5.1 except that each phase is shorter so that two peaks are possible. All of the other elements of training are similar to those in figure 5.1.

The plan illustrated in figure 5.3 is similar to that illustrated in figure 5.1: the same regression from long tempo to short tempo, culminating with specific speed for August and September. During these last two months of the preparatory phase, athletes do most speed training by repeating specific technical and tactical drills or by doing speed-specific training for team sports (e.g., turns, changes of direction, and stop and go). This type of speed training has to train the players for playing a game, which is dynamic, and for quick changes of speed, from jogging to maximum acceleration. The progression for power training has to support gains in specific speed that the player must maintain throughout league games. You can easily adapt the example in figure 5.3 to team sports in which the competitive phase is in the spring and summer months (e.g., soccer, baseball). In such a case, plan the preparatory phase for the fall and winter months and the sport-specific speed and power training for March and April.

Exercises

In this chapter we present 26 exercises and games that will help young athletes develop speed. These exercises are appropriate for all ages. Keep in mind that the instructor or coach should insist on good running form while athletes are performing the relays in this chapter (see "Teaching Correct Running Technique earlier in this chapter") and should emphasize skills over winning.

One final point: When it comes to developing training speed, you don't have to do what is *new* but rather what is *necessary*. Many fallacies exist in speed training, from running techniques to equipment. To improve speed, we need to focus on improving strength and power by following a progressive, periodized strength-training program that is age specific and by applying full-body running and jumping drills with proper technique that challenge the neuromuscular system to react faster, contract muscles forcefully, and improve coordination. Relays and races, such as some of the exercises in this section, encourage competition and help keep fast runs fast as athletes try to outrun the other team. Speed training for kids should be fun and invigorating and—most importantly—help them improve performance in their chosen sport, be it individual or team sports. This can be achieved by performing some foundational exercises that require little equipment and that can be performed indoors or outdoors.

File Relay

Focus: running form, velocity

1. Organize a group of players in two or more relay teams of 8 to 10.
2. Players stand behind the starting line. At the instructor's signal, the first player in each line runs as fast as possible up to a cone placed 10 meters or yards in front of each team.
3. After turning around the cone, the player runs back toward the starting line and touches the hand of the next player in line. No player can start his run before touching hands.
4. When a player finishes running, he goes to the back of the line.
5. The winning team has to finish the relay faster than the other teams, and the players must be lined up in the order in which they started the relay.
6. You can organize relays so that the players perform skills such as running, carrying a ball, rolling a ball all the way, or hopping.

10 yd or m

Starting line

Slalom Relay

Focus: fast running with turns around cones

1. This relay is organized like the File Relay except that players perform a slalom run around several cones placed in front of each team in single file.
2. As in the File Relay, players can run, dribble a ball, or carry a medicine ball or any other object.
3. The rules of the File Relay apply to any relay race.

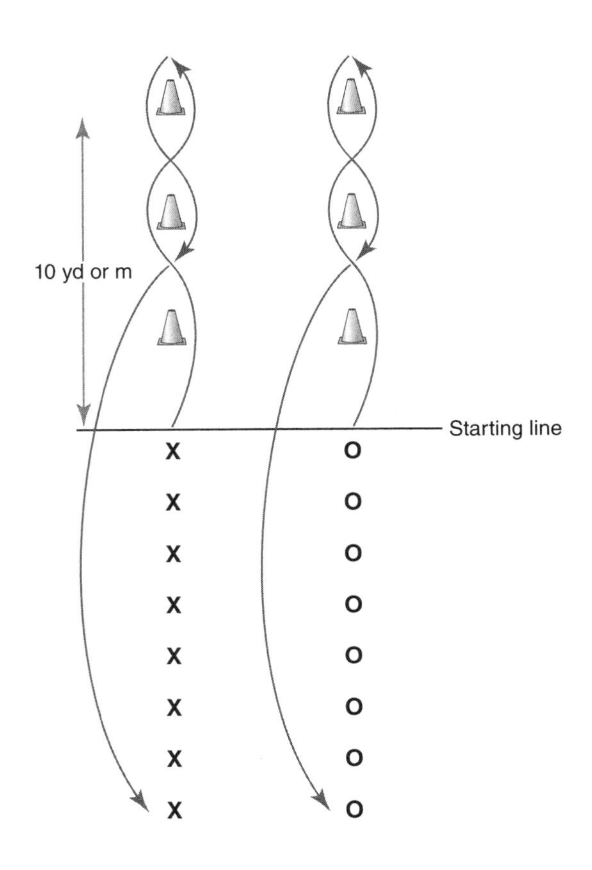

Fox and Squirrel

Focus: quickness, reaction time

1. Designate one fox and one squirrel.
2. The remaining children pair up and hold hands, facing each other with arms raised. They are designated as trees and spread out around the play area.
3. The fox chases and attempts to tag the squirrel. The squirrel can avoid being tagged by hiding in a tree. If the squirrel hides in a tree, the person facing the squirrel's back becomes the squirrel.
4. The game proceeds until each player has had a turn at being either the fox or the squirrel.

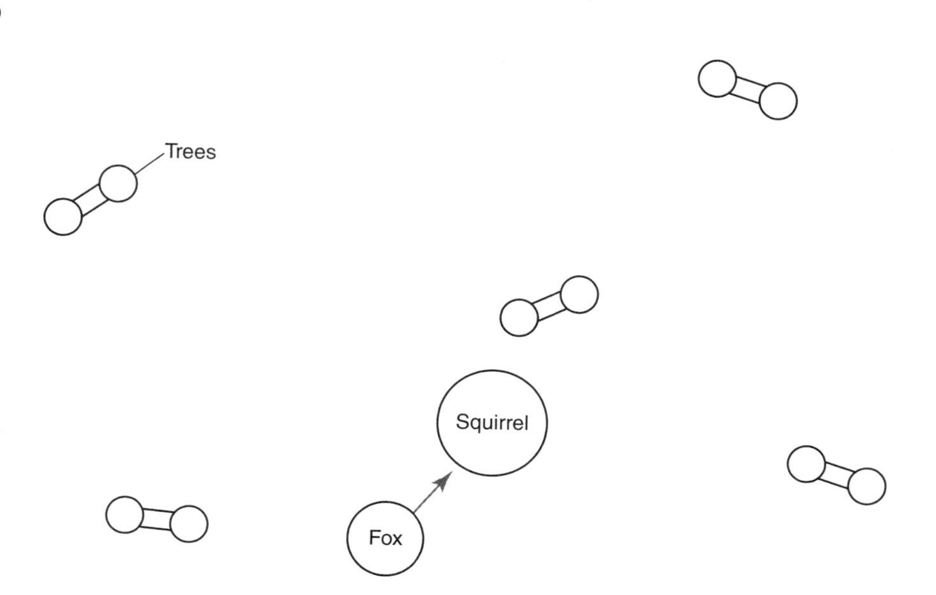

Partner Tag

Focus: quick reaction time, fast running around a circle

1. Designate one tagger and one chasee. The remaining participants pair up and form a circle.
2. The tagger chases the chasee. If the tagger tags the chasee, they reverse their roles.
3. If the chasee joins a pair before being tagged, the player she taps on the shoulder becomes the chasee.
4. If the tagger begins to tire, the instructor designates a new tagger.

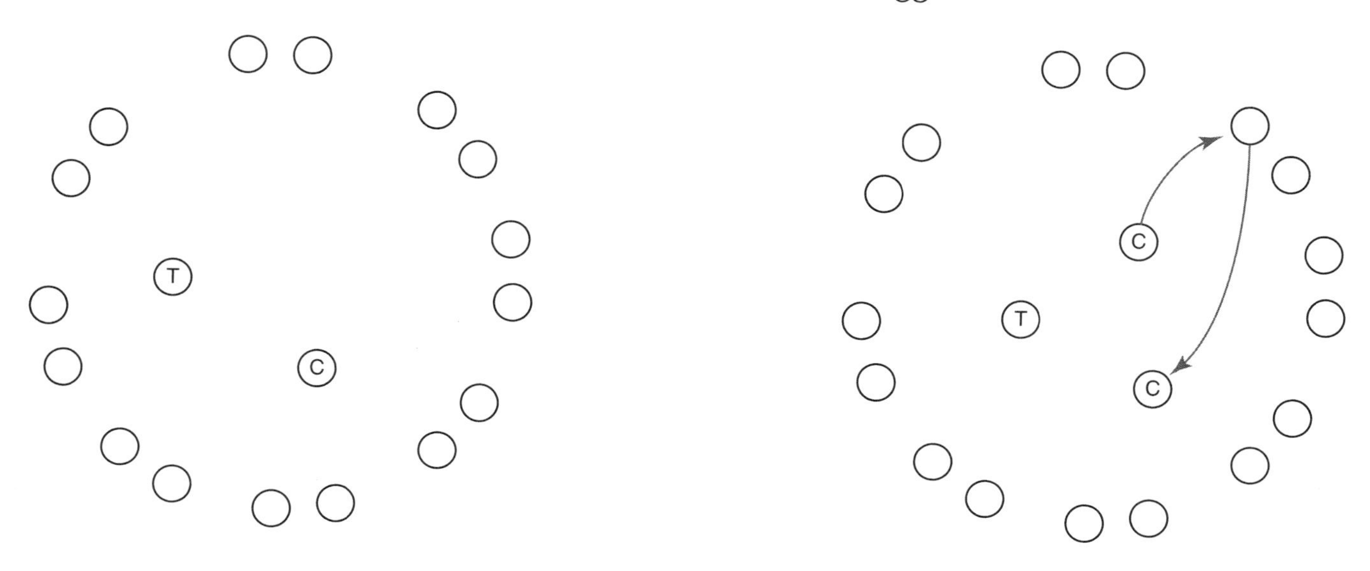

Octopus Tag

Focus: reaction time, high speed with changes of direction

1. Form a large group of 20 to 30 participants. Designate one or two participants as the octopus. The remaining participants line up against one wall.
2. The octopus yells "Octopus!" and the participants run to the opposite wall.
3. If the octopus tags a participant, the participant turns around on one foot to help tag others.
4. Game ends when all participants have been tagged.

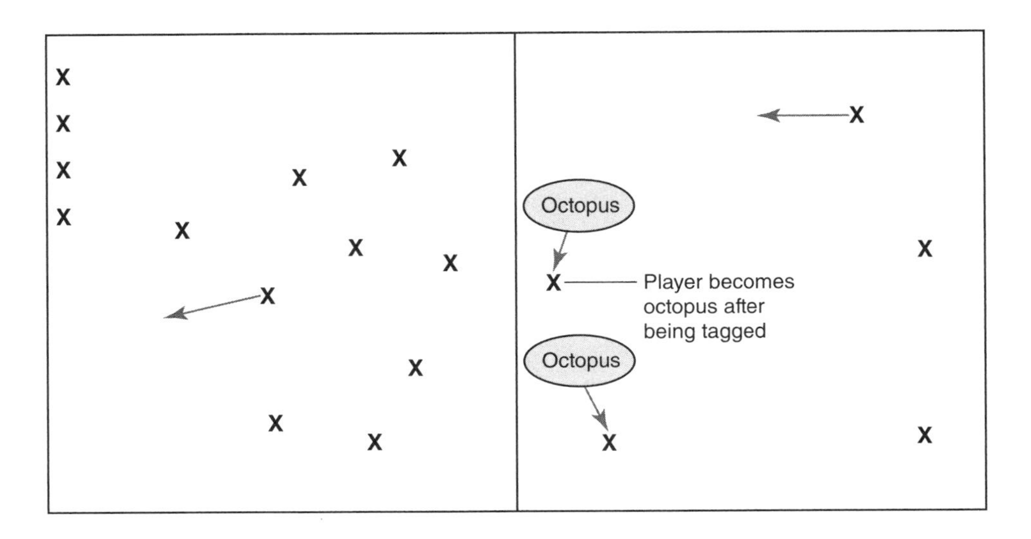

Arm Swing

Focus: arm drive, arm coordination

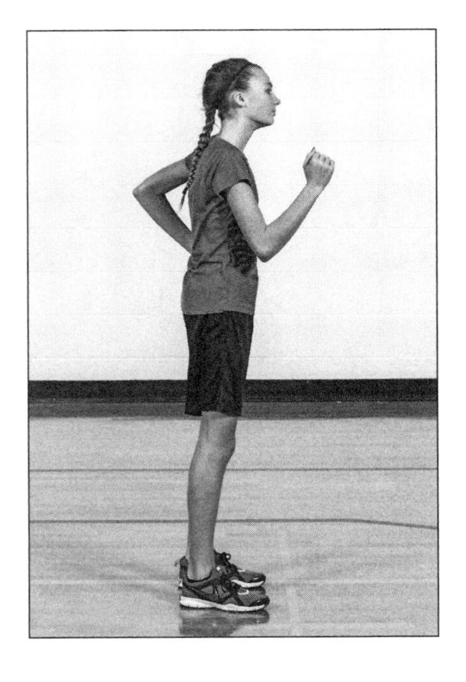

1. Stand with the feet parallel and six inches (15 cm) apart. Bend the elbows approximately 90 degrees.
2. Without changing the position of the body and elbow angle, swing the arms forward and backward. The shoulders should be down and relaxed while swinging the hands up to the level of the face.

Standing Start

Focus: quick acceleration from a standing position

1. In many sports, especially team sports, the ability to accelerate quickly is desirable. Standing start drills, therefore, train athletes to quickly start a fast acceleration in a given direction. Stand with the feet apart in a ready position.
2. At the instructor's signal, the player attempts to quickly accelerate in the desired direction.

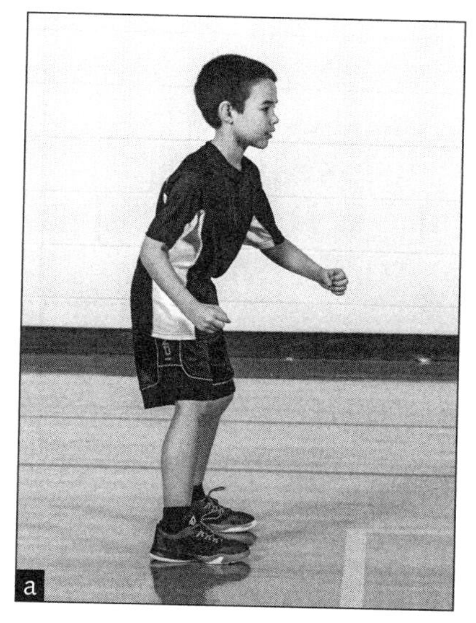

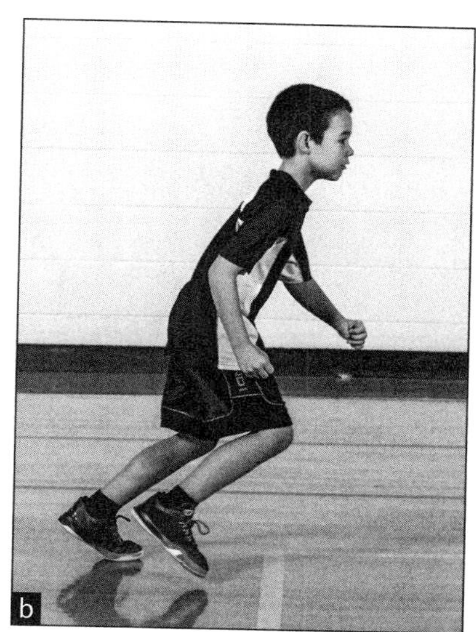

Variation

Perform the same exercise with turns around a cone or a series of turns or slalom around four or five cones.

Falling Start

Focus: quick acceleration from a falling-forward position

1. Begin in a standing position.
2. At the command "On your mark," move to the start line.
3. At the command "Set," place one foot back and the opposite arm forward, with both arms at approximately 90-degree angles. The body should be about to tip over from a slightly forward-leaning position.
4. At the command "Go," swing the forward arm back vigorously and the back arm forward and drive the back leg through to make the first stride.

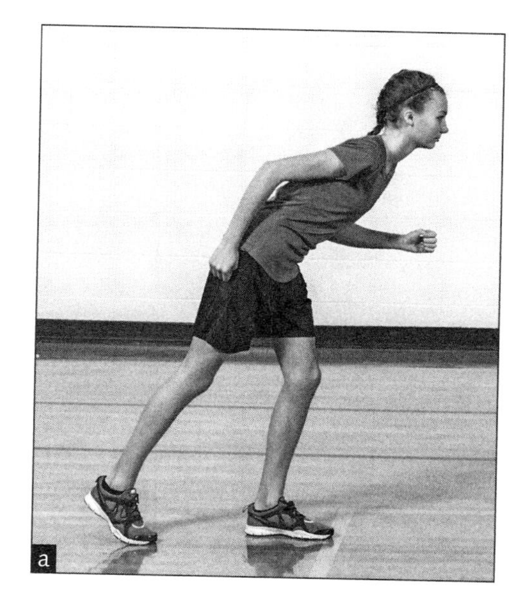

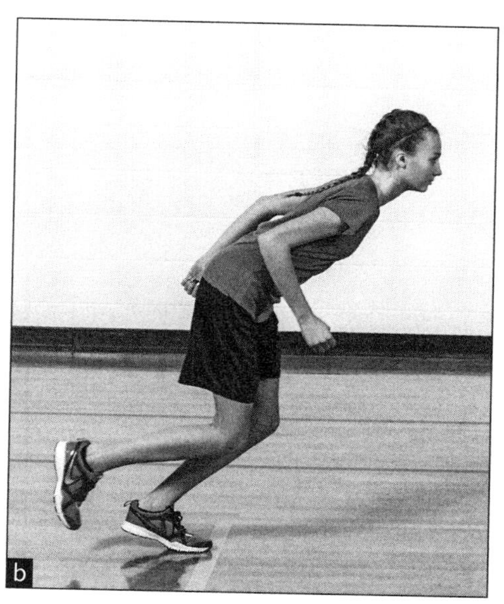

Quick Steps

Focus: quick acceleration with short and quick steps

1. Take either the standing or falling starting position.
2. Perform quick steps from the start for 10 to 15 meters or yards, always landing the front foot below the knee of the front leg. This will result in an acceleration with short and quick steps.

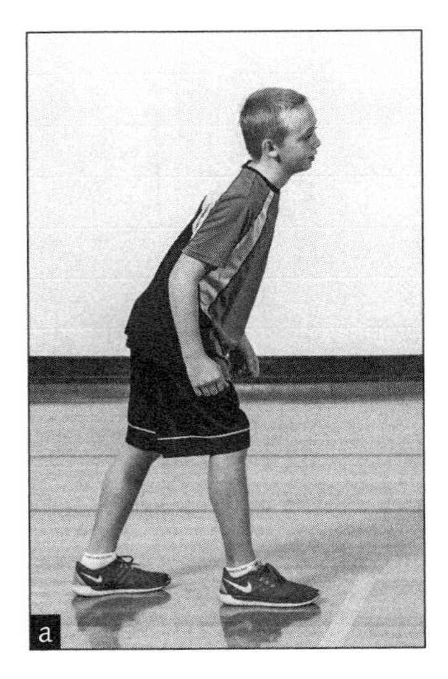

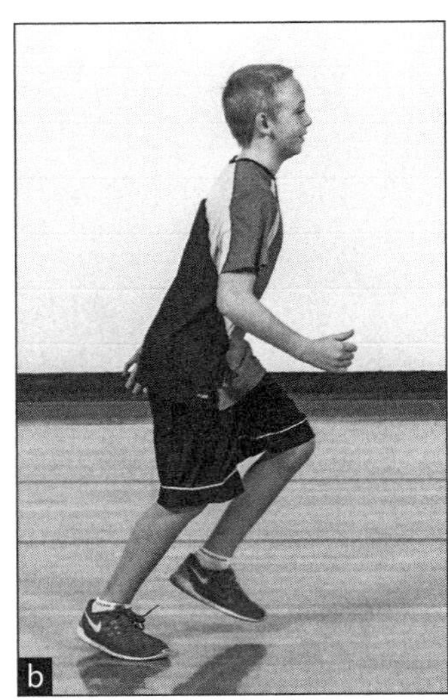

High Knees

Focus: calf and hip flexor strength

1. Walk, driving the knee of the front leg above horizontal and rising up on the toes of the supporting leg.
2. Bend the arms 90 degrees and drive them back and forth in coordination with the legs.
3. Do repetitions of 20 to 25 meters or yards.

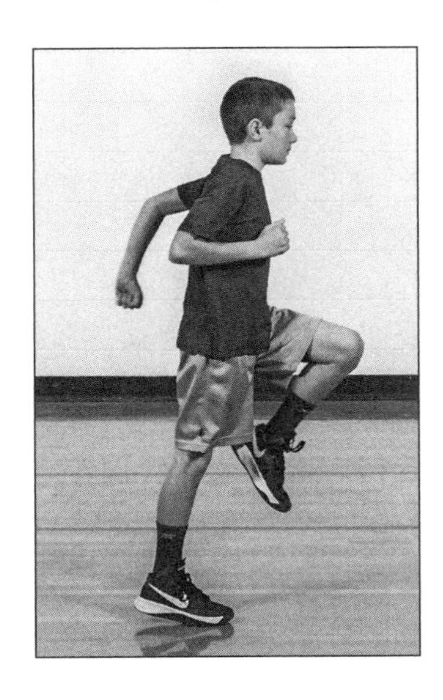

Harness Running

Focus: arm drive, leg power development

1. The instructor or partner places a rope or ribbon around the athlete's shoulders under the armpits (like a rucksack).
2. The instructor or partner holds the ends of the rope and opposes the athlete's forward drive with a slight resistance.
3. To overcome the resistance, the athlete has to push forcefully against the ground, slightly inclining forward and driving the knees forward powerfully.
4. Repeat for a 10- to 15-meter or yard run.

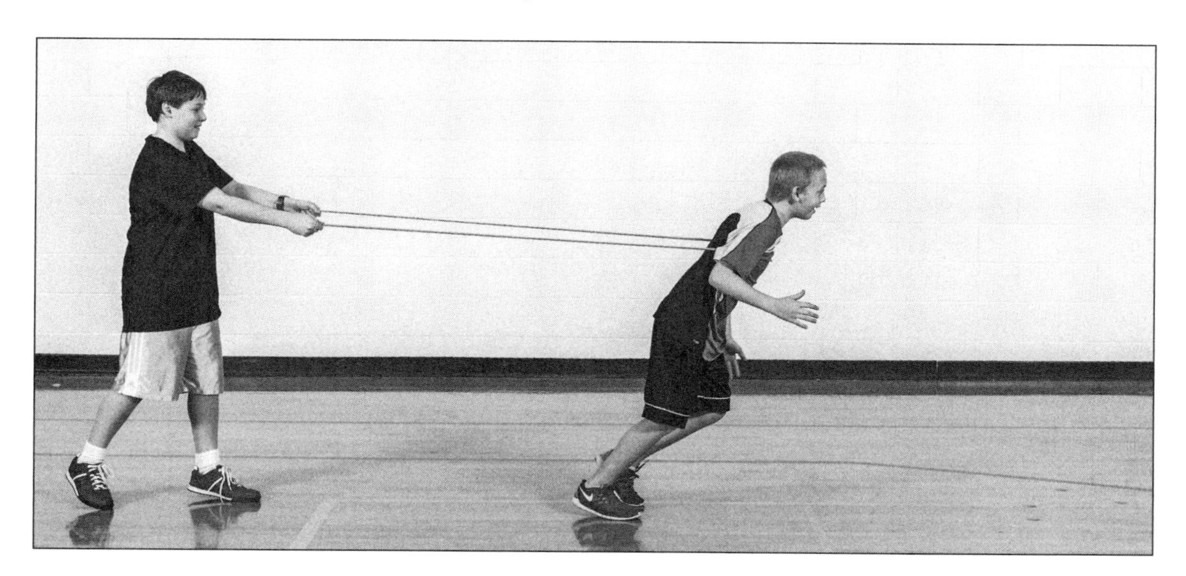

Big Steps

Focus: leg power, long strides

1. The athlete begins in a standing position.
2. The instructor makes 10 to 15 marks or circles on the ground at a distance that will force the athlete to perform big steps (strides).
3. The athlete performs long strides and always places the feet in the circles. When finished, the athlete walks back to starting point.

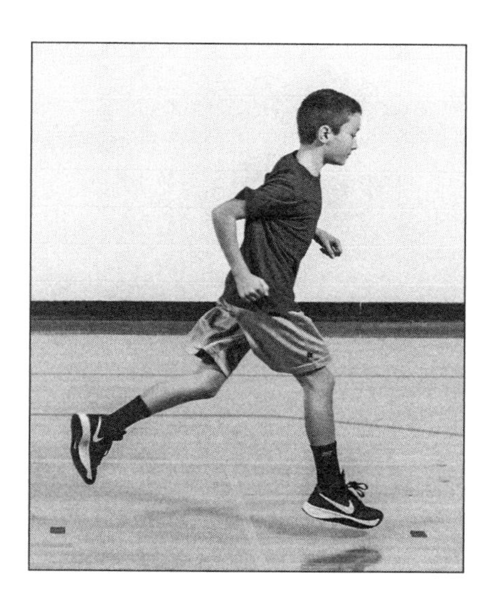

Acceleration Run

Focus: fast acceleration

1. Begin standing, one leg forward, in a ready position.
2. Repeat acceleration runs by sprinting as fast as possible while observing good form: running tall, arms and legs coordinated, arms bent, heels coming up to the buttocks, eyes forward, shoulders relaxed.

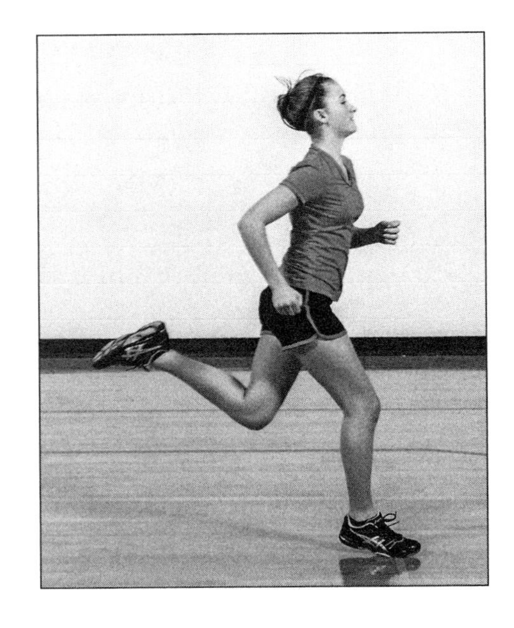

Beanbag Relay

Focus: acceleration, deceleration, leg power

1. Two teams line up single file facing each other, a maximum of 65 feet (20 m) apart.
2. The front athlete from one team runs with a beanbag and hands it off to the front athlete of the other team, who becomes the next runner. The first athlete sits down at the back of the line.
3. The relay ends when all members have run with the beanbag and are seated.

Beanbag Shuttle

Focus: fast acceleration

1. A run-and-fetch game with teams running to pick beanbags out of a box. Create two lines with an even number of players lined up in single file. Place the box of beanbags directly in front of each team, at a distance of 20, 30, or 40 meters (66, 98, or 131 ft).
2. The first runner takes a beanbag and places it in a box. The next player runs to the box as fast as possible, picks up the bag, and returns to her team, giving the beanbag to the next player in line.
3. The game ends when the last team member gets the beanbag and returns to the start.

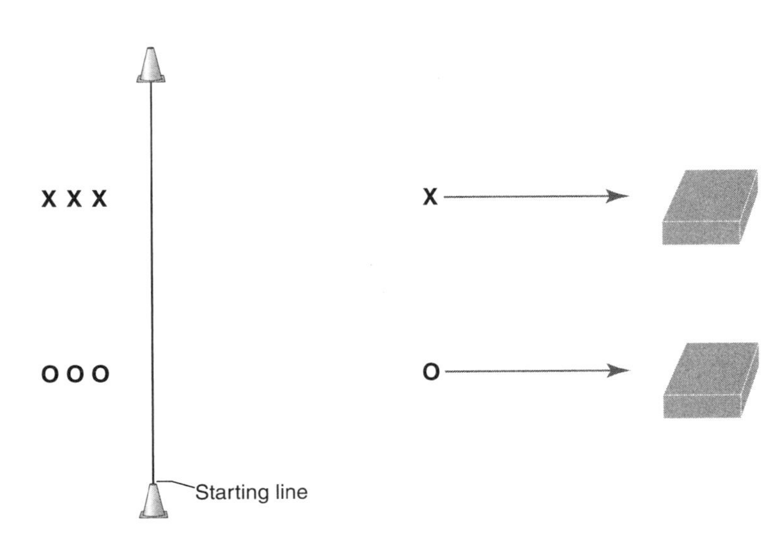

The Loop

Focus: start, fast run forward and around a loop

1. Divide the group into small teams of six or eight athletes. From a standing position, the athletes fall forward and start to run a loop around a cone. Place cone directly in front of the athletes a distance of 20, 30, or 40 meters (66, 98, or 131 ft) away from the start.
2. After running around the cone, the athlete walks rapidly back to the start.

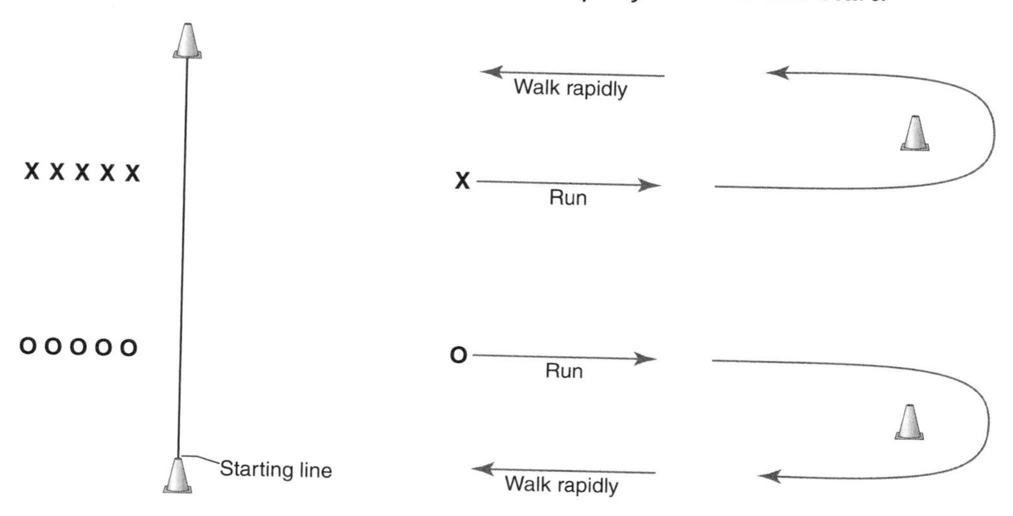

Rabbits and Roosters

Focus: fast acceleration with quick changes of direction

1. Two teams stand four meters or yards apart. Each team has a three-meter or yard safety zone in front of its home wall.
2. The instructor names one team Rabbits and the other team Roosters.
3. The instructor calls one team's name (either Rabbits or Roosters) to chase the other team to their safety zone.
4. Those tagged join the other team.
5. The game ends when players from one team have all been tagged.

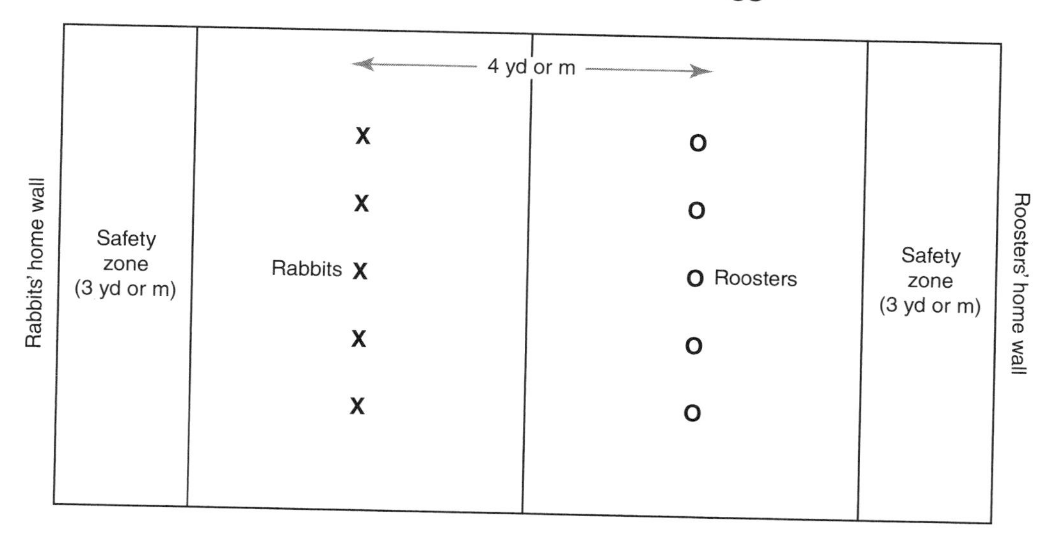

Finders Keepers

Focus: acceleration, deceleration, leg power

1. Divide the athletes into teams of four or five. Place two hoops on the floor 15 meters or yards apart, and place four beanbags or balls in each hoop. One team stands to the right of and behind each hoop; this is the team's "home hoop." The objective is to have six beanbags in the home hoop.
2. At the start command, the first runner runs to the opposing team's hoop, picks up a beanbag or ball, returns to the home hoop, and drops it.
3. Once the beanbag or ball hits the floor, the second team member goes to find a beanbag in the other team's hoop.
4. Both teams are simultaneously trying to get beanbags from the other team's hoop.
5. End the round when a team has six bean bags.

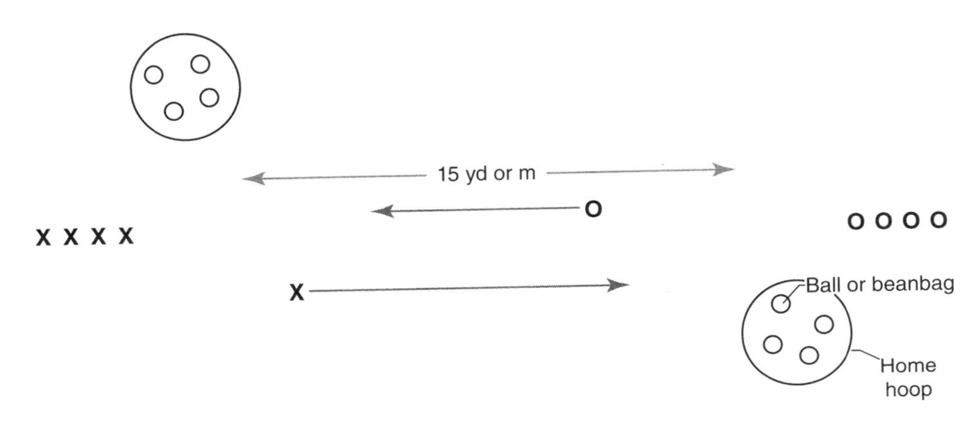

Tents and Campers

Focus: reaction time, acceleration

1. Athletes pair off and form one or more circles 15 to 20 meters or yards in diameter. In each pair, one athlete is a tent who stands with the feet apart, and one athlete is a camper who sits in front of the tent.
2. The instructor calls out words that begin with "t" or "c" sounds. When the instructor calls out *tent* or *camper*, the appropriate member of each pair runs around the circle and then either stands behind the camper or crawls under the tent.
3. Anyone moving when the instructor calls out anything but *tent* or *camper* has to wait out one run.

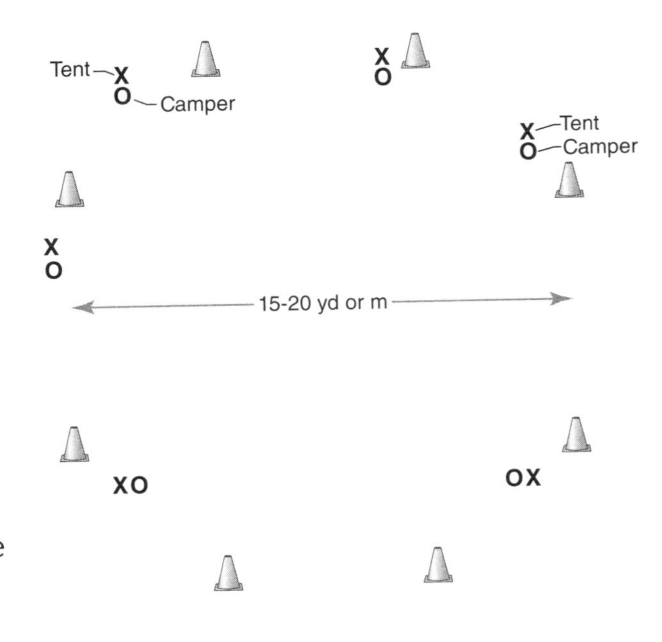

Obstacle Course

Focus: leg power, running around and over obstacles

1. Set a slalom course with benches to step over, cones to run through, hoops to step in, mats for front rolling, and saddle horses or boxes for ducking under or climbing over.
2. The athletes start with a walk-through and increase speed as capability increases. Leave enough room between athletes on the course (especially for doing front rolls).

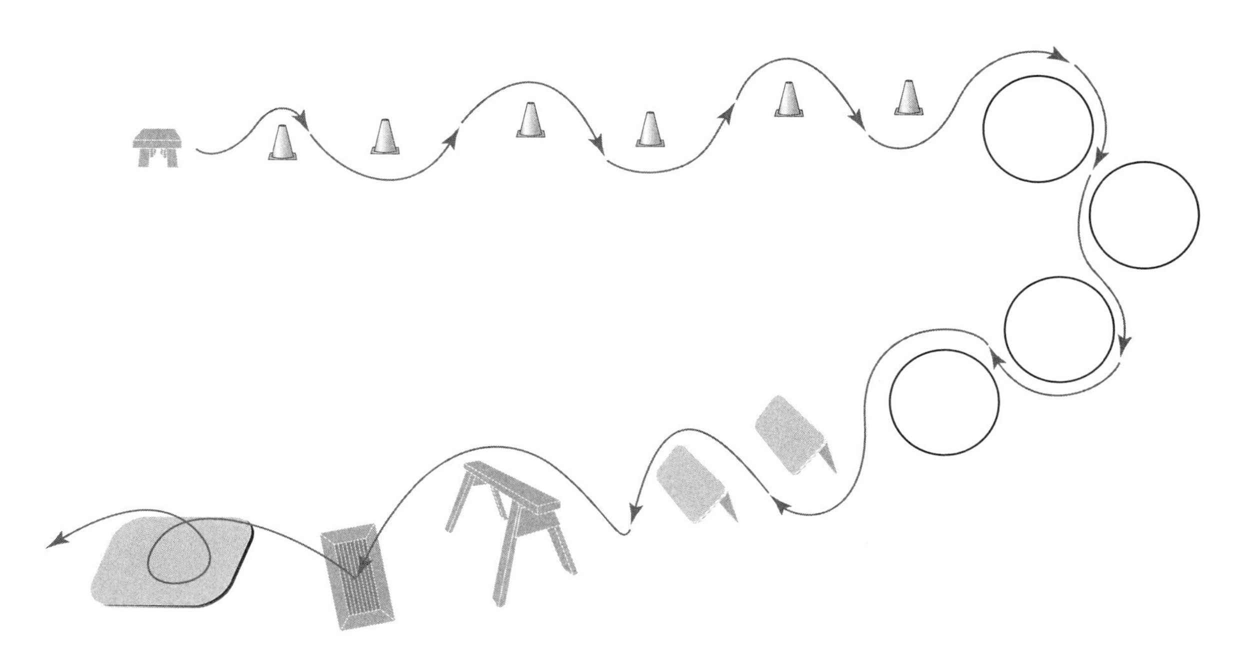

Low-Obstacle Relay

Focus: acceleration, leg power

1. Set out one or more straight courses with a cone as a turnaround point. (The fewer athletes per course the better.) The course should have low obstacles that athletes can run over, not leap or hop over. Placing the obstacles close together encourages quick steps, and placing them farther apart encourages longer or more steps.
2. Have the athletes run the course with two steps between the obstacles. Then spread the obstacles out and have the athletes run it again with three or four steps between the obstacles.

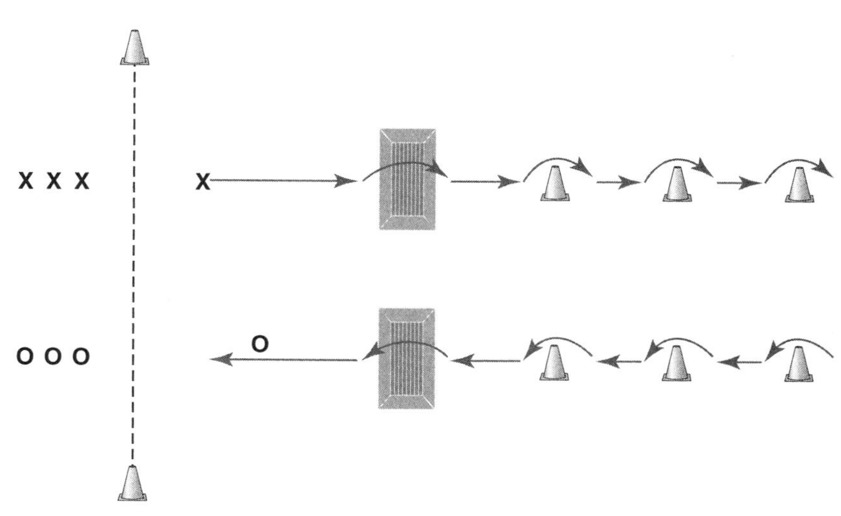

Note: The scope of these exercises is to improve quick footwork, which is important in many team sports.

Forward Crossover

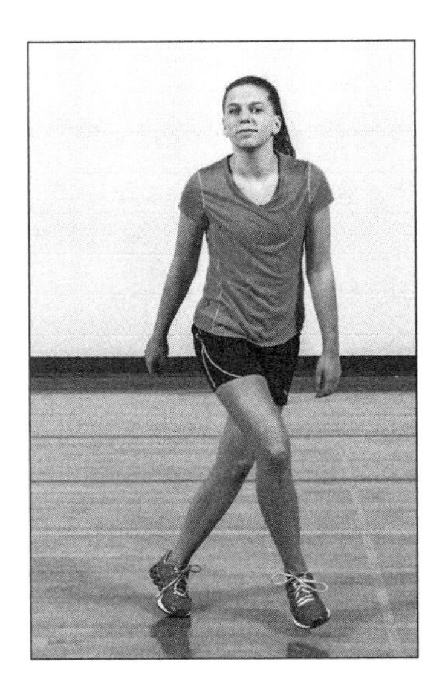

Focus: quick leg action, agility

1. Moving left, the right leg crosses in front of the left leg for 10 meters or yards in each direction.
2. Repeat.

Backward Crossover

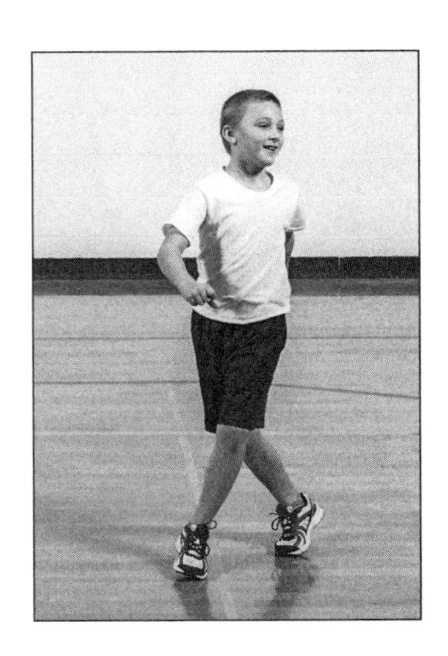

Focus: quick leg action, agility

1. Moving left, the right leg crosses behind the left leg for five to eight meters or yards in each direction.
2. Repeat.

Carioca

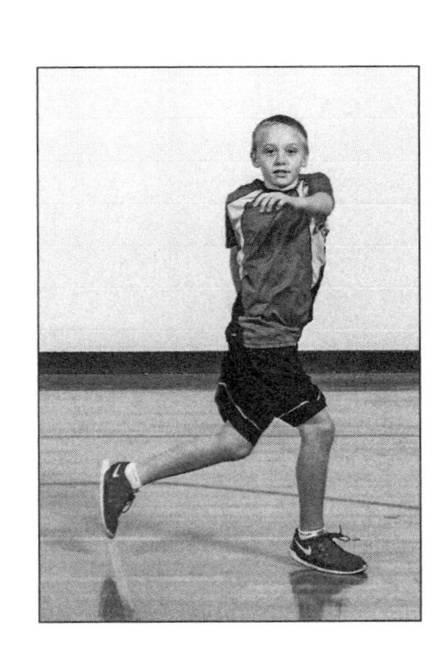

Focus: agility, quick feet

1. Quickly shuffling sideways facing in one direction, perform 3 to 4 forward crossovers, followed by 3 to 4 backward crossovers. You should cover a distance of 8 to 10 meters sideways, facing one way, forward crossover, backward crossover.
2. Quickly turn around at the end of the 10-meter distance and repeat the same actions facing the other way.
3. Complete at least 2 to 3 sets facing both ways.

Foot Touches

Focus: quick footwork, agility

1. While standing, perform these movements by lifting the feet to meet the hands. touch the left hand to the right heel in front of the body, then the right hand to the left heel in front of the body, then the left hand to the right heel behind the body, then the right hand to the left heel behind the body.
2. Repeat as quickly as possible.

Note: Simple reaction-time training should be part of most activities the children perform. Reacting to the demands of play will result in a reaction-time training effect.

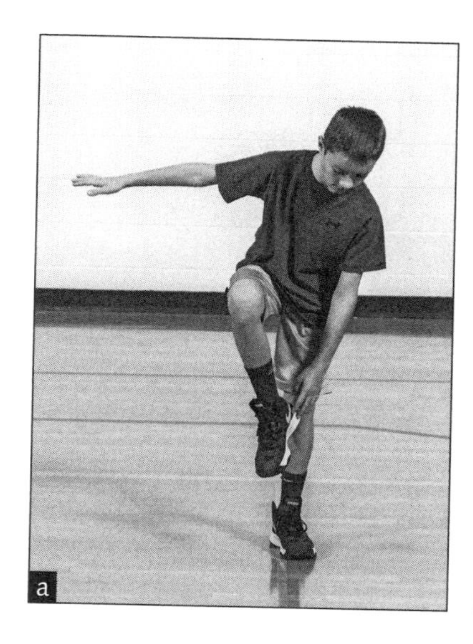
a

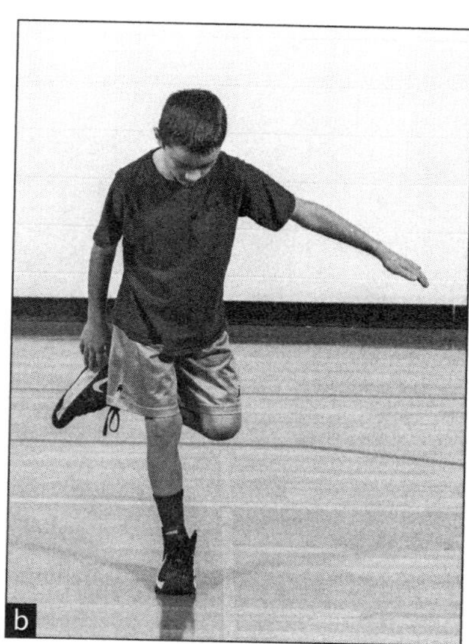
b

Go, Go, Go, Stop

Focus: reaction time, acceleration, deceleration

1. An athlete stands 10 meters or yards ahead of the remaining participants, facing away from the group.
2. The caller calls out "Go" as many times as he likes and then calls out "Stop."
3. At "Go," the runners run toward the caller, and at "Stop," they freeze on the spot.
4. After calling out "Stop," the caller turns to see whether anyone is still moving.
5. The last person caught moving becomes the caller for the next round.

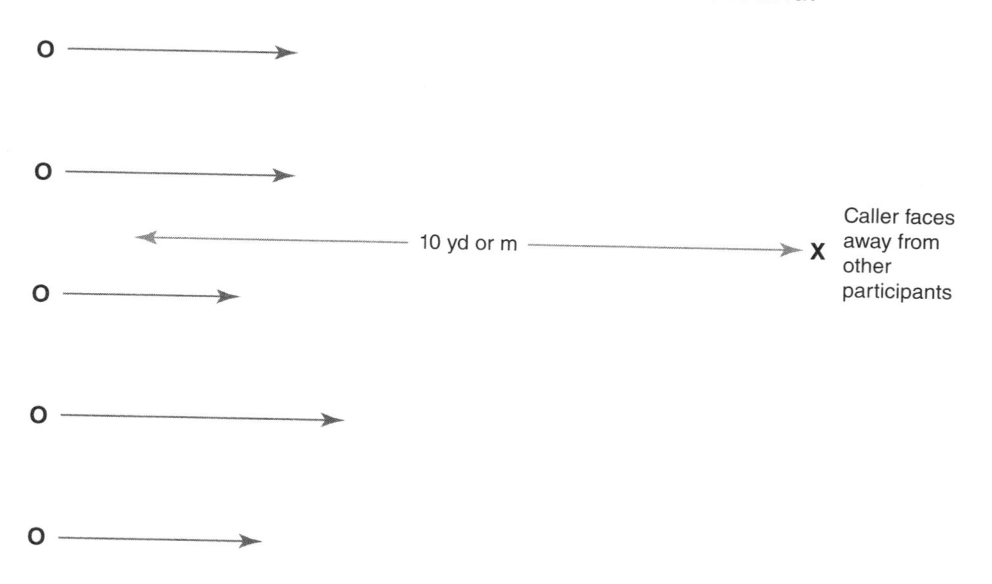

chapter 6

Agility and Quickness Training

A young athlete who is able to quickly change directions or rapidly vary movement patterns is referred to as agile. High-frequency footwork or quick feet, speed of reaction and movement, and the rhythm and timing of players' movements are important intrinsic elements of agility. Agility does not exist independently but rather relies on the development of a host of other abilities (e.g., those just described) in which power is a determinant factor.

The qualities of speed, agility, and power are visible in many team and racket sports and martial arts. Just watch how quickly basketball players move their legs on defense to stay in front of the players they are guarding. Their legs are always moving to be ready to react to any game situation that arises. Quickness, quick feet, and high-frequency footwork directly depend on the power of the calf muscles. Powerful and therefore quick players are able to initiate tactical actions consistently faster than their opponents, which can offer a great tactical advantage during a competition.

Some training specialists view agility and quickness as evolving from speed. This is a myth! The reality is that speed strictly depends on the force the athlete applies against the ground or floor. Therefore, a fast athlete is expected to be a strong and agile athlete. This is why coaches, especially in soccer, say, "We need to find fast players." Fast players can be individuals who have inherited genetic qualities that predispose them to agility, such as those born with a higher percentage of fast-twitch muscle fibers than slow-twitch muscle fibers (fast-twitch fibers have a very high contraction time, whereas slow-twitch fibers do not) or can be individuals who have been previously exposed to strength-training programs.

Training programs in which agility drills are performed year-round do not guarantee performance improvement because players may very soon reach a plateau. After a while, improvement in agility will stagnate simply because the load (i.e., distance and intensity of a drill) is constantly the same. Because speed directly depends on a player's leg power, it can be said that only a powerful athlete can be a fast athlete. The same can be said about agility: Only a powerful athlete can be an agile athlete.

Agility has been trained as a separate physical quality for only the past 30 to 40 years. It started with American football and, in the past few years, several so-called agility instructors have been promoting exercises and drills that are appropriate for American football but fail to meet the physiological requirements of other team sports in Europe. Some of these instructors do not seem to understand the physiological differences between American football and other team sports. A simple comparison of American football and the most popular sport in the world—soccer—shows why agility has to be sport and position specific.

American Football

- The average duration of a play in the game is between 4 and 12 seconds, depending on the position played. The intensity, therefore, of such a play is constantly very high.
- The dominant energy systems used are anaerobic lactic (50 percent), alactic (40 percent), and aerobic (10 percent).
- The limiting factors for performance are power and maximum strength.

Soccer

- The duration of a play in the game is often several minutes.
- The dominant energy systems used are aerobic (70 percent), anaerobic alactic (15 percent), and lactic (15 percent).
- The limiting factors for performance are power endurance and speed endurance.

The difference between these two sports is so visible that one may ask how it is possible for a sport instructor not to see the differences between the physiological requirements of the two sports. The duration and intensity of agility drills used in American football differs from the duration and intensity of those used in soccer, rugby, or handball. Using an agility drill of four to six seconds in soccer will work for a defender but not as much for a midfielder, who often runs nonstop for 5 to 10 minutes during a soccer game. The same is true for rugby or handball players. In agility training the coach must plan and practice skills and exercises that emphasize and improve an athlete's ability to both accelerate and decelerate.

Deceleration–Acceleration: The Essential Elements of Agility

To change directions quickly, players must first slow down and then move quickly in another direction. In other words, the action is performed in two phases: deceleration followed by acceleration, or deceleration–acceleration. Deceleration, or slowing down almost to a stop, results from the eccentric loading (lengthening) of the quadriceps muscles. The elastic energy stored in the muscles during deceleration is then used during the acceleration phase when players begin to run quickly again.

Effectively performing these two movements requires a specific technique that involves both the legs and the arms. In the case of deceleration, the arms move in coordination with the legs but with reduced amplitude and force. In other words, the arms have a very slight action that influences deceleration. A quick deceleration is invariably dependent on the strength of the legs. Athletes who want to decelerate fast must improve the strength of the quadriceps muscles, which contract eccentrically when an athlete attempts to decelerate.

Acceleration, on the other hand, is greatly influenced by the movements of the arms. To initiate the acceleration part of an agility movement or quick feet, the arms must move first! If the legs are to move fast, the arm drive back and forth has to be performed powerfully.

Muscular Sources of Agility

Athletes who want to reach a high level of quickness and agility have to first improve the strength and power of the major leg muscles (gastrocnemius, soleus, and tibialis anterior) and major thigh muscles (quadriceps). The ability to quickly decelerate and accelerate relies heavily on the ability of these muscles to contract powerfully, both eccentrically and concentrically. In deceleration–acceleration, deceleration appears to be the determinant and the limiting factor for performance. Deceleration–acceleration will be slow if power is not trained adequately.

All actions requiring agility or quick feet rely on leg power. The fast leg actions required when defending against offensive players or eluding a defender depend on two important elements: how skillfully the athlete performs the first step and how strongly the athlete pushes off against the ground.

Technique for the First Step of an Action

How quickly a player performs the first step of an action depends on how quickly the player moves the opposite arm. For example, if a player initiates a forward step or crossover with the left leg, the quickness of that step will depend on how fast the player moves the right arm. In both sprinting and agility runs, the arms and legs should alternate in perfect coordination. The movement of the arms and legs is performed in the following sequence: (1) arm action and (2) leg reaction (i.e., reaction to the arm motion). The interval between the arm action and the leg reaction is just a fraction of a second.

Force Applied Against the Ground

The stronger the push-off against the ground or floor, the more powerful the ground reaction force that works in the opposite direction. As the eccentric action (i.e., flexion or bending of ankles, knees, and hips) is performed, the leg muscles are loaded eccentrically. The dynamic movement of the push-off (the propulsion phase of the running step) depends on the amount of force loaded during the eccentric contraction. The higher the eccentric load, the more explosive the propulsion. Coaches concentrate so much on strength and power training because a strong push-off against the ground is so important.

The laws of physics have to be applied carefully in athletes' training. In this case we bring to your attention Newton's third law of motion: Every action has an equal and opposite reaction. During the propulsion or push-off phase of the running step, an athlete exerts force onto the ground, and the ground simultaneously exerts a force back onto the player. The higher the force applied against the ground, the higher the reaction, which in turn visibly benefits the power of the push-off—and the reactivity of the muscles during any agility exercises.

Periodization of Agility and Quickness Training

Agility training has to be viewed as a long-term solution to addressing the limiting factors of many team sports' quality in athletics. Agility training must be divided into two phases:

1. *The learning phase.* The focus of any agility drills used in children's training, especially during the initiation phase (6-11 years) and even the athletic formation phase (11-14 years), should be learning the skills involved in the drill rather than quickness and fast feet. These will come later as a result of improving strength and

power. However, after many repetitions of simple agility drills, play, and games, children will experience some degree of quickness because, as explained earlier, muscles learn to work together (i.e., muscle synchronization) and become more efficient.

2. *The development phase.* Performing agility drills helps athletes improve in quickness by developing maximum strength and power, especially after the specialization stage (15-18 years).

The role of maximum strength in the development and improvement of agility is poorly understood and greatly underutilized. Most instructors rely on the method of repeating agility drills without understanding that in order to move fast the athlete has to apply the highest force possible against the ground. When the athlete learns a drill and improves maximum strength, he will also become very agile. Relying only on the repetition of agility drills will result in improvement for only a short while, but improving maximum strength and power will result in maximum improvement of agility!

Long-Term Development of Agility

Long-term improvement of agility is achieved as a result of continuous repetition of agility drills—following a progression from simple to complex agility movement patterns—during the early years of training. A limited degree of leg power is also developed during the learning phase (i.e., junior, young players); however, performance plateaus are common once athletes reach the higher levels of competition. At this point, improvements in agility are hard to come by unless periodization and planning principles of strength training are implemented. Improvements in agility remain limited if maximum strength and power are not included as integral components of overall training.

A long-term annual plan is a strong necessity for developing well-trained athletes. Any agility training organized for children has to be planned for the long term and should be based on the background created by strength and power training. The periodization of long-term agility training has two main aspects: a long-term plan and a short-term plan. Table 6.1 presents an example of a long-term periodization plan. Table 6.2 suggests a short-term program that illustrates how to incorporate the periodization of agility into an annual plan.

Table 6.1 Long-Term Periodization of Strength and Agility Program

Stage	Types of training	Training benefits
Initiation (6-10 yr)	Simple games and participation in fun sports	Learning agility drills
Athletic formation (11-14 yr)	Anatomical adaptation and simple agility drills	Agility skill acquisition
Specialization (15-18 yr)	Strength training: 40-70 percent, power, and agility	Improved agility
High performance (19+ yr)	Maximum strength: ≥80 percent, power, agility, and agility endurance	High-quality agility and quickness

Table 6.2 Periodization of Strength and Agility Training (Annual Plan)

Specifics	Training phase				
	Preparatory			Competitive	Transition
Number of weeks	3	6	4-5	Rest of the season	4-5
Periodization of strength	Anatomical adaptation	Maximum strength	Power, power-endurance	Maintenance of maximum strength and power	Anatomical adaptation
Duration of a drill (sec)	8-10	15-20	20-90	Position-specific agility	General training and activities unrelated to sport
Progression of exercises	Individual	Individual	Individual and combined (group)	Individual and group agility drills	General individual or group activities unrelated to sport

Initiation and Athletic Formation Stages (Early Teen Period)

As illustrated in table 6.1, we propose using agility training beginning at the athletic formation stage (11-14 years). During the initiation stage (6-10 years), sport training should be informal and fun should be the main objective. However, practicing different games and simple athletic skills does improve basic agility. Changing directions and rhythm of walk and run also develops some power and agility, mostly as a result of neuromuscular coordination (i.e., the muscles learning to work in unison).

During the early years of training (11-14 years), the main goals of training are to adapt the body to basic strength training (e.g., anatomical adaptation) and to learn simple agility skills. As athletes become progressively more adept at reproducing agility skills in training and during games, their athleticism improves as well. However, athletes at this age do not develop dramatic gains in strength, which means that agility improves mainly as a result of neural adaptation in the form of intermuscular coordination. Therefore, the repetition of agility drills at this early stage of development is critical because it enables progressive improvements in agility as the muscles learn to work together.

Specialization Stage (Middle and Late Teen Period)

As children grow older, strength-training programs can become increasingly complex. Beginning at the age of 15 years, maximum strength training can be progressively and carefully introduced using loads below 80 percent. An improved level of maximum strength translates into an enhanced ability to recruit fast-twitch muscle fibers into action when performing agility exercises. Improvements in maximum strength also result in gains during power training because the discharge rate of the fast-twitch fibers increases.

Beginning of High-Performance Stage (Postteen Period)

Because in many sports high-performance athletics start at the end of the teen years (19+ years), heavier loads (>80 percent of maximum strength) can be progressively and carefully introduced during this stage to facilitate further gains in strength. Gains in strength will result in improvements in power and agility. From this age on, agility and quickness become more specialized, based mostly on the energy systems used in the selected sport. Such training leads to improvements in the quality of play.

Progression of Agility and Quickness Training During an Annual Plan

Like any other element of training, an agility-training program is planned for the duration of a year (see table 6.2). This plan assumes that players have a background of two to four years of basic strength training, power, and agility training. Strength and power training usually follow a traditional periodization plan in which the goal is for players to achieve maximum levels of power and power endurance just before the competitive season begins. This all but guarantees that players will have the physical support necessary for technical and tactical play throughout the season.

When designing an annual training plan, the instructor should consider the progression of agility training according to the main training phases: preparatory, competitive, and transition. Table 6.2 presents a set of training objectives and the progression from individual to group exercises for each of the three main training phases of an annual plan.

Initially, agility training should focus on individual exercises—learning and performing short agility drills that enhance quickness, explosiveness, quick changes of direction or exercise patterns, and quick feet. However, as training continues toward the competitive phase, various drills focusing on agility, quickness, speed, and power should be combined to create sport- or position-specific exercises (e.g., an attacker vs. a libero in volleyball, a goalie vs. a forward in hockey or soccer, a wide receiver vs. a lineman in football). The duration of a drill must also reflect the specific dynamics of a game (e.g., the duration of a rally, shift, or tactical combination).

Training Guidelines for Agility

This section provides important guidelines for organizing a successful agility-training program for young athletes. The best results are obtained when these suggestions are adapted to suit the training environment, players' individual skills and abilities, and the facilities available. Keep in mind that using personal experience and imagination are also key to creating the best program possible.

Intensity

Except for the agility exercises in which the focus is learning the drill, most if not all agility and quickness exercises have to be performed with a high intensity—from 80 to 95 percent of the athlete's best performance. To make gains in the performance of agility exercises, athletes have to apply dynamic force against the ground. Lower intensities will not result in visible gains in agility, and, as such, there will be little positive transfer to athletic performance. To figure out the ideal intensity to use in training, coaches must regularly test players to determine their maximum capacities for performing a given drill.

Because elevated intensity levels are taxing on the neuromuscular system and because the quality of agility exercises depends on the neural responses and reactivity of the neuromuscular system, agility type of training is often referred to as neuromuscular training. The ability of the central nervous system to send fast, powerful, and high-frequency impulses to the fast-twitch muscle fibers involved in performing agility exercises dictates the discharge rate (i.e., rate of muscle contraction) of fast-twitch fibers—and, consequently, the intensity and quality of an agility or quick-feet drill.

Duration

To get the greatest efficiency and gains from training agility, the instructor must organize agility training and the duration of the drills based on the dominant energy system used in the given sport. We suggest that instructors classify agility drills as follows:

- *Anaerobic alactic system.* Duration of 5 to 10 seconds with very high intensity (>90 percent) of application of force against the ground and quickness of actions; a rest interval of 1 to 2 minutes
- *Anaerobic lactic acid system.* Duration of 20 to 90 seconds with high intensity (80-90 percent); a rest interval of 2 to 3 minutes

Note that agility drills with medium intensity and short duration (4-12 seconds) are often promoted by coaches. The intensity of the drills and application of force against the ground are so low that the benefits of these drills are very questionable. Such drills might be useful for young athletes or for warming up, but they are quite useless for high-performance players. During the specialization stage, intensity needs to be high if agility is to be increased.

To avoid the potentially detrimental effects of fatigue on the performance of high-intensity agility exercises, the total time per training session should be between 5 and 10 minutes. When rest intervals (often lasting 2-3 minutes) are considered, the total time of agility training per session can be as high as 35 minutes. For instance, if during an agility-training session the total number of repetitions of alactic- and lactic acid-system drills is 10 drills of 10 seconds, 5 drills of 15 seconds, and 5 drills of 30 seconds (totaling 5 minutes and 25 seconds), then the sum of the rest intervals would be approximately 27 minutes (1 minute for the 10-second drills, 1.5 minutes for the 15-second drills, and 2 minutes for the 30-second drills). It is the coach's responsibility to properly monitor player backgrounds and progression, drill durations, number of repetitions, and number of sets per exercise.

Position-Specific Agility Drills

Because racket-sport athletes and team-sport athletes play specific positions in which the technical, tactical, and physical requirements are very specialized, agility training has to match the physiological requirements of a given position. The differences between certain positions in rugby, soccer, American football, handball, and volleyball are quite visible. Take, for instance, the difference between a sweeper and a midfielder in soccer. The sweeper's role requires more power, agility, and reaction, whereas a midfielder is often the leader on the field, the one who organizes the plays and is seen running up and down the field, playing various roles on the team. The dominant energy system of a sweeper is alactic–lactic, whereas the dominant energy system of a midfielder is aerobic. These differences demonstrate the need for agility training that is based on energy systems. Coaches must recognize such differences and train players according to their physiological requirements, especially from the specialization stage (15-18 years) on to the high-performance stage (19+ years).

Placement of Agility Training in a Workout

High-intensity agility training should be conducted immediately after the warm-up when the central nervous system is still fresh, well rested, and able to respond quickly to various stimuli. However, coaches can also plan agility drills in which the scope of training is to train quickness and reaction time under conditions of fatigue. In such a case, agility exercises should be conducted at the end of the training session. Although fatigue interferes with the reactivity of the central nervous system, players can adapt progressively to high levels of fatigue and still perform fast and quick movements, as is required in most games. Drills with this training objective must remain short (4-12 seconds) and be performed as quickly as possible. This approach must be employed if players are expected to be as sharp, fast, and explosive at the end of a game as they are at the beginning.

During agility and quickness training, the neuromuscular system is the first to experience fatigue as the neural reactivity of the fast-twitch muscle fibers and the effectiveness of the myotatic stretch reflex (the stretching reflex of the muscle spindles that causes a muscle to contract) diminish. Fatigue manifests in the visible deterioration of technique—athletes struggle to perform the agility drill effectively. Players look sloppy, and foot contact becomes noisy and lasts longer as the heel of the foot touches the ground. These responses clearly demonstrate a high level of neuromuscular fatigue. Under these conditions, coaches should stop the drill and provide a longer rest interval (e.g., 4-5 minutes) or, if necessary, terminate the agility-training session altogether.

Agility and Quickness Exercises

Coaches should always provide a variety of agility drills in training sessions. Although our suggested list of exercises is not exhaustive, these exercises should provide a solid base from which coaches can draw inspiration for designing their own training programs. It is not possible for players to perform all the following exercises in a single training session, so it is important that coaches select only three to six exercises for each agility session of a daily workout.

Coaches should keep the following points in mind when watching athletes perform agility or quick-feet exercises.

Watch foot contact. Foot contact should always occur at the balls of the feet to maximize the effect of the stretch reflex. This is called "light feet" and is characterized by springy actions that are generated by the muscles' elasticity. In contrast, hard landings on the soles constitute heavy feet. Any increase in the duration of the contact phase (i.e., contact between the foot and the ground) results in significantly slower movements. Therefore, athletes must perform agility exercises quickly by emphasizing light feet, thus maximizing the elasticity of the muscles and minimizing the duration of the contact phase.

Listen to the players' steps. It is just as important to listen to players performing agility drills as it is to watch them. Listening to the sound of a player's steps provides important feedback regarding the quality of execution. A clapping sound is an indication that players are landing on the soles rather than the balls of the feet, which significantly reduces the effectiveness of performing speed, quickness, and agility drills. The quieter the contact with the ground, the more fluid and elastic the movements and the higher the gains in power and agility. However, be aware that clapping or noisy feet—especially toward the end of a workout—can be the first indication that players are experiencing neuromuscular fatigue. When this happens coaches should know that the agility training is of questionable benefit and, as such, should terminate the session.

Observe the height of steps. The height of a player's steps should remain as low as possible so the player can quickly get the foot back in contact with the ground for another push-off. Athletes should do the following:

- Step below the height of the ankles. Upward movements are inefficient and lead to a loss of quickness.
- Move as quickly as possible between the two points of the agility step (i.e., the push-off and landing phases). The dynamic element of movements requiring speed and quickness is the push-off, or propulsion, phase. The more frequently an athlete pushes against the ground, the faster she moves.

Examine body mechanics. Athletes should maintain the correct body posture or stance: feet shoulder-width apart, feet pointing forward, and the weight of the body equally distributed on both legs. The vertical projection of the center of gravity (straight line of center of gravity at core to the ground) should fall within the base of support (i.e., between the feet). However, to improve dynamic body mechanics that more closely reflect those used in game situations, some agility drills should be performed from an unbalanced position, where the player's center of gravity falls outside the base of support.

Maximize the power of the push-off phase. Although agility is often characterized by light feet, sometimes (e.g., at the start of an agility drill or when changing directions) it is beneficial for coaches to instruct athletes to have the heels of the feet in contact with the ground. This takes advantage of the powerful calf muscles and allows for a more powerful push-off. If the heels are raised, propulsion power can decrease by as much as 50 percent of maximum force.

The power produced during the push-off phase depends on the angle between the top of the foot and the leg. The smaller the angle, the more potential for powerful forward propulsion. Many players find it difficult to maintain this acute angle due to a lack of ankle flexibility.

Team-sport players in particular must consistently and continually execute actions requiring power during a game. Although the benefits of power development are well known, many coaches are still unaware of the strong links between power and maximum strength. Coaches and players wish to see year-by-year improvements in power, speed, agility, and quickness. It is important to realize that these abilities cannot be improved consistently without similar improvements in maximum strength.

The best method for developing power, agility, and quickness involves applying science to training. For optimal improvements in athletic abilities, team-sport players need to incorporate (a) a maximum-strength phase in which the goal of training is to increase the recruitment of fast-twitch muscle fibers and (b) a power-training phase, which results in the increased discharge, or firing rate, of the fast-twitch muscle fibers recruited. This is the only way to consistently increase the game-specific physical qualities of power, speed, agility, and quickness. If this strategy is not followed, players will lose power, which then directly and negatively affects the development of speed, agility, and quickness. Of course, the volume and intensity of agility drills depend on the skill level and stage of athletic development. Kids in the initiation phase cannot be expected to perform precise agility drills at a level of intensity that is recommended for those in the athletic formation stage; their limited motor skill development would make performing the exercises very difficult. The key to strong and powerful movements (i.e., agility) is to properly train the athlete at her current level of development. As the athlete's strength and speed work slowly and progressively increase in volume and intensity, so will her ability to apply force against the ground, thus developing and improving her agility. Agility is not a stand-alone program or set of exercises but rather an important skill that must be complemented with an appropriate program in strength, flexibility, power, and speed training.

The following agility exercises can be used for both the athletic formation and specialization stages. The volume and intensity of the drills can be modified according to the phase of training and the athlete's skill base.

Slalom Jump and Sprint

Areas worked: triple extensors (calf muscles—gastrocnemius, soleus, and tibialis anterior; knee extensors—quadriceps; and hip extensors—gluteus maximus)

1. Tape or draw a line approximately 10 to 15 feet (3-4.5 m) long on a gym floor or field.
2. Players jump in a zigzag pattern (like slalom skiing) for the entire length of the line and then forward sprint for 30 to 45 feet (9-13.7 m).

Suggested Program

1 to 3 sets of 3 to 5 reps; rest interval = 2 minutes

Variations

- Players perform the sprint in a different direction each time.
- Players perform the jumps backward followed by a sprint in a different direction each time.
- When performing the sprint portion of the exercise, players accelerate for 15 to 30 feet (4.5-9 m), stop, immediately change direction, and accelerate for another 15 to 30 feet.

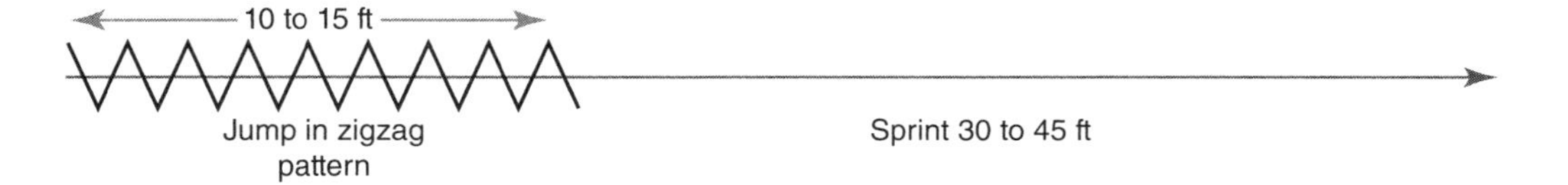

Scissor Splits

Areas worked: triple extensors

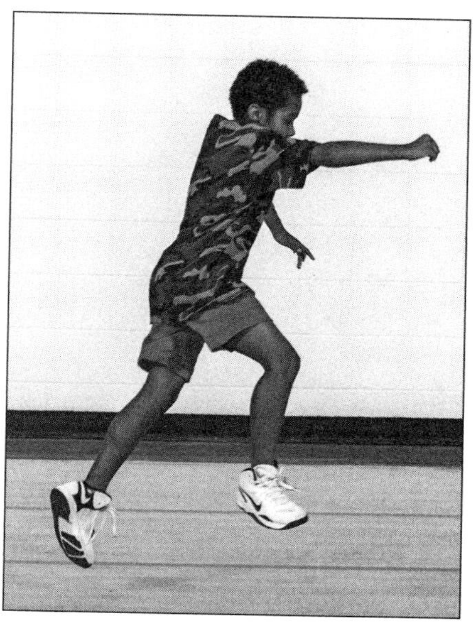

1. Athletes begin by standing with one leg forward and the other leg back.
2. Athletes perform a vertical jump, switching legs (drive right leg forward and left leg back; land and repeat other side) quickly in midair. They jump again immediately upon landing and repeat this pattern for the duration of the drill. Athletes should emphasize the height of the jump and minimize the duration of foot contact with the ground.

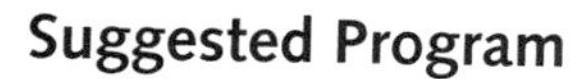

Suggested Program

2 or 3 sets of 5 to 10 continuous jumps; rest interval = 2 minutes

Variation

The players may turn in a given direction (e.g., to the right or left, slightly forward or backward) during each jump performed.

Cone Jumps

Areas worked: triple extensors, shoulders, hip flexors (iliopsoas muscles)

1. Set up a row of 8 to 10 cones, placing each cone 10 to 13 feet (3-4 m) apart.
2. Players run at a high frequency (i.e., take short strides) between cones and jump over each cone using a single-leg take-off (like in a long jump), minimizing the duration of foot contact with the ground. Players return to the starting line after jumping over all of the cones.

Suggested Program

2 to 4 sets (a set is considered one length of the agility drill); rest interval = 2 to 3 minutes

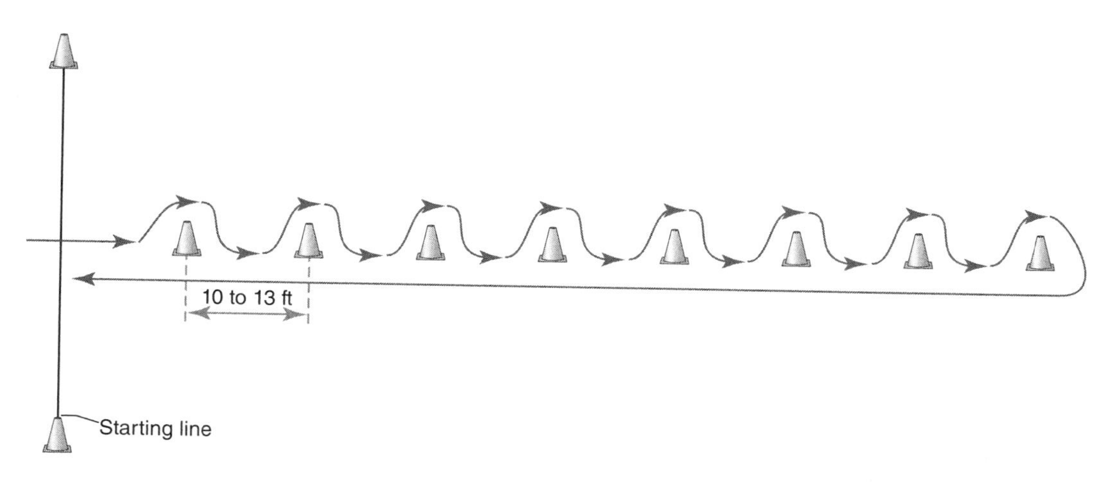

Crossover Steps

Areas worked: calf muscles, quadriceps (to a lesser degree)

1. The athlete moves left for about 30 feet (10 m), crossing the right leg in front of the left leg.
2. The athlete repeats the sequence in the opposite direction.

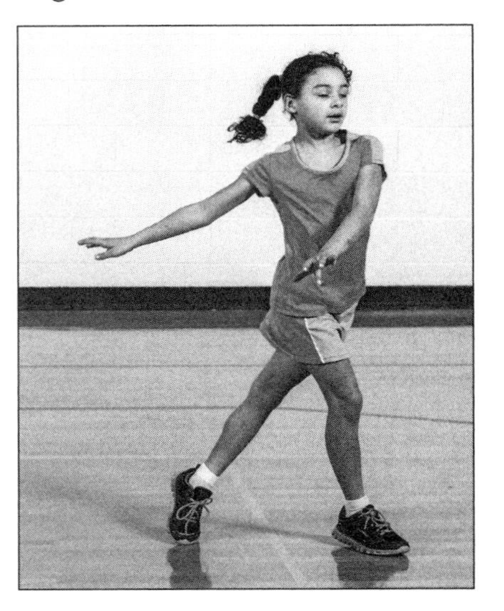

Suggested Program

3 to 5 sets in each direction (a set is considered a 30-foot line of crossovers); rest interval = 1 to 2 minutes

Single- or Double-Leg Jumps

Areas worked: triple extensors, tibialis anterior

1. Tape or draw a 20-inch by 20-inch (50-cm by 50-cm) square on the floor. Draw or tape four equal squares within the larger square. Simply place a vertical and horizontal line down the middle creating four equal squares.
2. The athletes jump from square to square inside the larger square. Jumps can be performed on either one leg or two legs.

Suggested Program

2 to 4 sets of 10 to 12 jumps performed continuously; rest interval = 2 to 3 minutes

Variation

Athletes can jump from square to square forward, backward, or sideways.

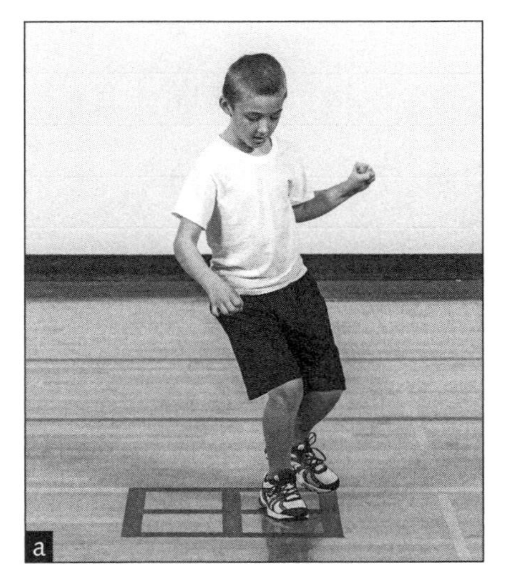
a

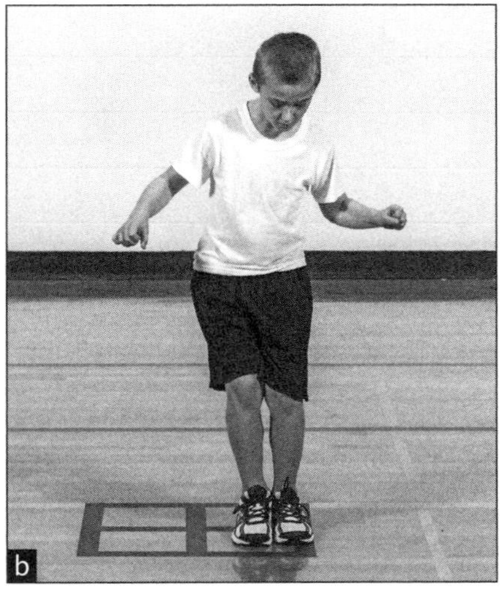
b

Inside-Out Jumps

Areas worked: triple extensors

1. Tape or draw four squares, each 20 inches by 20 inches (50 cm by 50 cm), on the floor as shown in the Single- or Double-Leg Jumps drill.
2. Players stand at the "1" marked on the square and hop, feet together, in and out of the square to each of the eight numbered points sequentially.
3. Examples of possible hops can be: 1 to side 2 to forward 3 to center, back to side 3 to forward 4 to side 5 to back to center, to forward 5 to side 6 to back 7 and side hop to center to side 7 to back 8 to side hop to 1.

Suggested Program

2 to 4 sets (a set refers to jumping once around all four squares); rest interval = 1 to 2 minutes

Variations

- Players perform the same sequence but jump on only one leg.
- Players change direction based on instructions called out by the coach.

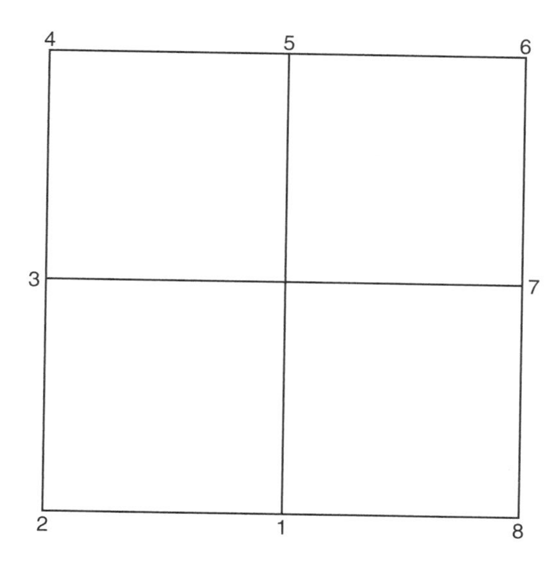

Ladder

Areas worked: triple extensors, tibialis anterior

1. Draw or secure a rope ladder on the floor or field. Each square of the ladder should measure approximately 20 inches by 20 inches (50 cm by 50 cm); make the squares slightly smaller for elite athletes.
2. Players move in and out of each square using different techniques. Players can use a side step out of the ladder or a single or double leg hop in and out of the ladder. Each action in and out of the ladder should be performed with a powerful push-off.

3. Players should emphasize contacting the ground with the balls of the feet and maintaining a fast, rhythmical pattern. Foot actions should be performed as close to the ground as possible to emphasize fast footwork. Athletes should avoid stepping on the markings of the ladder at any time.
4. Although the ladder is a very popular training element, unless the push-off is powerful the ladder is not as efficient for training agility as many coaches believe.

Variations

- Players begin with one foot in the first square of the ladder and the other foot outside of the ladder. At a given signal, players run forward with very short, high-frequency steps on the balls of the feet. The feet should not be lifted higher than 4 to 6 inches (10-15 cm) off the ground.
- Players stand perpendicular to one end of the ladder (i.e., with one shoulder facing the ladder) and perform crossovers over the lines marking the squares (i.e., the rungs of the ladder).
- Players stand facing the first square at one end of the ladder. They run (using very short and quick steps on the balls of the feet) into the first square, turn around, run out of the square, back to the starting position, turn around again, and do the same thing running through the first square and into the second before turning around and running out to the starting position. Continue until they complete all the squares of the ladder.
- Athletes complete the first and second variations but instead of running they perform low, high-frequency jumps over the lines with either one leg or two legs.
- Athletes perform single- or double-leg jumps over the lines and perform a 45-degree rotation when crossing over each line.
- Athletes combine quick and low runs with jumps on one or two legs.
- Athletes perform any of the variations while running backward (i.e., backpedaling).

Suggested Program

Perform each of the ladder exercises for 3 to 5 sets, emphasizing the push-off phase. Best performed in groups, so the athletes have a 30- to 60-second recovery time between sets.

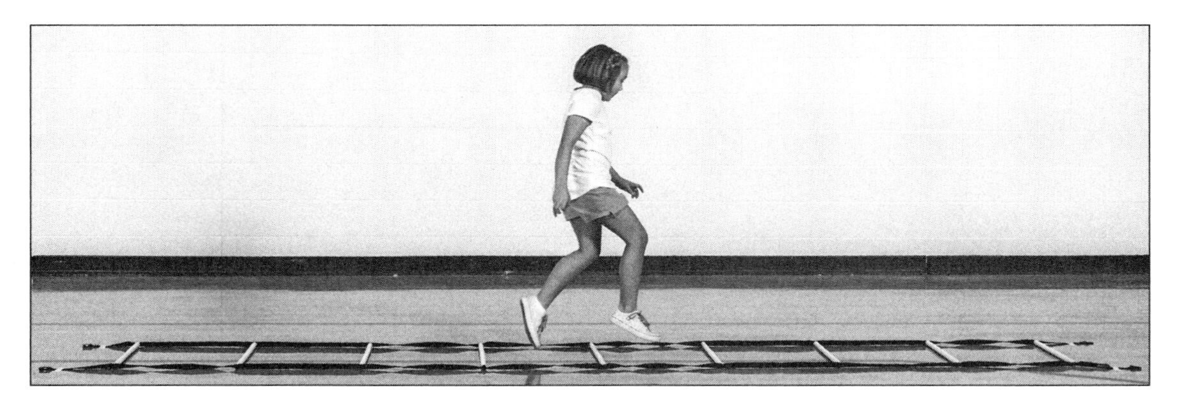

Agility Wheel

Areas worked: triple extensors, arms, shoulders (to develop fast arm drive)

1. Using cones, create a "wheel" on the floor or field. Mark eight stations 10 to 15 feet (3-5 m) from the center of the wheel as shown in the diagram.
2. Players start at the center of the wheel and run as quickly as possible to each station in numerical order, returning to the center after reaching each station.
3. The players can either touch the cones or go around the cones when completing the circuit.
4. Players should emphasize working on the elasticity of the muscles when performing quick changes of direction and quick footwork. The actions should look easy and should have good flow. Players should show no contraction of the facial muscles (grimacing). Grimacing indicates uneasiness in performing the exercise and results in unnecessary contraction of the trunk and shoulder muscles, which inhibits the efficient contraction of the leg muscles and ultimately reduces a player's level of agility in performing the drill.

Variations

- Players run tall without bending the knees or hips too much.
- Players assume a low position—ankles, knees, and hips slightly flexed.
- Players run forward, run sideways, or backpedal.
- Players perform side shuffling, crossovers, or low and fast jumps of 1 to 2 feet (.3-.6 m).
- Players change directions according to the call of the coach.
- Players dribble a ball from station to station of the wheel. In this variation the cones can be 15 to 30 feet (4.5-9 m) away from the center.
- Players perform all running possibilities during a single repetition of the exercise.

Suggested Program

Perform 2 to 4 sets, emphasizing technique and a powerful push-off at each turning point. Rest 2 to 3 minutes between sets, so each set involves maximum effort.

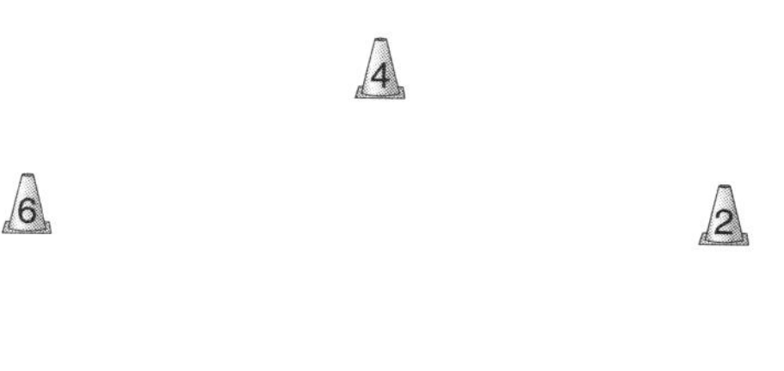

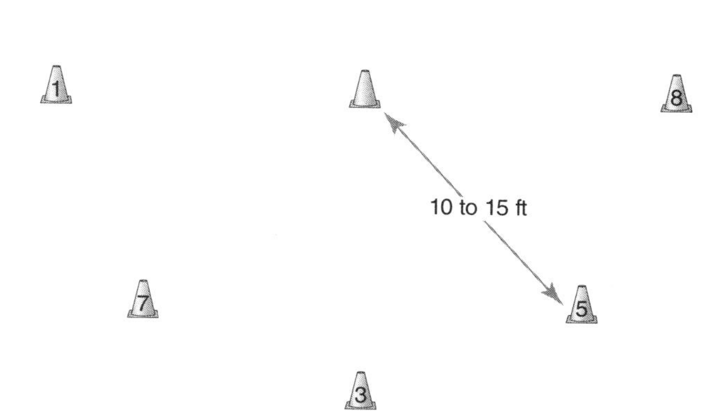

Relay Game

Training sessions can become monotonous over time. Relays and games can provide some fun and excitement for players, especially toward the end of a long training session. They also add an element of competitiveness, which most athletes appreciate. More importantly, relays and games continue to train agility, reaction time, speed, and power—the objectives set out in training—in an exciting atmosphere that keeps the players motivated and interested. See chapter 5 for additional relay exercises and games.

Over–Under Bridge Relay

Areas worked: trunk muscles (erector spinae and lumbar muscles), gluteus maximus, abdominals, quadriceps

1. Divide the players into two or three teams of equal number. Players line up in single file in a line, standing approximately 1 to 2 feet (.3 to .6 m) apart depending on leg and arm length.
2. Each team passes an 8- to 12-pound (4-6 kg) medicine ball down the line. The players alternately pass the ball over the head and between the legs.
3. The last player in line runs quickly with the ball to the front of the line and starts the sequence again.
4. The team that finishes first is the winner. The coach can decide how many full rotations constitute a win. For instance, the team that completes two full rotations (meaning that the last player in the line receives the ball and runs to the front two times) is the winner.

Suggested Program

3 to 5 sets (a set is considered a relay completed by all players on a team); rest interval = 1 minute

Variations

- To challenge the muscles, increase the distance between players to 10 to 15 feet (3-4.5 m). The players throw the medicine ball to the next player rather than handing it off.
- Players throw the ball sideways over the head, bending the trunk sideways as the ball is thrown.

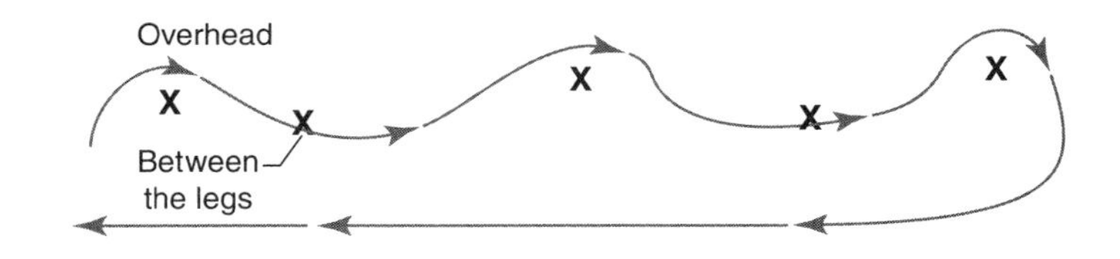

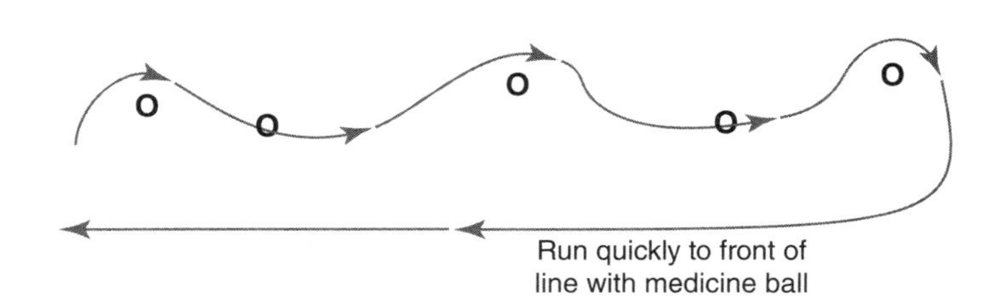

Simple Tumbling Exercises

Simple tumbling and space-orientation exercises such as side rolls and shoulder rolls can be used effectively to develop agility in players. Try combinations of the following exercises to add variety.

Forward Roll and Vertical Jump

Areas worked: triple extensors, triceps

1. Athletes begin in a low crouch position with the hands flexed at knee level.
2. The athlete tucks the head under the body and initiates the forward roll, landing in a half-squat position. Finally, the athlete extends the legs powerfully to perform a vertical jump coming out of the roll.
3. The athlete lands and then repeats the roll and jump.

Suggested Program

6 to 10 repetitions (a repetition is performing the roll and jump twice); rest interval = 30 seconds to 1 minute

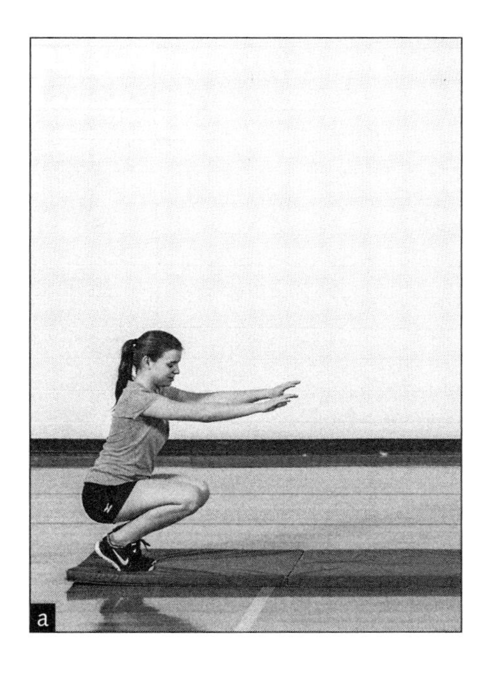
a

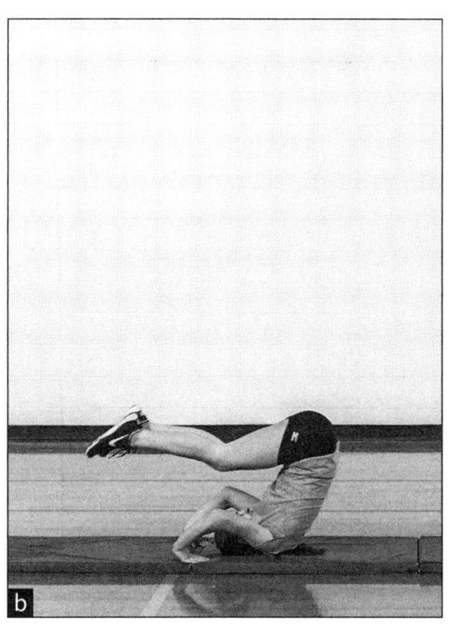
b

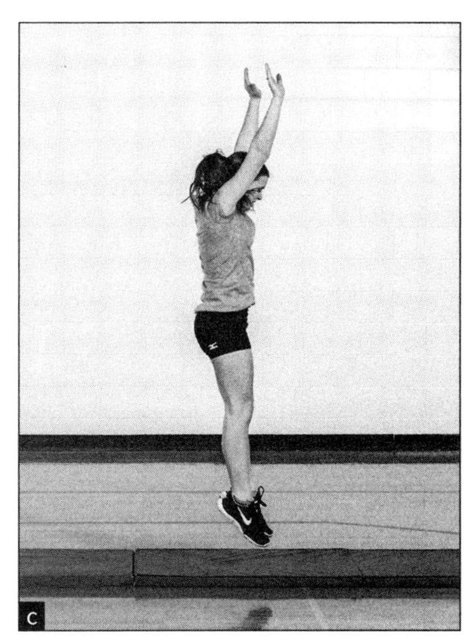
c

Backward Roll Into a Handstand

Areas worked: trunk muscles, triceps, trapezius

1. The athlete begins in a low crouch or pike position with the chest above the knees.
2. The athlete quickly swings the upper body backward, rolling onto the shoulders, and places the palms of both hands on the ground below the shoulders.
3. When approaching vertical during the rollover, the athlete extends the arms powerfully into a handstand and holds the position as long as possible.
4. The athlete lowers the legs back into a low crouch and repeats the movement.

Suggested Program

6 to 10 repetitions; rest interval = 30 seconds to 1 minute

Backward Roll Into a Vertical Jump

Areas worked: trunk muscles, triceps, triple extensors

1. The player begins in a low crouch position with the chest above the knees.
2. The player swings the upper body backward, rolling onto the shoulders, and places the palms of both hands on the ground below the shoulders.
3. The player rolls backward into a full squat position (full bend of the knees whereby the heels of the feet are in close contact with the buttocks) and then performs a powerful vertical jump from the squat position.
4. The player lands and repeats the movement.

Suggested Program

8 to 10 repetitions; rest interval = 1 to 2 minutes

Explosive Cone Drill

Areas worked: legs, arms and core

1. Set up four cones. Cone 1 is set at the starting position. Cone 2 is directly in front of the cone at a 10-meter distance. Cones 3 and 4 are diagonal to cone 2, at approximately a 10-meter distance from cone 2. The distance between cones 3 and 4 is also approximately 10 meters.
2. The athlete starts by lying on his stomach with arms extended directly in front of him at cone 1.
3. The athlete gets up quickly and sprints to cone 2, touches the top of the cone and returns back to cone 1, touches the top of cone 1 and sprints to cone 3, touches top of cone 3 and turns around and rushes back to cone 1, touches top of cone 1 and turns and sprints to cone 4, touches cone 4, and sprints back to cone 1.

Suggested Program

5 to 8 repetitions; rest interval: 2 minutes

chapter 7

Strength and Power Training

Parents of young athletes often ask whether strength training is safe and necessary for their children. Our answer is yes, strength training is both necessary and safe provided that parents or coaches follow the information and training programs suggested in this chapter.

Numerous studies in the past 20 years have highlighted the important role that strength training can play in the physical and emotional development of young athletes. Benefits include improved bone density, self-esteem, strength, power, and speed and increases in fat-free mass (Dahab and McCambridge, 2009). Concerns regarding injury and growth plate issues have been set aside as recent publications and updated papers clearly summarize the efficacy and benefits of strength training for young athletes (Behm et al., 2008; Faigenbaum et al., 2009). In addition to improving performance, strength training decreases the chance of sport-related injury and creates a foundation for maintaining an active lifestyle and protecting against the onset of diseases as children mature (Barbieri and Zaccagni, 2013).

Children can begin to strength train as early as 7 or 8 years of age. The intensity of the training sessions should be very minimal. Sessions should focus on multilateral development, and body-weight exercises should be the foundational exercises used in training. Although epiphyseal plate injuries are common in sports that involve repetitive impact such as gymnastics and baseball (Cahill, 1998), most injuries in youth strength training are not caused by strength training itself but rather by the misuse of equipment, lifting too much too fast, inadequate instruction, and poor technique (Caine et al., 2006; Ratel, 2011). In other words, with proper supervision and an age-appropriate program, children of all ages and both sexes will benefit from a strength-training program.

Depending on the level of training, young athletes can use free weights, resistance bands, medicine balls, and weight machines. Athletes should perform multijoint exercises, which train the major muscle groups. Olympic lifts (e.g., clean and jerk, power clean), if desired, should be geared for athletes in the later teen years. What is of grave importance is that the program focuses on the well-being of the athlete, helps them mature physically, and helps them gain confidence in their abilities on and off the field, ice, or court. This is achieved by following proven principles of physical development, not by training the young body based on fads, marketing gimmicks, or state-of-the-art training equipment. Once again, you don't have to do what is *new* but what is *necessary* to achieve success in training and athleticism.

In simple terms, strength is defined as the ability to apply force against resistance. Strength enhances the performance and execution of many athletic skills. All the skills athletes must perform against resistance will benefit from improving strength. In sport, resistance is produced by water in swimming and rowing; by the force of gravity in running, jumping, and team sports; and by an opponent in wrestling, martial arts, and team sports.

Strength training for children has been a controversial topic. In the past, children were discouraged from using weights for fear of injury or prematurely stopping the growth process. Most injuries in athletics occur at the ligaments and tendons. A well-designed strength-training progression will strengthen the ligaments (which hold together the bones that form joints) and tendons (which anchor muscles to bones) and, as a result, allow the athlete to better cope with the strain of training and competitions. Strength training not only helps prevent injuries in the present but also provides a strong foundation for the later stages of high-performance athletics. Following a progressive program of multilateral development in which the exercises, movement patterns, and equipment vary helps challenge the body to adapt and grow as the athlete improves in the skills of the sport or event.

Another misconception about strength training is that it applies only to bodybuilders or powerlifters. As demonstrated in the past few decades, many athletes improve their performance faster using strength training rather than simply performing the skill of the chosen sport. Strength training is an integral part of athletes' training in many sports, including football, baseball, track and field, rowing and canoeing, wrestling, and tennis. The philosophy has so drastically changed that some people now accept the notion that no one can be fast before being strong, no one can increase the height of a jump or take-off without strength training, and no one can throw a ball without arm and trunk strength. Indeed, strength training has gained an important role in most sports. In one study, researchers divided boys and girls aged 7 to 12 years into three groups: one group that did 1 day of strength training per week, one group that did 2 days of strength training per week, and a control group that did not participate in the program. Participants in both strength-training groups performed 1 set of 10 to 15 repetitions on 12 exercises. All exercises were performed on age-appropriate machines. Researchers measured one repetition maximum (1RM) for the chest press and leg press, hand grip strength, long jump performance, vertical jump performance, and flexibility both before and after 8 weeks of training. Participants who trained twice per week improved significantly in chest press strength compared with the control group. Both strength-training groups improved in leg press strength. Training frequency did not influence changes in other measured outcomes. Overall, the participants who trained once per week failed to achieve the strength improvements seen in the group that trained twice per week. Regardless of age, the young participants were able to improve strength. Like in adults, increasing the frequency of strength-training sessions from once to twice per week can significantly improve strength in children (Faigenbaum et al., 2002).

In addition to improving performance and safeguarding against injuries, strength training has health benefits. Strength training increases the mineral content of the bones, thus serving as a preventative measure against osteoporosis later in life. According to medical data, women are more prone to osteoporosis; therefore, strength training should be part of the physical education and training program of young girls (American Academy of Pediatrics, 2008). Strength training can also have social and psychological benefits including enhanced discipline, mental determination, self-esteem, and self-confidence. Finally, strength training should be part of a healthy lifestyle because increasing the body's proportion of lean muscle mass also increases metabolism and, in the process, burns calories.

Strength training can be a positive component of a child's active lifestyle; however, the coach must carefully design the program for a specific age or sport (Bompa and Buzzichelli, 2015; Faigenbaum, 2000). Before participating in a strength-training program, young athletes must be ready physically and psychologically and must understand proper lifting technique and the role of strength in performance improvement. Both the instructor and the child should be aware of safety factors, including spotting and how to use different types of equipment. Equally important, the supervising instructor must be competent in strength training, both in the technique of lifting and in training methodology.

Before beginning a strength-training program, a child should have a thorough medical examination. This will detect any potential illness (e.g., heart problems) that may prevent the child from doing strength training or any type of physical training. With clearance from a physician, children with certain physical or mental disabilities can participate in a safe and professionally conducted strength-training program. Thankfully, in recent years medical advances in research have eliminated certain barriers to sport participation. For instance, parents of children with asthma were once encouraged to limit the amount of physical activity their child participated in to avoid triggering the symptoms of asthma. Today, with proper medical attention, medication, and inhalers, children with asthma are encouraged to exercise, play, and enjoy many sporting activities. In fact, regular participation in exercise and sporting activities can help strengthen a child's airways and improve breathing mechanics.

Terminology

The literature uses several terms—*weight training, resistance training, power training*, and *strength training*—interchangeably. Because an individual can develop strength without using weights or applying force against resistance, we use the term *strength training* to refer to force produced by a group of muscles.

Strength can also be combined with other factors such as speed and endurance. Strength and speed result in power, or the rate at which an individual can generate force. The force generation is usually fast and explosive, such as in batting or jumping. The second combination, strength and endurance, is called muscular endurance, which results in the ability to perform many repetitions against resistance, as in rowing, swimming, and cycling. Chapter 8 discusses the development and progression of endurance training as well as program design.

Sport skills are performed by a specific group of muscles. The larger and more powerful muscles that are primarily responsible for performing technical skills are called prime movers. Other muscles that cooperate in accomplishing the movement are called synergistic muscles. Antagonist muscles, which are mainly on the opposite side of the bone, act in opposition to the synergistic muscles. All motions are influenced by the contraction of synergistic (also called agonistic) muscles and a balanced, controlled relaxation of the antagonistic muscles.

While an athlete performs a motion with this critical interaction between agonistic and antagonistic muscles, other groups of muscles support the limb so the needed muscles can produce the motion. During pitching, for instance, the abdominal muscles contract to stabilize the lower part of the trunk so the arms can throw the ball. These supporting muscles are called fixators, or stabilizers, because they keep one part of the body or limb stable while another part contracts to perform the motion.

The load in strength training is expressed in pounds or kilograms and is calculated as percentage of 1RM, or the highest load an individual can lift for only one repetition. A coach can easily test an athlete's 1RM using the bench press exercise. The athlete starts with a small load, such as 60 pounds (27 kg). If the athlete lifts this easily, the coach makes the next load heavier, such as 80 pounds (36 kg). The highest load the athlete lifts for only one repetition is called 1RM, or 100 percent. Use this load to calculate the percentage for training, which in most cases is between 30 percent and 95 percent of 1RM.

The number of repetitions refers to how many times to repeat an exercise in a set. Use the following guidelines:

- For a load of 100 percent, the athlete performs just 1 repetition.
- If the load is 95 percent, 2 to 3 repetitions are possible.
- At 90 percent of 1RM, 3 to 4 repetitions are possible.
- For a load of 85 percent, an athlete can do 5 or 6 repetitions.
- If the load is 80 percent, an athlete can do 8 to 10 repetitions.
- For a load of 75 percent, an athlete normally performs 12 repetitions.
- For 70 percent of 1RM, an athlete can do 12 to 15 repetitions.
- If the load is between 60 percent and 70 percent, a trained athlete can easily perform 18 to 20 repetitions.
- If the load is 50 percent, an athlete can perform more than 25 repetitions per set.

During a strength-training session young athletes can perform 1 to 2 sets per exercise. Athletes in late postpuberty can perform up to 3 sets in a progressive way, increasing the number of sets over 2 to 4 years. Young athletes have no reason to perform more than 2 or 3 sets. By performing a higher number of sets, the number of exercises has to be low (i.e., 5-6). Between sets, athletes should always take a rest interval to replenish the spent energy and relax the muscles before performing the next exercise. The suggested programs in this chapter always have a rest interval of 2 to 3 minutes.

Laws of Strength Training

Three basic laws underlie a good strength-training program. These rules apply to anyone involved in strength training during the stages of growth and development but are especially important to the young athlete who has just started along the road to high performance.

Law One: Develop Joint Flexibility

Most strength-training exercises, especially those employing free weights, use the whole range of motion of major joints, particularly the knees, ankles, and hips. For example, in deep squats the weight of the barbell compresses the knees and may cause strain and pain if the athlete does not have good flexibility at the knee joint. If deep-knee squats are used in children's training, the load must be very low in order to avoid strain in the joints. However, considering the age groups we are referring to (i.e., athletes in the initiation and athletic formation stages), for the purpose of injury prevention we suggest that the athletes perform half squats (until thighs are parallel to the floor) rather than full squats.

In a low squat position, the lack of good ankle flexibility forces the performer to stay on the balls of the feet and toes rather than keep the feet flat on the floor, which ensures a good base of support and balance. Therefore, developing good ankle flexibility during prepubescence and pubescence must be a major concern. Simply participating in running and jumping activities and hill running will help facilitate better ankle flexibility and overall lower-body strength. Start developing flexibility during prepubescence and pubescence and maintain it in the later stages of athletic development.

Law Two: Develop Tendon Strength Before Muscle Strength

Muscle strength always improves faster than the tendons' abilities to withstand tension and the ligaments' ability to prevent injury and to preserve the integrity of the bones forming the joints. Faulty use of specificity and the lack of a long-term vision cause many training specialists and coaches to constantly stress only the specific exercises for a given sport. Consequently, they do not pay attention to the overall strengthening of ligaments, particularly at an early age when time is not pressing.

Athletes strengthen tendons and ligaments through a program designed to attain anatomical adaptation (discussed later in this chapter). As we note earlier, tendons attach the muscles to bones. Their main function is to transmit the pull or force that muscle contraction generates against the bone so that motion is possible. Vigorous strength training without proper anatomical adaptation of tendons and ligaments can result in injuries of muscle attachments (tendons) and joints (ligaments). Tendons and ligaments are trainable, and their enlargement (i.e., increase in diameter) increases their ability to withstand tension and tearing. Parents and coaches must stress the development of full-body strength using low to moderate loads and numerous exercises so that the skeletal muscle system develops in its entirety. Simply following a program or placing a child into a camp that encompasses sport-specific training at a high intensity level can result in injury and place undue stress on a sensitive system. This is not to say that all sport-specific camps are bad or that they place children in physical danger; that would be a very generalized statement. However, we are saying that parents and coaches alike should be aware of the long-term goals and critically analyze if a sport-specific camp is the right option, given the athlete's age, physiological preparedness, and current focus. For example, if a 12-year-old soccer player is training for improvements in general strength and aerobic endurance, a sport-specific camp that stresses agility drills and power training may not be appropriate or required at the time. Attending camp A, which performs a thorough, 12-exercise workout with 2 sets, and a few weeks later attending camp B, a hockey camp that promotes high-intensity training in which young athletes work out until they drop, may not be in the best interest of a developing athlete. Progression is the key to achieving anatomical adaptation and properly preparing the body for the higher demands of sport in later years.

Law Three: Develop Core Strength Before Limb Strength

Training specialists often misunderstand the principle of specificity and direct most of their attention toward developing strength in the arms and legs. Athletes play most sports with the arms and legs. Therefore, many trainers concentrate on strengthening these two segments of the body, believing that the stronger they are the more effective they will be.

Although it is true that the legs and arms perform all athletic skills, the trunk is the link between them. The legs and arms are only as strong as the trunk! A poorly developed trunk leads to a weak support for the hardworking arms and legs.

Long-term strength-training programs should not focus only on the arms and legs but rather should include the musculature of the abdomen, lower back, and spinal column. Consequently, in training programs for young athletes, especially during prepubescence and pubescence, exercises should start from the core section of the body and work toward the extremities. In other words, before strengthening the legs and arms, concentrate on developing the link between them: the core muscle groups of the trunk.

The abdomen and back comprise an array of muscles whose bundles run in different directions and surround the core area of the body. This provides a tight and powerful support for a wide range of physical moves. Back muscles are the long and short muscles that run along the vertebral column and work with the rotator and diagonal muscles as a unit, taking part in sideways bending, turning the trunk, and rotating. The abdominal muscles which comprise the anterior and lateral compartments of the torso enable the trunk to bend forward and sideways, rotate, and twist. The abdominals play important roles in many sport skills; therefore, weak abdominal muscles can restrict athletes' effectiveness in many activities. All trunk muscles can work as a unit to stabilize the trunk during movements of the arms and legs, especially in throwing activities.

It is best to have the athletes perform a number of core-strengthening exercises. They needn't rely only on the basic crunch exercise to develop core strength. Full-body exercises such as jumping on a trampoline, crab walks, and wheelbarrow or simply playing on the playground are great for training the abdominals to support the body and its wide range of physical movements.

Adapting Strength Training for Young Athletes

Scientific studies have demonstrated that both boys and girls gain in strength after strength training (Bar-Or and Goldberg, 1989; Behringer et al., 2010; Carpinelli et al., 2004). Comparisons of children in all three stages of growth and development (prepubescence, pubescence, and postpubescence) show that postpubescent children make the greatest gains—often as much as two or three times those of prepubescent children and almost twice those of pubescent children.

Most gains in postpubescent children are the result of growth in muscle mass (hypertrophy) and of nonmuscular factors such as neuromuscular adaptation to training. Although gains in strength are visible in prepubescent and pubescent children, gains in muscle mass are not because these children have an immature hormonal profile. Strength improvements in early age are not, therefore, the result of muscle enlargement (hypertrophy) but rather of the ability of the central nervous system to activate or stimulate the muscles (Bompa, 1993; Sale, 1986). We see this in the improved ability of children to perform a skill efficiently and with force and power. Consequently, most muscles learn to cooperate, synchronizing their actions and contracting the chain of muscles involved in strength training. The result is increased force in the intended direction of movement. With kids becoming less active and spending more time at a desk or in front of a screen, it is very important that regular resistance training become part of their lifestyle. Children can no longer rely on life activities for proper neuromuscular development. The days of milking cows, carrying buckets of water, stacking hay, and walking two miles on a hilly dirt road to school are in the past for most kids. Playing organized sport one to two times per week is not enough for health and surely not enough to strengthen the body structures to full potential. Kids need to be encouraged to play and, with proper supervision, to participate in a structured strength-training program.

Strength gains for male athletes during postpuberty and maturation are mostly the result of muscle enlargement caused by large increments, from puberty on, of testosterone, estradiol, growth hormone, and insulin-like growth factor (Cooper, 1996). Female athletes cannot report similar gains during these periods because their testosterone levels are tenfold lower than those in males (Fox et al., 1989; Hansen et al., 1999). For this reason, even nonathletic males increase strength and size markedly compared with females. As a consequence, trainability of strength is rapidly increased in both male and female athletes during puberty and is maintained during the following development stages.

Strength training should not be seen as a one-off program or a set of plans that are classified as strength training, but have very little in progression, variety, and long-term goals. If the long-term goal is to increase maximum strength, then the short-term goal must be to strengthen the ligaments, tendons, muscles, and joints with lower loads so as to give the body an opportunity to heal, grow, and develop the neuro-coordination required to lift heavier loads. A long-term vision when planning a strength-training plan is important for best athletic improvement, improved confidence in one's athletic abilities, and prevention of injuries. Parents and instructors should consider creating a multiyear, long-term strength-training plan in which careful progression is a major concern. Such a plan is the best investment a parent or coach can make in a child's athletic success and healthy life.

Considerations for Prepuberty

The prepuberty years are characterized by constant growth that favors developing fundamental movements and basic skills. Motor performance among children varies greatly and can change over a short period of time. Heredity (the natural qualities children inherit from their parents) certainly plays an important role in individual performances and their variations, including strength and aerobic endurance (Bray et al., 2009).

Physique and strength are generally related for boys; overall body size influences physical achievement. Excess body fat, however, plays an adverse role in most motor activities.

Physical achievements increase markedly and linearly with age, but sex differences in average strength (particularly lower-body strength) do not seem to be drastically different. Boys seem to do better in strength-related activities for the upper body, such as throws, compared with activities for the lower body, such as sprinting. Girls tend to perform better in balance and flexibility activities (Duda, 1986; Raudsepp and Pääsuke, 1995; Smith, 1984).

Considerations for Puberty

Motor performance improves with age during puberty (Kakebeeke et al., 2012), but the development pattern is not uniform based on age, sex, and task (Flatters et al., 2014; Malina, 1984). For girls, strength performance levels off during puberty and does not visibly change afterward. For boys, strength increases with age at an average rate, with marked acceleration during growth spurts, when visible increments in muscle mass also occur. This probably reflects gains in testosterone, growth hormone, and insulin-like growth factor. In particular, normal levels of growth hormone during adolescence and puberty determine the increases in strength and lean muscle mass in both boys and girls (Hulthén et al., 2001). Also, from a social perspective, peer pressure seems to motivate boys to want to look bigger and be stronger. Because large increments in muscle size are not possible, especially during early puberty, it is important for everyone involved in children's sport to discourage young athletes from taking part in strength training solely to create big muscles. Doing so can result in fatigue, injury, and slow recovery. Dealing with an injury so early in life does not benefit a young athlete emotionally or physically. Such gains in muscle size are possible only after hormonal changes have occurred during this growth stage because increments in muscle mass parallel the development of sex organs (Bailey et al., 1985; Rogol et al., 2002).

From puberty on, boys are significantly stronger than girls in the upper body and arms. There appears to be less of a difference for leg strength. In general terms, strength visibly relates to body size and fat-free muscle mass, which gives boys an advantage because they tend to participate in more physical activities than girls do (Kraemer and Fleck, 1993).

Regarding power, the performance of boys and girls on tests such as the standing long jump is similar during prepuberty. However, from puberty on these sex differences in power change visibly. At the same time, gains in excess body fat appear to lower performance proficiency in some girls.

Considerations for Postpuberty

Postpuberty signals a large difference in motor performance relative to sex. During adolescence, the difference between girls and boys in tasks and performances related to strength seems to accelerate due to boys' adolescent growth spurt. From this stage on, few girls perform as well as boys in strength, which was possible during prepuberty. These differences reflect sex differences, especially because boys grow larger in size. Social and motivational factors are also important considerations in interpreting children's performances; for example, more boys than girls are directed toward involvement in physical activities.

Some boys decline in performance during peak increases in height. Often children at this stage grow two to four inches (5-10 cm) per year, which clearly affects performance. This is especially true for girls, who experience a greater decrease in strength due to growth and changes in leverage (Bailey et al., 1985; Micheli, 1988; Wild et al., 2013). Most strength and power scores start to improve again after this phase of fast growth in height, demonstrating good adaptability to challenging training loads. Boys begin to steadily increase body weight with an increase in height, a decrease in body fat, and gains in lean muscle mass. These physical changes combined with peer pressure to be strong and look big make it difficult for some boys to resist the temptation to use drugs that increase muscle size. Parents, educators, and coaches must explain the dangers of drugs and demonstrate that better alternatives, such as the periodization of strength training, exist.

Some children grow faster (early maturers) than others of the same age (late maturers). Girls who experience menarche at an early age (i.e., during puberty) are slightly stronger than those who experience it later. By the time girls reach postpuberty, early maturers are less strong than late maturers because of gains in relative body fat combined with decreased activity in the upper-body region. Early maturers tend to be heavier and taller than late maturers. In early maturers, the upper body and abdominals are weaker because they grow more quickly. Their strength in relation to body size decreases because their growth spurts are quicker compared with those of late maturers. When the growth spurt is over and training gains become visible again, early maturers seem to have a strength advantage over late maturers, particularly in the legs, the strength of which girls sometimes retain during maturation.

Early-maturing boys perform better than average and late maturers. Average-maturing boys increase strength linearly until late adolescence. From this stage of development on, differences in strength performance between early- and average-maturing boys are negligible. Boys who reach early sexual maturation, however, perform better in strength-related movements (Borms and Hebbelinck, 1984; Malina, 1984, 2006; Round, 1999). Later maturers, on the other hand, rarely catch up with early maturers in most strength- and power-related motor tasks. Again, body size seems to significantly influence performance. However, athletes in later phases of athletic development (high-performance stage) may not retain any advantages or disadvantages of the early growth and development stages. It is important, therefore, to understand and follow a long-term periodization of athletic development, which guarantees a gradual and complete development of the abilities necessary for all sports.

In conclusion, training programs for children have to consider the dynamics of growth and development for each stage. Programs for both boys and girls should be similar and well-balanced for the first two development stages but completely separate for postpuberty. As part of a well-rounded training concept, strength is a major factor in general fitness. For girls to maintain strength proportionately in the upper and lower body from puberty and especially postpuberty on, programs should emphasize upper-body, trunk, and shoulder-girdle strength because girls tend to be weaker in these areas.

Preventing Injuries

Children may experience injuries from lifting heavy weights during growth, especially during prepuberty and puberty. Parents should always be cautious regarding instructors or coaches who expose children to bodybuilding, Olympic weightlifting, and powerlifting programs. The strain resulting from these techniques could, at times, be hazardous for young athletes. The enthusiasm of some instructors for some lifting techniques, and especially for using heavy loads, should instead be directed toward learning the techniques of lifting with low loads. Children, especially prepubescents, cannot activate their muscles as adults do and are therefore more prone to certain injuries than adults (Dotan et al., 2012; Fleck and Falkel, 1986; Rovere, 1988). Often, the size of young athletes does not equal their capacity to generate strength and power. Children lack endurance and cannot recover as quickly from exhaustive exercise as adults (Dotan et al., 2012). Understanding the aerobic, anaerobic, and neuromuscular limitations of young athletes may deter coaches and parents from suggesting that their children engage in full-body explosive-strength exercises such as the clean and jerk or power clean. Young, immature bodies cannot recruit the high-threshold Type II muscle fibers that allow the safe movement and control of heavy and explosive loads. A lack of knowledge in training and appropriate load progression, improper posture during lifting, and weak abdominal muscles are in most cases the culprits in children's injuries. Young athletes experience lower-back problems and knee injuries.

Growth plate injuries (compression injuries in the shaft of the bones) are the most serious injuries. A growth plate fracture during childhood may result in shortness of a limb. These injuries occur most often in contact sports. Strength training appears to be safe for the growth plates; however, bone and muscle injuries have been recorded (Blimkie, 1993). Most injuries have been the result of poor instruction on proper technique, excessive loading, rotation, and ballistic movements (Ramsey et al., 1990). Young children are extremely susceptible to serious damage from sudden violent forces because the ligaments that protect major joints are stronger than the growth plates. Consequently, trauma that would cause ligament damage in adults will often cause growth plate fractures in children. Coaches should focus on repetition and variety in exercise selection and lessen loading, which may only contribute to injury and provide little gains in strength. Muscle overload can create serious injuries in children. Extreme muscle contractions transmitted along the tendons, which can cause muscle tearing in adults, can cause the muscle and tendon to separate from the main structure of the bone in children. If such injuries stop growth, the result could be deformity and functional impairment.

Injuries such as strains, sprains, and soft tissue damage are far more common, and yet much more difficult to prevent, than growth plate injuries. These injuries occur frequently in highly organized competitive sport programs. Although they are not necessarily serious, they can slow the overall development of athletic talent.

Bigger, stronger children are more likely to experience injuries, especially during late puberty and postpuberty, because they feel ready for heavy loads. What these young adults don't understand, however, is that the ossification process is not yet completed. As a result, muscles should not pull against connective tissue with maximum force.

A well-structured strength-training program that is designed with long-term periodization, like the ones in this chapter, is safe for children. Among the most effective injury-prevention techniques are the following:

Use strength-training programs that are designed to prevent injuries. A well-planned, long anatomical adaptation phase, as suggested by the models in this chapter, can help build injury-free athletes. Athletes who do not participate in a weight-training program have three times the number of injuries compared with athletes who do.

Poor coaching, high intensity, and lack of progression in training volume and intensity can result in injuries. To prevent injuries, use a variety of training modes such as body weight (i.e., push-ups and pull-ups, abdomen and arm curls), medicine balls, and free weights (i.e., light barbells, dumbbells, rubber tubing, simple weight machines with low loads, and lighter power balls).

Always start a training program with a warm-up of 10-15 minutes of easy running, stretching, and body-weight exercises. In addition, a few repetitions using loads that are lighter than those used in the actual program prepare the young athletes for the training session. Performing a thoroughly structured warm-up before each training session and competition can significantly decrease the number and severity of injuries, especially injuries to the knees and ankles.

To prevent shoulder pain, design a compensation strength-training program for all muscles (especially for the abdomen) to balance the strength of the lower back and the rotator cuffs. These areas tend to be neglected in training.

Do not abuse specificity in training programs for children by only using exercises specific only to your sport. Multilateral (overall) training at an early age will pay off at maturation. Specificity of training at an early age has a greater chance of creating overuse injuries (Caine and Maffulli, 2005). The National Athletic Trainers' Association estimated that approximately 50 percent of overuse injuries could be prevented if fundamental fitness skills and exercises are developed first (Valovich McLeod et al, 2011).

Do not expose athletes to maximum loads greater than 70 percent to 80 percent of 1RM or to explosive lifts with free weights during prepuberty, puberty, and early postpuberty. This is too strenuous for anyone, let alone for a young body with immature anatomical development. Discomfort should not be part of the early years of training, period!

Young athletes should not participate in competitions in weightlifting, powerlifting, or any maximum lifts until they achieve skeletal maturity (ossification), which occurs around age 18 to 20 years.

Thorough instruction in lifting techniques, especially free weights, must be part of any strength-training program. Any instructor with a long-term vision will require an adequate phase of learning lifting technique with no weight or light weights.

Close guidance and supervision are necessary at all times for a problem-free gym. Children, especially prepubescent and pubescent children, have short attention spans and may not be highly motivated to strength train. Have equipment serviced regularly, and always return weights to a safe place.

Never use faulty or worn equipment. Before lifting with free weights, such as barbells, make sure that the collars are secured to prevent the discs from falling off and harming someone.

Allow children to be children. Don't rely solely on modern forms of strength training in the belief that machines will make children faster, stronger, and healthier. The human body adheres best to a level of force that promotes adaptation and progressive stimulation, not to intense activities that require active recovery and create undue fatigue and muscular pressure. Allow kids the freedom to play, jump, kick, climb, and move their bodies in various planes and directions while challenging their muscles to greater heights and strength levels. This is best achieved by exercising the body and allowing the chronological and biological age of the individual athlete to determine the level of force output and muscle activation.

Periodization Models for Strength Training

Table 7.1 provides a long-term periodization model for strength and gives an overview of the development stages, training method, volume (quantity), intensity (load), and means of training. Use the suggested circuit-training programs as a model. You may alter some exercises based on your athletes' needs, but make sure that the exercises address all parts of the body.

Table 7.1 Periodization Model for Long-Term Strength Training

Stage	Forms of training	Training methods	Volume	Intensity	Means of training
Initiation (6-10 yr)	• Simple exercises • Games or play	Informal circuit training	Low	Very low	• Own body • Partners • Light medicine balls
Athletic formation (11-14 yr)	• General strength • Relays/games	Circuit training	Low to medium	Low	• Medicine balls • Light free weights
Specialization (15-18 yr)	• General strength • Specificity	• Circuit training • Power training • Low-impact plyometrics	• Medium • Medium high	• Low • Medium • Submaximum	• Free weights • Medicine balls • Body-weight exercises
High performance (19+)	Specificity	• Maximum strength • Power/plyometrics • Muscular endurance	• Medium • Medium high • Maximum	• Medium high • Submaximum	• Free weights • Machines

Note: The progression in volume, intensity, and training methods should be properly monitored by the coach with special consideration given to the transition from simple exercises, such as in the initiation phase, to general exercises and then exercises that are sport specific..

Strength-Training Model for Initiation

View the suggested strength-training model for prepuberty as preparatory time in which the athlete develops the foundation for high performance in an enjoyable, playful environment. High performance at athletic maturation does not depend on strength training during prepubescence. At this stage, the body is susceptible to injury with excessive stress. Regimented, stressful strength training using machines not only puts prepubescent athletes at serious risk for injury but also leads to burnout and hurts the careers of potential high performers. Therefore, view strength training for prepubescent children only as an addition to technical work and general skill development and limit it to body-weight or medicine ball exercises.

Remember that multilateral development is the major scope of training for prepuberty. By playing sports (the more varied the better), children develop basic strength, general endurance, short-distance speed, and good coordination. For instance, if a child participates in a recreational swimming program, she can also take a few gymnastics classes to develop basic flexibility and balance. While playing games, a young athlete develops endurance, speed, coordination, agility, and space orientation and performs a variety of skills. This will result in a harmonious physical development rather than a sport-specific narrowness.

Although children spend most of the time performing their chosen sport, they should dedicate 20 percent to 30 percent of their training time per week to physical training, both strength and flexibility. They should perform such a program informally, free from regimentation and rigidity and full of enjoyment and fun.

The purpose of the strength-training program for prepubescent and pubescent athletes is to prepare the muscles, tendons, and joints for the training stress of high performance at maturation. The aim of the program is overall, harmonious, proportional body development, as called for in the principle of multilateral development. Athletes should prepare during the six to eight years of carefully progressive development so that they are injury free in the later development stages.

Circuit Training

Instructors can use simple circuit training (named as such because the stations are organized in a circle), consisting of six to nine stations, to develop basic strength. Tables 7.2 and 7.3 provide example circuit-training programs. Consider the following when organizing a circuit-training program:

- Training should last between 15 and 20 minutes and can progressively increase to 30 minutes toward the end of prepuberty.
- Arrange the exercise stations so they alternate limbs, body parts, and muscle groups worked. We suggest the following order: legs, arms, abdomen, and back.
- The program should comprise between six and nine exercises.
- For new exercises, teach the proper technique. Correct execution should take priority over the number of repetitions performed.
- Do not demand that the children complete an exercise or circuit as fast as possible. At this stage of development, speed is not important. For children to enjoy performing a circuit of exercises, they must do the exercises at their own speed.
- Children should be able to perform the movements smoothly and without experiencing discomfort. A grimace during a stressful activity is a sign of discomfort. At this stage of development, stress is categorically undesirable. Where there is stress

Table 7.2 Circuit Training With Six Exercises

Exercise	Reps or duration*	Rest interval (sec)
Push-up	4-6 (8)	30
Medicine ball scoop throw	10-12 (15)	30
Dumbbell curl	8-10 (12)	30
Hanging hip flexion (from monkey bars)	5-8	60
Dumbbell shoulder press	8-12	30
Tuck jumps	60 sec	120

Note: Depending on the abilities of the athlete involved, a child may perform one to two circuits, or even three circuits toward the end of puberty. You may use other exercises as needed for your athlete.

* The maximum number of reps that should be completed is in parentheses.

Table 7.3 Circuit Training With Nine Exercises

Exercise	Reps or duration*	Rest interval (sec)
Push-up	6-8 (10)	30
Hip thrust	6-10	30
Single-leg burpee	8-10/leg	60
Medicine ball twist	6-8	30
Medicine ball scoop throw	10-12 (15)	30
Abdominal crunch	6-8	30
Dodge the rope	60 sec	60
Dumbbell curl	8-10 (12)	30
Squat	90 sec	120

Note: Start with one circuit and over time progressively increase to two and then three. You may use other types of exercises as needed.

* The maximum number of reps that should be completed is in parentheses.

there is no fun! Stop any activity before children experience discomfort. Do not push! Let children have a positive physical experience.

- As much as possible, introduce exercises into the circuit that are enjoyable and that the children will be interested in performing.
- Choose exercises that require equipment that is easy to carry, such as medicine balls, rubber bands, and dumbbells. If possible, plan the circuit outdoors and include playground equipment and partner exercises.
- Provide constant rewards and encouragement for good technique and individual improvement. Circuit training should be an environment for individual improvement, challenge, and personal satisfaction, not for competition among children. However, children should know from the beginning that they cannot expect improvements all the time. The road to a good performance is full of both gratification and frustration, and performance does not always improve constantly. Consistent and persistent work is always rewarded in the long run.

Remember that children should not lift heavy loads during prepubescence. No child should attempt to know their 1RM. All strength-training programs should be age specific, prescribed under the supervision of a qualified instructor, and matched to the developmental characteristics of the young athlete (Faigenbaum et al., 2009).

The exercises and training guidelines we suggest previously are adequate to build the base for future phases of strength development. With the activities children perform during puberty, they will build the foundation for the training to come during adolescence and maturation. To do it any other way would mean burnout for the young athletes, and they will lose interest in sport before they reach their best performance at the time of physical and psychological maturation.

Strength-Training Model for Athletic Formation

A training program for pubescence continues to build the foundation of training necessary for an athlete to specialize in a sport. Such a base is paramount for the success many athletes aspire to during the high-performance phase. Therefore, view puberty as an important stage in the equation for producing high-quality athletes.

Although pubescent children grow rapidly during this stage, sometimes 4 to 5 inches (10-12 cm) per year, adequate strength training is essential for the young athletes. Recent research touts high-intensity resistance training as being safe and beneficial for youths. Studies in which athletes perform 1 to 2 sets of 10 or more exercises for 8 reps at high intensity have shown increases in strength without injury (Ratel, 2011) and with improvements in body composition (Benson et al., 2007). We do not recommend that children and adolescents use maximal loads. Maximal loads require low repetition counts and open up the possibility of numerous injuries, including soft tissue injuries and joint problems caused by the athlete's inability to maintain proper technique when performing the heavy lifts. The American Academy of Pediatrics (2008) endorses the use of submaximal loads for youth strength training until the time that the athlete's neuromuscular system has matured to a level that can progressively handle and recover from maximal loads.

From puberty on, boys and girls will have different gains from strength training. The development of sexual organs in boys results in high levels of growth hormones, including testosterone levels that are 10 times higher than those in girls. For this reason, boys get bigger and stronger than girls.

Scope of Strength Training

View strength training as part of overall development. Multilateral training—developing a high variety of skills and basic motor abilities, such as flexibility, endurance, and speed—is still an important goal.

The aim of a strength-training program is the proportional and harmonious development of the body and musculature. Except in sports in which athletes achieve high performance during late puberty and early adolescence, resist falling into the trap of specificity. Do not stress training methods and especially do not employ exercises that are specific for only selected sports. Stressing specificity at this early stage will mean rapid adaptation, causing the athletes to reach good performance at an unnecessarily young age. As children improve fast, the temptation increases to push them higher, use heavier loads, and demand better performance. This stress in training is often exacerbated by entering the young athlete into more difficult competitions. The result of this approach is predictable: high stress and burnout. The goal of strength training in pubescence is to further the base of strength for the high-performance phase. During the 2008 and 2012 Olympic Games, most medalists were in their late 20s and early 30s. Avoid specificity; work for multilateral development; build a solid base for the future; and, most importantly, create an environment that is enjoyable and a positive physical experience. Remember the Roman dictate "Festina lente," which means hurry up slowly!

Program Design

A strength-training program designed for pubescence should continue to apply the three basic laws of strength training. Work further on developing joint flexibility, strengthening the tendons, and improving the core area of the body.

Developing a good strength base, with harmonious muscles, is a major goal of strength training at this stage. This will prepare the athletes anatomically for the training stress they will face during postpubescence and maturation. The direct benefit of such long-term progression is the creation of injury-free athletes. With good progression this is a possibility.

A training program for pubescence is a vital step in preparing the athlete for high-performance training. Although an athlete may use similar means of training and use the same types of equipment (e.g., exercises that require body weight and a partner), the number of repetitions and resistance will be slightly more challenging during the pubescence stage. To develop speed and power, use the athlete's body weight and continue performing exercises with medicine balls, mostly throws and relays. Increase the weight of the ball slightly, from five to nine pounds (2-4 kg). Numerous types of medicine balls are available on the market today, including balls with one or two handles. Use exercises that incorporate dumbbells, barbells, heavy bags, and resistance bands as well as devices such as the TRX (a suspension training system) or the Lebert Equalizer to develop the strength base and adapt the tendons and ligaments. These products are relatively inexpensive (when compared with gym equipment) and mobile and can be effectively used in a circuit.

Because they are slightly increasing the total amount of work, children will experience some fatigue. This will be especially true if they perform skills of a given sport and 30 minutes of circuit training for strength development in the same day. The instructor should constantly observe the young athletes and learn how much they can tolerate before they feel discomfort. Cease activity before the athletes feel pain.

A sign of comfortable physical exertion is that training still looks effortless. To prevent muscle strain, children should focus on the task while being relaxed. They should understand that although the agonistic muscles contract, the antagonists should relax.

At this stage of training, children can use free weights such as light, simple barbells and dumbbells. However, this does not mean that they should begin using Olympic weightlifting techniques. Rather, this stage is the time for them to learn what kinds of exercises they can perform with a barbell. The main reason for suggesting dumbbells and barbells rather than sophisticated machines is that athletes can perform a greater variety of movements in different positions and planes using free weights. It is easier to mimic a skill pattern that an athlete will perform during postpubescence and maturation. Before thinking about training, however, the instructor should thoroughly teach correct lifting techniques. This is crucial for preventing possible injuries. Most gym machines are not designed for the length of children's limbs.

Consider the following key elements of basic technical instruction:

- Teach the basic stance: feet parallel and shoulder-width apart. This position will guarantee a good support base, giving the child controlled balance.
- Teach proper technique for all movements. Show the athletes how to engage the core muscles of the body to stabilize the lifts and how to properly breathe to maximize strength and focus.

Most concerns should address multijoint movements—exercises that require the engagement of, for instance, both the lower and upper body. Because half or deeper squats are popular exercises, the progression for learning this exercise is as follows:

1. Learn the correct technique without any weight (free squats).
2. Learn to balance the barbell that will be used in the future by placing a stick on the shoulders and positioning the hands toward the ends of the stick.
3. Go through the motions of the exercise using one dumbbell in each hand, lifting them on the sides of the body.
4. Use just a barbell with no additional weights attached.
5. Use slightly increased loads while concentrating on correct technique.

Any instructor who is not aware of the correct technique should learn it from a specialist. In any case, understand that this progression is a long-term proposition. It usually takes a couple years before the athlete uses a heavier load. Normally, this occurs in late postpuberty.

As children develop a better training background, they should progressively experience slightly more challenging demands on skills for technical development, speed, agility, and strength. This helps their adaptation reach higher ceilings, illustrated by their growing capacity to tolerate work and progressively increase their physical potential. To achieve this, the total training demand has to progressively increase following a certain methodology, such as the following:

1. Increase the duration of a training session. Assume that the athlete trains twice a week for one hour. To slightly increase the training capacity, the instructor adds 15 minutes to each session. Now the child trains twice a week for 75 minutes—an additional 30 minutes per week. Over time, such increments may progress to up to 90 minutes per session. The 90-minute session does not include just strength training. Rather, it includes technical and tactical work, speed, agility, and, toward the end of the session, strength training.

2. Increase the number of training sessions per week. Considering that a 90-minute session is long enough for training, a new training challenge will come from increasing the number of sessions from two to three per week.

3. Increase the number of repetitions per training session for all types of activities and skills, including technical, tactical, and physical. If for a certain period the coach feels that training three times per week for 90 minutes is what the children can tolerate, the next training increment will come from performing more work in the 90 minutes. This means more technical drills or exercises for physical development. Consequently, slightly decrease the rest interval between drills and challenge the children to adapt to high training demands.

4. When you exhaust the previous three options, higher training demand will come from increasing the number of repetitions of drills or exercises performed per set. In this way, the new training task is to progressively adapt a child to performing the increased number of repetitions without a rest interval between them.

You must apply this proposed progression carefully over a long time. It may take two or three years to increase the training load from two 60-minute sessions a week to three 90-minute sessions a week. An experienced instructor will certainly make a smooth and careful transition.

The strength-training increment can be from 20 to 30 and even 40 minutes per session toward the end of pubescence. The circuit-training method still satisfies the needs of strength development, except that the number of exercises can increase progressively up to 10 or 12, with 8 to 15 repetitions per exercise.

Strictly adhere to individualization so that training programs match individual potential. Similarly, the child must choose—without pressure from the instructor—the speed at which to perform an exercise. This allows the child to find his way according to his individual rhythm of growth and development, which can differ drastically between two children of the same age.

The instructor may use rewards (e.g., praise for achieving a task) as a motivational tool. However, give any rewards for individual self-improvement rather than for being the best athlete in the group.

During pubescence, children should experience various track and field events with reduced weight for throwing implements (e.g., use tennis balls rather than a javelin) and shortened distance for sprinting (e.g., 50 meters rather than 100 meters). The advantage of learning basic skills and developing speed and power is that a valuable positive transfer will occur later—for example, from javelin throw to pitching in baseball or from good sprinting abilities to football, basketball, or soccer. Therefore, the multilateral base for prepubescence and puberty is not just a concept but a necessity for high athletic performance.

Training Program

A strength-training program for puberty can successfully use the circuit-training method. Use tables 7.2 and 7.3, which present circuits of six and nine exercises, respectively, as training guidelines. Parents or instructors can easily create other programs using many of the exercises in this chapter. Adjust the number of repetitions and the number of circuits according to the potentials of the children in the program.

Strength-Training Model for Specialization

From postpuberty on, the training program changes slightly compared with the first two stages of growth and development, when the major scope was multilateral training. With the foundation athletes create during prepubescence and pubescence, training during postpubescence becomes progressively specific to the needs of the selected sport. Strength training diversifies to include power and to progressively use the periodization model for each competitive year.

As a result of increasing growth hormones, mostly in boys, muscle size and strength will be noticeably greater during postpubescence. From this stage of development up to maturation, boys will increase the proportion of muscles from about 27 percent of total body mass to about 40 percent (Richmond and Rogol, 2007). Under such circumstances, strength certainly improves drastically. Girls' strength also improves to much higher levels (Faigenbaum et al., 2001; Hebbelinck, 1989; Malina, 1984; Seger and Thorstensson, 2000).

Scope of Strength Training

Postpubescence is a development phase that includes young athletes who differ in chronological age by two or three years. Therefore, instructors must carefully and progressively monitor the introduction of training specificity according to the needs of the sport.

Maintain multilateral training during postpubescence, although the proportions between it and sport-specific training will progressively change in favor of specificity. Of equal importance is maintaining work for strength and functionality of the core area of the body. Although many types of strength machines are available on the market, young athletes benefit most from using free implements such as medicine balls, dumbbells, resistance bands, and kettlebells, which train the neuromuscular system to perform and adapt in an unbalanced environment and thus improve the trainability of the core muscles. If training at a gym or fitness center, coaches should use a variety of equipment, including cable machines, lat pull-down machines, squat racks, dip bars, and, of course, free weights. Avoid using the Smith machine. Although it is deemed a safer alternative to squats, performing movements on the Smith machine is unnatural and forces the body into fixed positions that could cause more harm than good.

Specificity of strength training incorporates exercises that mimic the motion that the prime movers (agonistic muscles) perform. The athlete must angle and plane the motion so that it is specific to the technical skills of the selected sport. However, instructors should implement specificity so it does not disturb the harmonious development of the other muscles (antagonists).

Because strength training diversifies to address the specific needs of a sport, the athlete will develop different components of strength, such as power and muscular endurance. Instructors should use specific training methods to address such needs and must understand and implement periodization of strength each competitive year.

Program Design

After the first one or two years of postpubescence, when pubescent-specific training still applies, training becomes progressively sophisticated. Athletes may use additional training methods and more sophisticated equipment. As training becomes more complex and strength plays an important role, monitor the stress in training. As athletes add more power and heavier loads, training intensity takes a toll and they experience fatigue. To prevent a critical level of fatigue and potential injury, the instructor should know how to appropriately increase the intensity in strength training. We suggest the following progression:

1. Decrease the rest interval between sets from 3 minutes to 2.5 minutes. Although athletes may find it difficult to sit, stretch, and wait for the next set, advise them on the importance of rest for optimally improving strength and, ultimately, performance.
2. Increase the number of sets per training session, especially for the higher percentage of 1RM. When doing so, taking an appropriate rest interval is of paramount importance because various energy systems will be fatigued by the increase in both volume and intensity.
3. Increase the training load. According to the principle of progressive increase of load, increase the load in steps, usually three, followed by a regeneration week. (Refer to chapter 1 for an explanation of the step method.) To adapt to the new load, the athlete must maintain a training program of similar intensity for approximately a week before increasing to a new load increment.

Figure 7.1 illustrates a hypothetical load increment over four weeks. The training load increases from step to step by approximately 10 percent except during the regeneration week, when it decreases by 20 percent. Note that the load per step refers to the training program for one day, which the athlete must repeat two or three times, depending on the number of training sessions per week. After two to three workouts at the same training load, the athlete can move to the next load and to further adaptations.

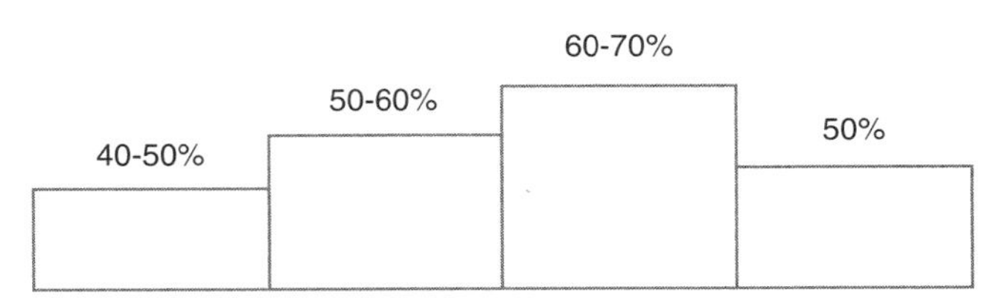

Figure 7.1 Percentage increase of training load for a four-week cycle.

Apply this progression over a long time. In doing this, it is normal to expect that athletes will use high percentages (close to 100 percent) at the end of postpubescence and during maturation. Similarly, the number of sets can increase to three, four, or more to challenge the muscles for adaptation and improvement.

As the complexity of training increases, instructors may be tempted to use sophisticated strength machines or Olympic weightlifting moves, such as the clean and jerk and the snatch, with the belief that doing them will quickly improve strength for the selected sport. We strongly discourage using these methods because they are technical, sometimes dangerous, and not sport specific.

In using more sport-specific exercises and methods, specificity in strength training becomes dominant as the athlete approaches the stage of high performance. Therefore, the instructor has to select the type of equipment that best suits the needs of the sport. Although some machines can be used in certain training phases (i.e., maximum-strength phase), free weights seem to be more practical. They are more mechanically similar to most athletic skills and coordinate different muscle groups. Although proper technique is more difficult to learn, free weights allow the athlete to perform moves in various directions and planes. The athlete can duplicate most of the dynamic nature of sport actions to create a sport-specific acceleration throughout the range of motion. In fact, this is one of the most important advantages of free weights.

Free weights are popular but can cause injury if improperly used. Besides teaching the technique, the instructor should ensure that a spotter is constantly assisting the performer. The main objective of spotting is safety and injury prevention.

The instructor should do the following when introducing a new movement:

- Explain the main elements of lifting.
- Demonstrate the correct technique.
- Have the athlete perform the movement with a low load and remark on the athlete's execution.
- Explain and demonstrate the role of the spotter.

An effective spotter, usually one of the instructors or an experienced athlete, should do the following:

- Know the techniques of lifting and spotting.
- Give the performer the necessary technical clues.
- Throughout the performance, know the program (e.g., number of repetitions) in order to be an attentive and effective spotter.

The methodology of developing strength changes and becomes more difficult as the athlete approaches maturation. The athlete is now seeking to train for maximum strength or one of its components (e.g., power or muscular endurance) rather than for general strength.

Training Programs

Postpuberty includes young people aged 13 to 18 years, or the beginning of maturation. Because so many biological and psychological differences exist among young people in this age range, we divide the training program into two parts: early and late postpuberty.

Training Program for Early Postpuberty

Because the biological and psychological potentials of children in early postpuberty (approximately 14-15 years of age) are closer to puberty than adulthood, a training program can still use circuit training to benefit continuous athletic improvement. The great difference between circuit-training programs for puberty and for early postpuberty lies in the following:

- Exercises are more difficult.
- The load for some exercises will be higher.
- The rest interval between exercises will be lower.

Tables 7.4 and 7.5 present two examples of circuit training. The example in table 7.5 is more difficult and has more power exercises and a few simple plyometrics exercises (e.g., cone jump, vertical hop, scissors splits).

Use the suggested load and number of repetitions flexibly. They might be too difficult for some athletes and too easy for others. Adjust the program to individual potentials.

Training Program for Late Postpuberty

Late postpuberty includes athletes aged approximately 16 to 17 years. Assuming that strength training follows technical work, strength training is a complementary activity that can last for 30 to 60 minutes, especially during the competitive phase. During some

Table 7.4 Circuit Training for Early Postpuberty

Exercise	Reps or duration*	Rest interval (sec)
Pull-up	4-8	30
Leg press or dumbbell squat	10-12	30
Medicine ball twist	8-10	30
Lat pull-down	8-10	30
Slalom jump	30 sec	60
Dumbbell preacher curl	6-8 (10)	30
Medicine ball trunk raise	6-8	60
Push-up	6-8 (10)	30
Cone jump	30 sec	120

Note: Do two circuits. Adjust weight based on children's potential.

* The maximum number of reps that should be completed is in parentheses.

Table 7.5 Circuit Training for Early Postpuberty (More Challenging)

Exercise	Reps or duration*	Rest interval (sec)
Leg press	12-15	20
Pull-up	4-6	30
V-sit	4-6 (8)	30
Vertical hop	30 sec	30
Dumbbell or barbell chest press	6-8	20
Supermans	6-8 (10)	20
Scissors splits	30 sec	30
Lat pull-down	6-8 (10)	20
Cone jump	30 sec	120

Note: Do two circuits. Modify the program based on individual potential.

* The maximum number of reps that should be completed is in parentheses.

segments of the preparatory phase, a strength-training session can be conducted apart from technical or tactical training. Regardless of when strength training occurs, the instructor should make sure that the athletes have a comprehensive warm-up.

Table 7.6 presents an annual plan in which the competitive phase occurs during the summer months. Using this model, coaches can create a plan in which the competitions occur in either fall (e.g., football) or winter (e.g., skiing, basketball). Table 7.6 can easily be applied to an endurance sport in which the volume is high but the intensity (load) is low to medium. Note that below each training phase we indicate the type of strength to train in that phase.

Table 7.7 presents a training program for maximum strength for this age. Anatomical adaptation is the only strength-training phase for which coaches can organize circuit training, as mentioned earlier. Power training is discussed later in this chapter, where specific power-training programs are suggested. Note that strength-training programs for athletes aged 19 years and up are not included in this book. Because training for this age is very specialized and dedicated to high performance, we suggest you refer to *Periodization Training for Sports, Third Edition* (Bompa and Buzzichelli, 2015).

Coaches should adjust the program in table 7.7 according to the environment, the equipment available, and, most important, the abilities and backgrounds of the athletes. Parents or coaches who organize their own programs should consider the following important points:

- For exercises where the load is expressed as a percentage of 1RM, a one-repetition test should be performed with the particular exercise before calculating the actual amount of weight planned for a given training session.

Table 7.6 Periodization Model for Strength Training: Annual Plan for Late Postpuberty

	Month											
	Nov	Dec	Jan	Feb	Mar	Apr	May	Jun	Jul	Aug	Sep	Oct
Training phase	Preparatory							Competitive			Transition	
Periodization of strength	Anatomical adaptation			Maximum strength <80 percent				Maximum strength and power			Anatomical adaptation	

Table 7.7 Strength-Training Program for Maximum Strength (<80 Percent)

Exercise	Load (percentage 1RM)	Reps*	Sets	Rest interval (min)
Leg press	70-80	6-8	2	2
Dumbbell or barbell chest press	70	8	2	2
Dumbbell swing	—	8-10 (12)	1	1
Supermans	—	12-15	1	1
Dumbbell squat	60-70	10-12	2	2
Drop push-up	—	6-10	1	1
Leg curl	50	10-12	2	3
Pull-up	—	Maximum	2	2
V-sit	—	8-10	1	2

Dash indicates no load for that exercise; use own body weight.

* The maximum number of reps that should be completed is in parentheses.

Table 7.8 Training Log

		Sets					
	Exercises	**1**	**2**	**3**	**4**	**5**	**6**

Enter exercise load and number of repetitions per set (example: 180 × 6).

From T. Bompa and M. Carrera, 2015, *Conditioning young athletes* (Champaign, IL: Human Kinetics).

- Do not use loads greater than 80 percent of 1RM. The athlete may not be ready for such loads.
- Alternate each week workouts for maximum strength and power.
- In any program, try to include two exercises that work the arms and two exercises that work the legs.
- Athletes must perform power exercises dynamically and explosively.
- Do not shorten the rest interval. If anything, increase it! Proper recovery is ideal for optimal gains in strength and for preventing fatigue or overuse injury.
- Do not push! The athlete still has a few years before using heavy loads (greater than 80 percent) or performing taxing workouts.

A training log is always convenient for keeping records of an athlete's training and monitoring her progress more efficiently. Refer to table 7.8 for a sample training log.

Power Training for the Young Athlete

As young athletes approach maturation, training programs must become more specific and be conducive to the needs of the selected sport. From late puberty and adolescence (17-18 years of age on), coaches should incorporate specific programs for the development of power. Power is a fundamental ingredient in producing a good athlete. More importantly, a specific power-training phase has to be introduced during the competitive phase (table 7.9). The scope of the power phase is to transform gains in strength into power. Power exercises have to be performed quickly and forcefully to increase the discharge rate of the nervous system and the contraction of the muscles performing the technical moves of the chosen sport.

Table 7.9 Periodization Model for Strength Training and Power During Late Postpuberty for a Team Sport

	Month											
	Nov	Dec	Jan	Feb	Mar	Apr	May	Jun	Jul	Aug	Sep	Oct
Training phase	Transition		Preparatory				Competitive					Transition
Periodization of strength	Anatomical adaptation		Maximum strength <80 percent				Power					Anatomical adaptation

Power training for young athletes has several benefits:

- It increases the athlete's power by improving intramuscular coordination. That means that the muscles contracting during a power exercise learn to work together in unison for best performance in a power exercise or athletic skill.
- It improves intermuscular coordination, meaning that the agonistic muscles—the muscle performing an action (e.g., the biceps during an elbow curl)—contract while the antagonistic muscles (e.g., the triceps) relax to allow a more effective, quick, and smooth contraction. The main muscles performing a technical skill are called prime movers. These muscles should be the main focus of strength and power training.
- Power is the main element for all sports that require high speed of movement and quickness in performing technical skills. In many team sports, racket sports, and martial arts, agility is also important. Like speed, the improvement of agility requires a high level of strength and power development. No athlete can be fast and agile before first being strong and powerful!

Research shows that an increase in power comes from higher force and not from a higher velocity of training (Bompa and Carrera, 2005; Enoka, 2002). In other words, athletes must develop strength and power with heavier implements before concentrating on training speed and agility.

Power training follows and benefits from the strength-training phase planned during the preparatory phase. For best power benefits, the equipment and methods used for power training have to be planned in a specific progression. Note that the suggested periodization (planning of training phases) of power training equipment, such as medicine balls and power balls, suggested in figure 7.2 follows the strength-training phase usually planned during the preparatory phase. Therefore, the use of power-training equipment should start with heavier medicine balls and power balls (late preparatory phase) followed by lighter loads before and during the competitive phase. The lighter loads facilitate a much faster application of force against the resistance encountered in sport (e.g., water, gravity, technical implements, and opponents), resulting in an increased application of power. However, if the competitive phase lasts longer than four to five months, power training can follow a ratio of 60 percent lighter loads to 40 percent heavier loads.

Late preparatory phase	Competitive phase
Heavier MB: 3-6 kg; 8-12 lb PB: 6-10 kg; 15-20 lb	Lighter MB: 2-3 kg; 5-10 lb Lighter PB: 3-6 kg; 8-12 lb

Figure 7.2 Periodization of power training using medicine balls (MB) and power balls (PB) for late postpuberty.

Because safety is always the primary concern, coaches should make sure that athletes are not overextending or snapping the elbows during, for example, the medicine ball chest throw. All power exercises should be performed as smoothly as possible with little jerking or uncontrolled movements. Coaches should consider the following to maximize the effectiveness of power training:

- The exercises for power training should be low in number and sport specific and should mimic as much as possible the skills of the selected sport. Performing too many exercises may result in an increased level of fatigue. Fatigue is the worst enemy of quickness and high-velocity performance.
- Discontinue the repetition of a power exercise when speed or quickness of execution declines. Fatigue during power exercises impedes the expected improvements in power, speed, and agility.
- For similar reasons, plan a low number of sets, especially for the athletic formation and specialization stages. For the high-performance stage (ages 19+ years), you can select a higher number of sets, depending on the physiological requirement of the sport and the training potential of the athlete.
- One of the key elements of an effective power-training program is the rest interval between sets. In order to develop the athletes' abilities to develop power, the rest interval should be two to three minutes or even longer. This will guarantee a high degree of recovery of the energy spent in previous sets and, as such, the ability to apply force as quickly as possible during the following sets.

Selected Power-Training Methods

The main scope of power training is to increase the athlete's ability to apply maximum force against the resistance of an implement, gravity, or opponent in the shortest period of time. When the athlete's force doesn't visibly exceed the weight of an implement, the motion occurs slowly. On the contrary, when the athlete's force visibly exceeds the weight of the implement, the motion is fast and dynamic. The action of a very powerful muscle contraction against an implement is described as ballistic. This section discusses some of the most effective power-training methods.

Ballistic Method

To optimize power development, coaches should use varied equipment in training such as medicine balls, power balls, shots used in track and field, rubber tubing (mostly for legs; e.g., squat jumps), and lighter balls. During a ballistic action the athlete's force against these implements is exerted dynamically; the goal is constant acceleration through the range of motion, culminating in the release of the implement. In order to throw the implement the maximum possible distance, maximum acceleration must be achieved at the moment of release. The distance the implement is thrown is proportional to the power applied against it. Knowing and monitoring the distance should motivate the coach and athlete because increased power translates into increased distance! Finally, increased distance results in increased athletic performance.

Program Design

Ballistic exercises can be performed at the beginning of the training session, immediately after the warm-up, or after technical or tactical training. For sports or positions in which power is the most important physical element (e.g., throwing and jumping events in track and field, diving, ski jumping, martial arts, baseball, or speed or power positions in football), ballistic training should be planned after the warm-up so that fatigue does not inhibit the display of power. For many other sports (e.g., most team sports, wrestling, boxing, and racket sports), ballistic training can be planned either (a) immediately after the warm-up so that maximum gains in power can be expected or (b) after technical and tactical training because in these sports athletes should train both power and power endurance, or the ability to repeat power exercises for the entire duration of the game or competition.

In ballistic exercise, the quickness of action is paramount. To achieve this, the athlete should recruit most of the muscle fibers of the muscles involved (i.e., the fast-twitch motor units), enabling him to apply maximum force against the medicine ball, shot put, discus, or whatever implement is used. The quickness of the contraction in each repetition, not how many repetitions an athlete performs in one set, is essential for realizing this explosive quality. Therefore, first analyze the specific requirements of the selected sport and then choose whether to concentrate on power, power endurance, or both.

The load in ballistic training is standard, meaning that medicine balls and power balls have a standard weight that is written on the ball. The normal weight for a medicine ball is between 4.5 and 13 pounds (2-6 kg) and for a power ball is between 22 and 70 pounds (10-32 kg).

The rest interval is essential for the ballistic method. The rest interval should be high (2-4 minutes) or as long as necessary to reach an almost-full recovery so that the athlete can repeat the same high-quality work. For power endurance the rest interval should be shorter (30 seconds-1 minute).

Training Program

The frequency per week (i.e., one to three times) of ballistic training depends on the specifics of the sport, stage of athletic development, and training phase. Power training is normally planned along with technical and tactical training or with other strength-, power-, speed-, and agility-training methods.

Table 7.10 suggests a three-week power-training program for an early postpubertal female basketball player. Consider this example as a guideline for other sports.

Table 7.11 provides a three-week power-training program for a postpubertal athlete. In this program, ballistic and maximum-acceleration exercises are combined.

Table 7.10 Suggested Three-Week Power-Training Program for Female Basketball Player in Early Postpuberty

Exercise	Week 1	Week 2	Week 3	Rest interval (min)
Medicine ball forward overhead throw	2 × 8	3 × 8	3 × 10	2-3
Vertical hop and medicine ball chest throw	2 × 6	3 × 6	3 × 8	2-3
Medicine ball backward overhead throw	2 × 10	3 × 12	3 × 15	2-3
Medicine ball twist throw	3 × 10	3 × 12	4 × 10	2-3

Table 7.11 Suggested Three-Week Power-Training Program With Combined Ballistic and Maximum-Acceleration Exercises

Exercise	Week 1	Week 2	Week 3	Rest interval (min)
Medicine ball forward overhead throw	2 × 10	3 × 12	3 × 15	2
Vertical hops and medicine ball forward chest throw	2 × 8	3 × 10	3 × 15	3
Medicine ball backward overhead throw	2 × 10	3 × 12	3 × 15-20	3
Medicine ball side throw (each side)	2 × 12	3 × 15	3 × 20	3
Medicine ball forward overhead throw	2 × 12	3 × 10-12	3 × 12-15	2-3
Medicine ball scoop throw followed by 15 m/yd maximum sprint	4 sets	6 sets	6-8 sets	3-5
Clap push-up followed by 25 m/yd maximum sprint	4×6 to 8 reps for clap push-up	6×6 to 8 reps for clap push-ups	8×4 to 6 reps for clap push-ups	3-5

Power Training With Plyometrics

To some individuals, plyometrics are dangerous, especially for children! Some instructors are quite cautious about using them. Have you ever seen a child climb and jump off a tree or off a swing in motion? In training we call this jump a drop jump. It is part of a group of plyometric exercises that increase tension in the muscles and, as a result, improve leg strength and power. Exercises should always begin at a very light level and slowly progress in difficulty and intensity. In reality, children perform plyometric-type exercises each time they play on the playground, play hopscotch, skip rope, or jump from the top level of the jungle gym. When training is properly performed and monitored, children will experience the benefits of hopping and jumping and the resulting increase in strength and power development.

Plyometric exercises are based on the reflex contraction of the muscle fibers in which the muscles are loaded eccentrically (lengthening) before the jump, followed immediately by a concentric (shortening) contraction that allows the jump to occur. For instance, an athlete can jump higher from a standing position if before the jump he bends the knees (lengthens the muscles, or activates the fast-twitch muscle fibers) and then takes off (shortens the muscles). This lengthening–shortening action activates the muscle fibers to such a degree that it transforms the strength of the muscles into explosive power.

A good strength-training background of several years always helps the young athlete to more easily adapt, progress through plyometrics training, and avoid injuries. From the stage of athletic formation (11-14 years) on, children can progressively be exposed to simple, low-impact plyometrics training, often in the form of play and games. Coaches shouldn't rush to show athletes all the exercises they know. Patience is essential in children's training. For the best adaptation to power and plyometrics training, coaches should design a long-term training program with a healthy progression. At the end of the athletic formation and specialization phases (15-18 years) children can be introduced to more demanding exercises in which both the weight and duration of particular exercises are increased, especially at the end of the strength-training phase. It is important to pay close attention to the onset of fatigue, which, in the case of plyometrics training, manifests in an increased take-off time or a sloppy take-off.

For the initiation stage of development, let the kids have fun and play on the local playground. There they will develop the necessary skills of strength, power, and endurance at their own pace and level of comfort. Activity on the playground is valuable preparation for sport training that will inevitably take place during the athletic formation stage of development.

Coaches should also consider these points when planning plyometrics training:

- If injuries are a concern, especially for younger children (under age 15 years), perform exercises on a soft, padded floor. However, for athletes in the late teens with a good background in strength training and conditioning, use a harder floor. Harder floors can enhance the ground reaction force and the reactivity of the neuromuscular system and, as a result, increase the muscle power that will add to performance improvement.
- The use of weighted ankles and vests is not recommended for athletes, especially younger athletes. This additional load can overly stress the legs of the young athletes and obstruct the reactivity of the neuromuscular system, thus negatively affecting the development of speed and agility.

Plyometrics exercises can be classified into three categories based on their degree of intensity and their effect on the neuromuscular system. This classification will allow coaches and parents to better plan plyometrics intensity and better alternate training demand throughout the week. Use table 7.12 as a guideline for planning the progression of the intensity of power training (using medicine balls and power balls) and plyometrics training. This program is proposed for athletes in the specialization (aged 15-18 years) and high-performance (aged 19+ years) stages.

Table 7.12 Suggested Plyometrics-Training Program for Late Specialization

Intensity level	Type of exercise	Training demand	Reps and sets	Reps/session	Rest interval (min)
1	Bounding exercises: Two legs One leg	Submaximal	8-15 × 5-8	50-75	3-5
2	Low reactive jumps of 20-40 cm	Moderate	6-10 × 5-8	40-60	3-6
3	Low-impact jumps and throws: On spot Implements	Low	8-15 × 6-8	40-75	2-3

Athletes use different training equipment and methods during the training phases of the annual plan. Table 7.13, which shows the periodization of strength and power, will help coaches better understand how strength and power training can be planned in the annual plan. The progression from basic strength training (anatomical adaptation) to maximum strength and then to power is easy to follow. This progression will ensure that the athlete achieves maximum performance toward the end of the competitive phase. This is the time when both coach and athlete will see the benefits of training and preparation throughout the year. Table 7.13 is suggested as a guideline for the stages of specialization and high performance. Note how the type of strength training and the weight of the implements progress throughout the year of training.

The program suggested in table 7.12 may be considered a minimum requirement, especially if the athlete's background in strength training is very good and, as a result, the athlete is ready for an increased challenge. Deciding the duration (in months) of each training phase and training method is essential for success in implementing the suggested program (table 7.13).

In addition to the exercises suggested in table 7.12, we propose using the following exercises:

- For intensity 1 (sub-maximal load): repeated standing long jumps and triple jumps; jumps with higher and longer steps, hops, and jumps; jumps over a rope or high bench (35 cm [14 in.] or higher); jumps on, over, and off of boxes (35 cm [14 in.] or higher)
- For intensities 2 (moderate intensity) and 3 (low intensity): skipping rope, rope jumps, hops and jumps over benches (25-35 cm [10-14 in.] high), medicine ball and power ball throws

Power training is a must for both individual and team sports that require speed, quickness, and explosive power. However, an athlete cannot be fast until he is strong, so any power-training program that includes the use of medicine balls, power balls, and plyometrics must be preceded by a well-structured strength-training program that maximizes loads and uses exercises that train the prime movers of the sport. The development of strength does not rely on variety but rather on focused movements that prepare the body for the needs, demands, and expectations of the sport or event.

Table 7.13 Periodization of Strength and Power Training

Integrating periodization models	Training phase			
	Early preparatory	**Late preparatory**	**Early competitive**	**Late competitive**
Periodization of strength	Anatomical adaptation	Maximum strength	Conversion to power Maintain maximum strength	Maintenance of maximum strength and power
Periodization of medicine ball and powerball (weight of the implements)	Heavy Medium	Heavy	Medium Medium/light	Medium/light
Periodization of intensity of plyometrics	3 (low intensity)	3 (low intensity) and 2 (moderate intensity)	2 (moderate intensity) and 1 (high intensity)	All 3 intensities (low, moderate, and high)

The following exercises can be useful in developing both the strength and power of young athletes in the different stages of athletic development.

Exercises for Prepuberty

The following exercises are guidelines only and are not restrictions. Coaches can use other exercises, depending on the training environment and facilities.

Dumbbell Squat

Area worked: legs

1. Begin standing with the feet apart and the arms at the sides of the body, holding a dumbbell in each hand.
2. Bend the knees and extend the hips back until the thighs are parallel to the floor.
3. Return to the starting position.

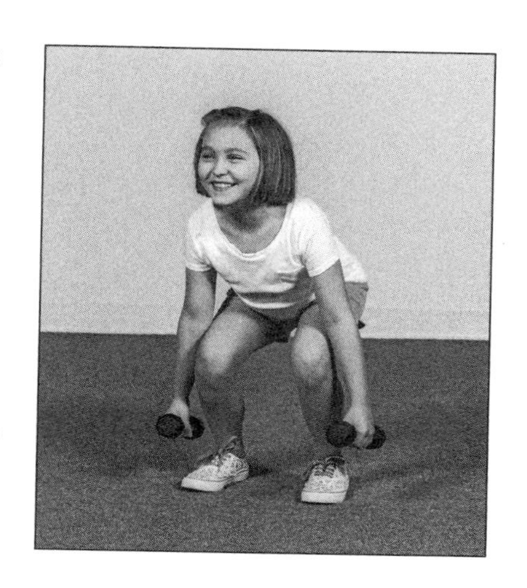

Variation

Using just body weight, bend the knees, drive the hips back, and touch the sides of the ankles with the hands before returning to the starting position.

Dumbbell Curl

Area worked: biceps

1. Begin standing with the arms extended down in front of the hips, palms facing up. Hold a dumbbell in each hand.
2. Flex the right elbow, lifting the weight toward the right shoulder.
3. Return to the starting position. Repeat with the left arm.

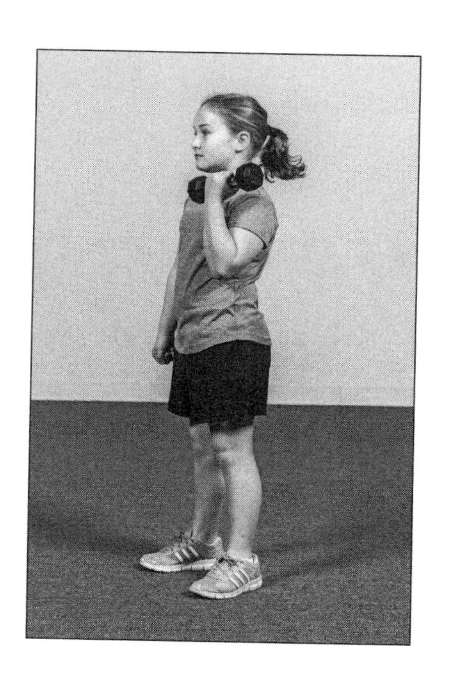

Dumbbell Shoulder Press

Area worked: shoulders (especially the trapezius)

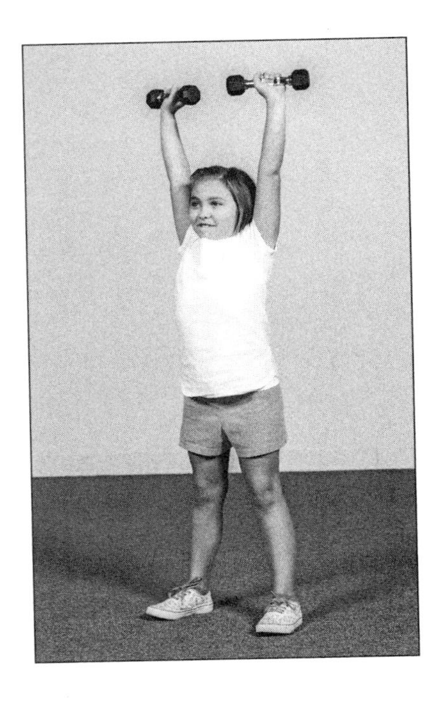

1. Begin standing, holding a dumbbell in each hand at shoulder level.
2. Press the dumbbells straight up and above the shoulders.
3. Return the arms to the starting position.

Dumbbell Pullover

Areas worked: back and shoulders

1. Lie on the back on the floor, grasping one end of a dumbbell with both hands.
2. Extend the arms back and to the floor (figure *a*).
3. Return to the starting position and repeat.

Variation

By holding one dumbbell in your hand, repeat the exercise with each arm alternately (figure *b*).

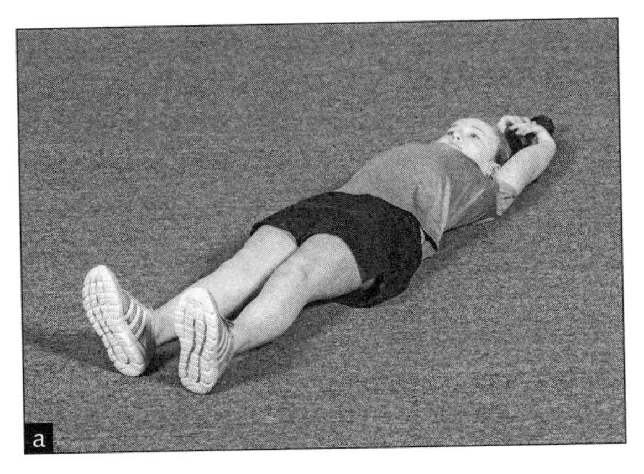
a

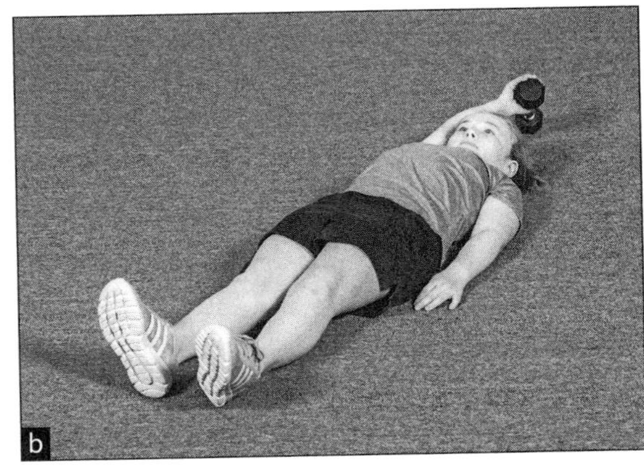
b

Dumbbell Fly

Areas worked: chest and shoulders

1. Lie on the back with the arms extended out to the sides, holding a dumbbell in each hand.
2. Raise both arms to vertical (above the chest).
3. Return to the starting position.

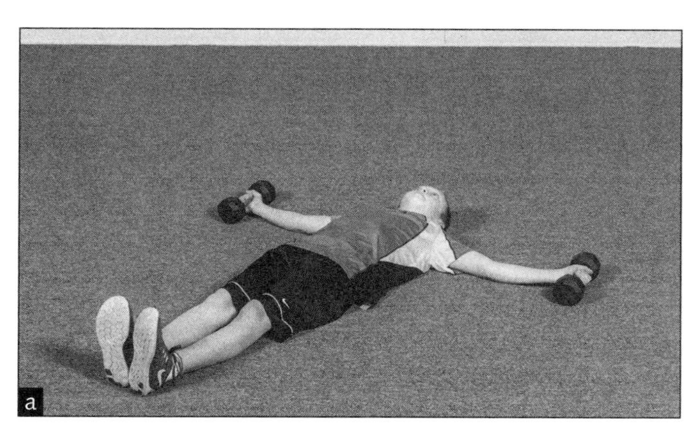
a

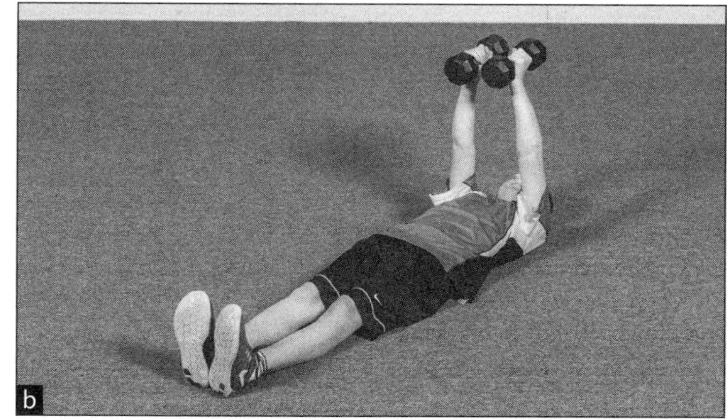
b

Band Row

Areas worked: back and arms

1. Grasp a resistance band with both hands. Hold the arms in front of the body and slightly bend the knees while seated on the floor. Place band around soles of feet as shown in photo. If standing, have a partner grasp one end of the band, wrap the band around a stable pole, or purchase a door attachment.
2. Pull the band until the hands are midline to the body or around the belly button. The bottom of the hands should be around the level of the belly button when arms are fully extended, and squeeze the shoulder blades together. Keep the stomach tight throughout the movement.
3. Slowly return to the starting position and repeat.
4. Minimize body sway and control the movement.

Variations

Try using different hand grips (i.e., palms facing each other, palms down, palms up). Have one partner hold one end of the band while the other partner pulls, or use a door attachment to perform the exercise.

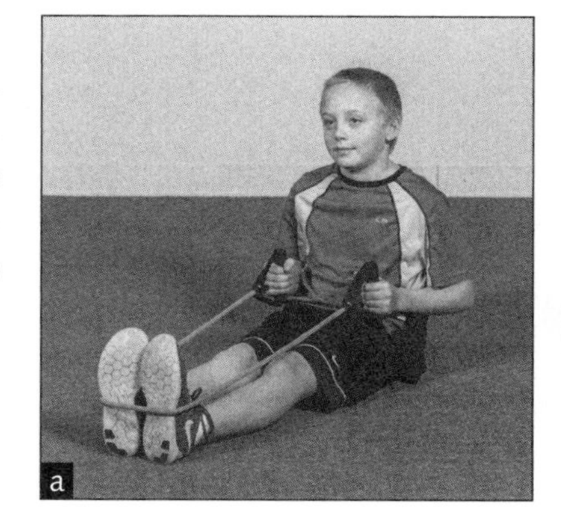
a

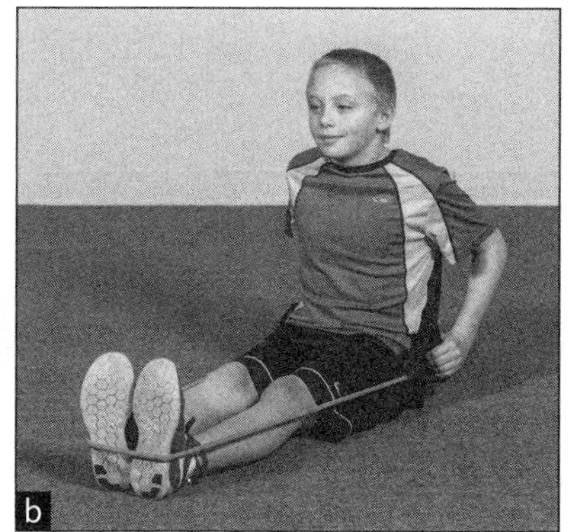
b

Athletes perform most medicine ball exercises by catching and throwing. The thrower performs the action progressively faster, achieving maximum acceleration at the end of the movement. The catcher anticipates the ball by extending the arms forward to receive it. As the athlete catches the medicine ball, the arms flex progressively to absorb the shock. After absorbing the shock, the athlete can maintain momentum by performing a semicircular motion. The speed of the ball accelerates, culminating in another throw. The suggested weight for the medicine ball is 4 pounds (2 kg) for prepuberty, 7 to 9 pounds (3-4 kg) for puberty, and 9 to 13 pounds (4-6 kg) for postpuberty.

Medicine Ball Chest Throw

Areas worked: shoulders and arm extensors (triceps)

1. Two partners stand facing each other 8 to 10 feet (2.5-3 m) apart. Partner A holds a medicine ball in front of the chest.
2. Partner A extends the arms up and forward, throwing the ball toward the chest of partner B.
3. After catching the ball, partner B throws the ball back to partner A.

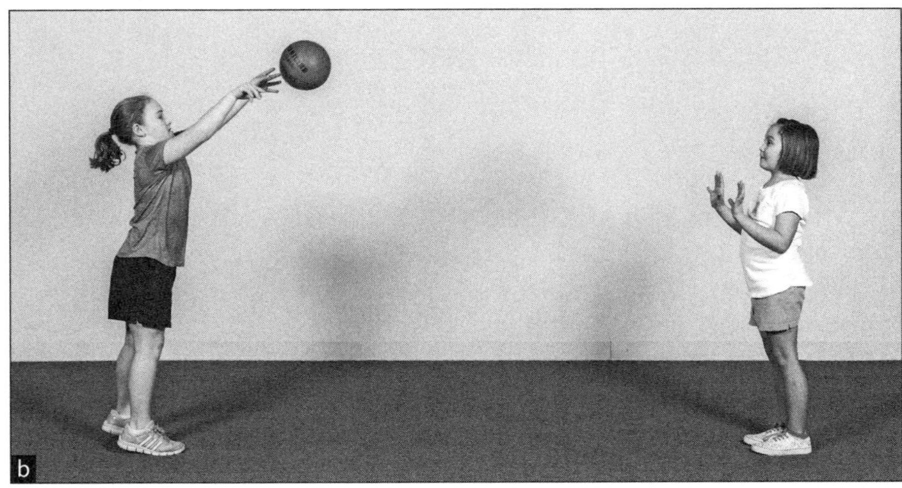

Medicine Ball Twist Throw

Areas worked: arms, trunk, and oblique abdominal muscles

1. Partner A faces partner B with the left side, holding the ball at approximately hip level.
2. Partner B faces partner A, anticipating the ball with the arms extended forward.
3. Partner A turns the body to the left, arms extended, and releases the ball to the side toward partner B.
4. Partner B catches the ball, turns so that the right side faces partner A, performs a rotation, and returns the ball to partner A in the same manner.

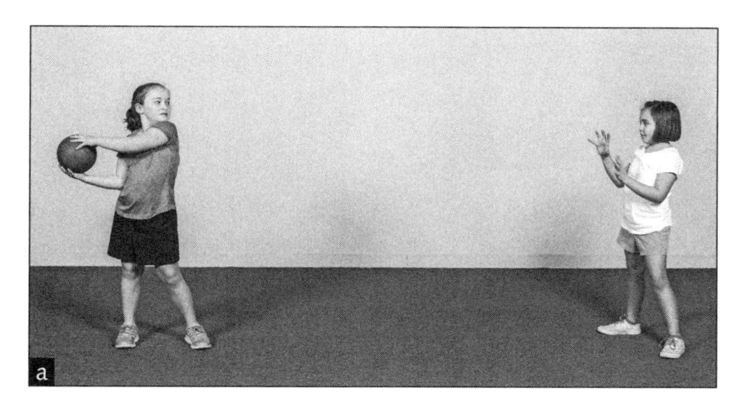
a

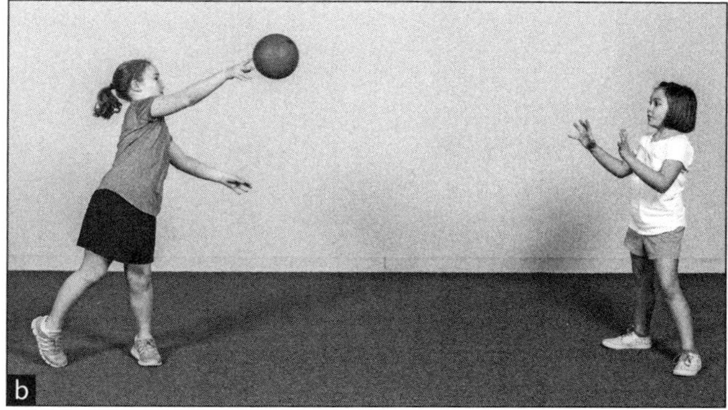
b

Medicine Ball Forward Overhead Throw

Areas worked: chest, shoulders, arms, and abdominal muscles

1. Partners stand facing each other 8 to 10 feet (2.5-3 m) apart, with partner A holding the ball above the head.
2. Partner A extends the arms backward, then immediately forward and over the head toward the chest of partner B.
3. Partner B catches the ball and then returns it to partner A with the same motion.

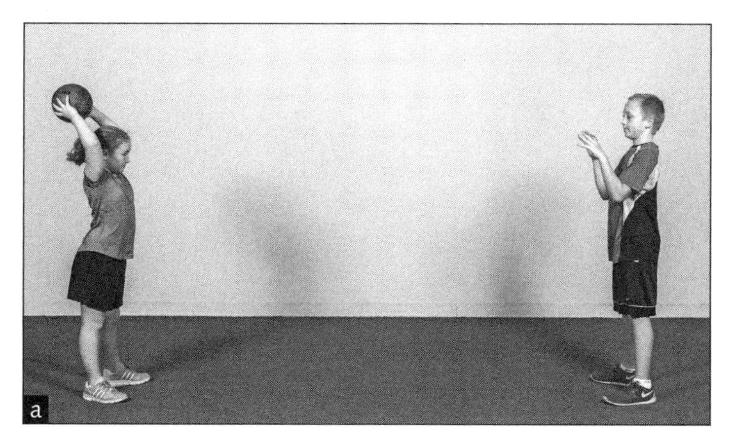
a

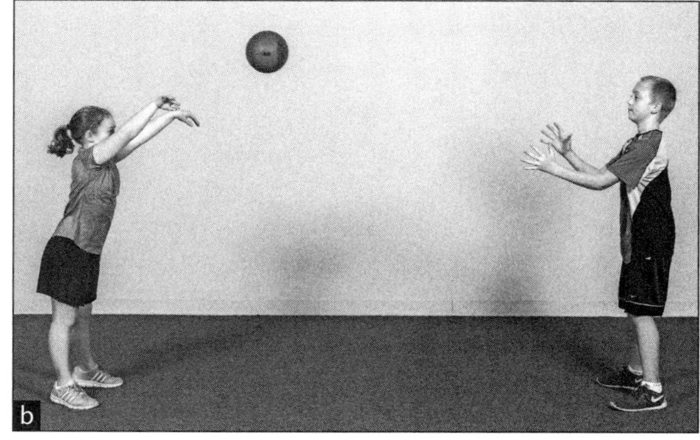
b

Medicine Ball Scoop Throw

Areas worked: ankles; knees; hip extensors; and arm, shoulder, and back muscles

1. Begin standing with the feet apart, holding the ball between the legs.
2. Bend the knees and then immediately extend the knees, throwing the ball vertically with the arms.
3. Extend the arms up to catch the ball, and return to the starting position.

Variation

Perform the exercise with a partner.

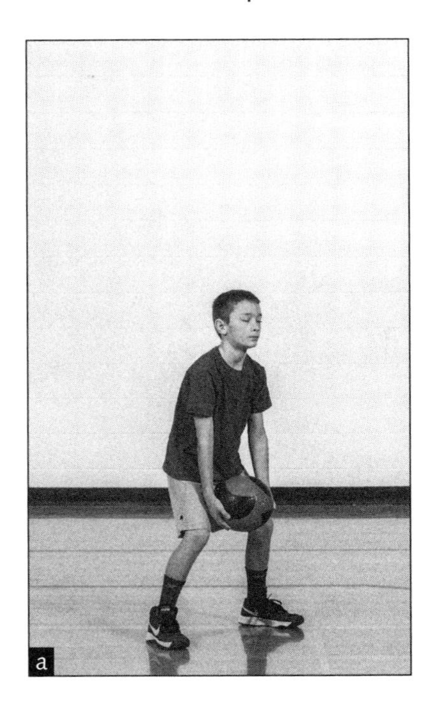

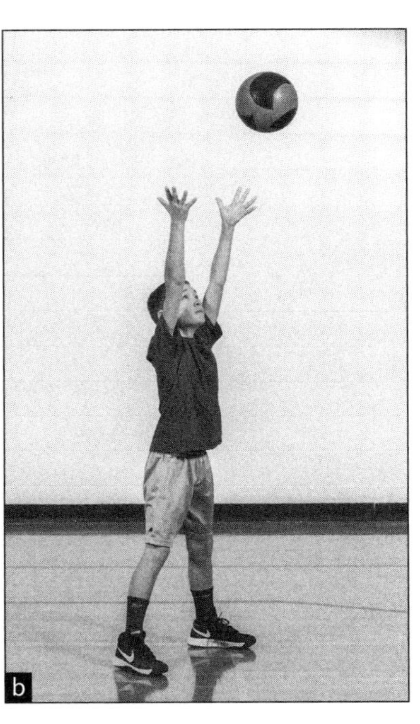

Medicine Ball Back Roll

Areas worked: abdominals and hip flexors

1. Lie on the back with the arms along the body. Hold a medicine ball between the feet, with the knees slightly bent.
2. Raise the knees up to the chest.
3. Lower the legs back to the starting position.

Variation

Perform the exercise with a partner, throwing the ball backward overhead.

Note: When the ball is above the face, place the palms over the face to catch the ball in case it falls toward the face or head.

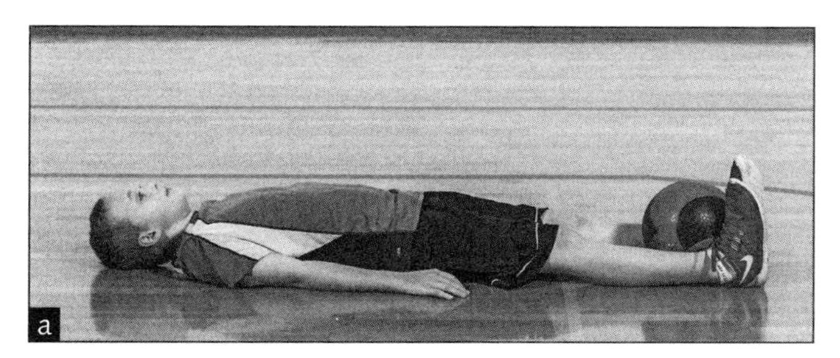

a

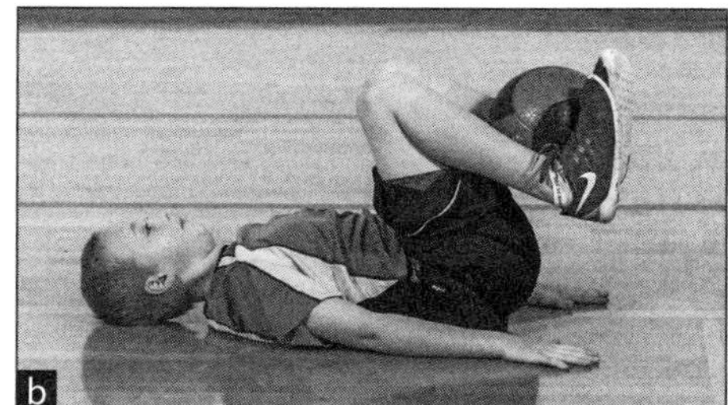

b

Medicine Ball Twist

Area worked: abdominal obliques

1. Lie on the back with the knees bent 90 degrees. Place a light medicine ball between the knees.
2. Rotate the legs to one side of the body and back to the center. Repeat for both sides.

Variations

1. Rotate the legs from one side to the other without stopping in the middle. Control the movement.
2. Lean slightly back, with the trunk in an oblique position. Turn the trunk to the left as far as possible. Return to the starting position and turn the trunk to the right as far as possible.

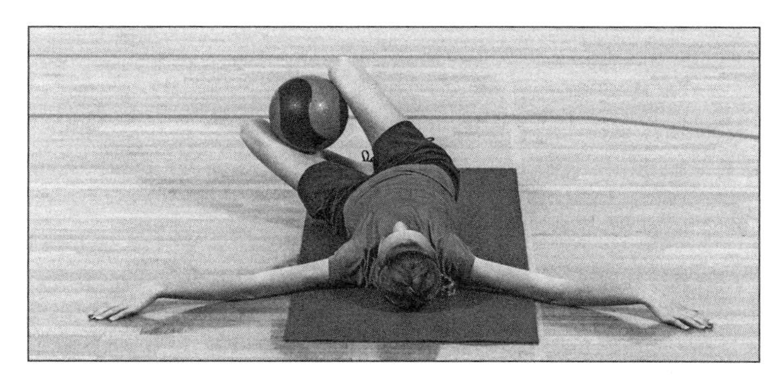

Medicine Ball Zigzag Throw

Areas worked: arms and shoulders

1. Four to six or eight players form a zigzag pattern with players standing 10 feet (3 m) apart. The instructor hands the ball to one player.
2. The player throws the ball down the line to one player, who catches the ball and throws it to another player.
3. Players continue to throw the ball in a zigzag pattern, using an overhead pass, underhand pass, or side throw.
4. Players can choose to throw the ball against ground and in direction of player or simply toss ball toward a player. The player receiving the ball should allow the ball to hit the ground before retrieving it.

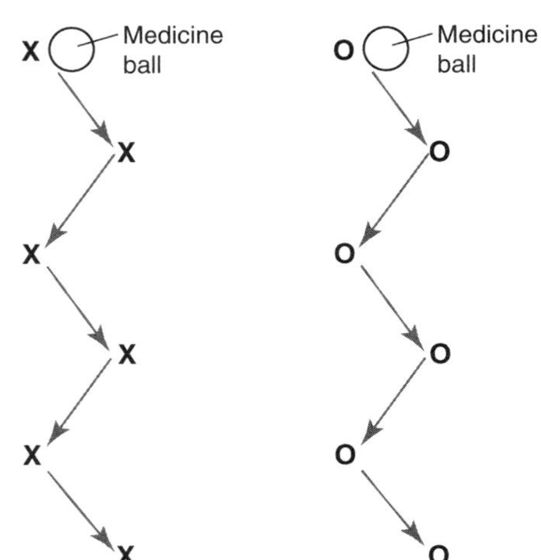

Variation

Players can throw the ball with one hand, overhead with two arms, and from the side.

Medicine Ball Side Pass Relay

Areas worked: abdominal obliques and shoulders (deltoids)

1. Two equal teams sit on the floor in a line with the feet apart. Players should sit so they can comfortably pass the ball to the next player in line. The first player holds the ball.
2. The first player rotates to the right, passing the ball to the next player.
3. Players pass the ball as fast as possible to the end of the line.
4. The last player stands up, runs with the ball to the front of the line as quickly as possible, sits down, and starts the sequence again.
5. The relay is over when the first player is at the end of the line. The winner is the team that finishes first.

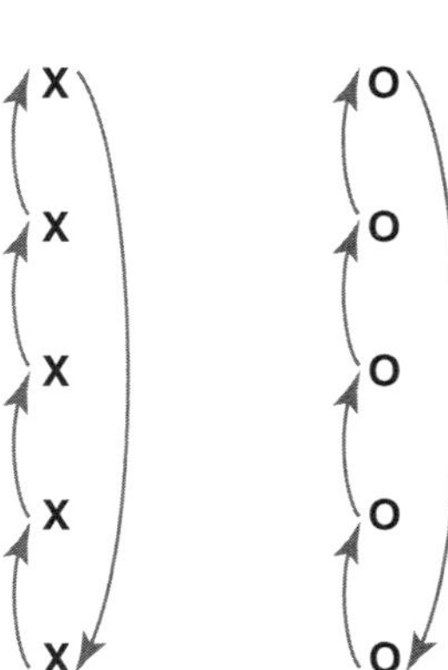

Variations

- Pass the ball alternately to each side.
- Pass the ball back over the head.
- Hold the ball between the feet, roll over, and pass the ball to the feet of the next player.

Single-Leg Back Raise

Areas worked: hip extensors and spine muscles

1. Lie on the stomach with the arms extended forward.
2. Lift the left leg upward as high as possible.
3. Lower the left leg to the floor and lift the right leg upward as high as possible.

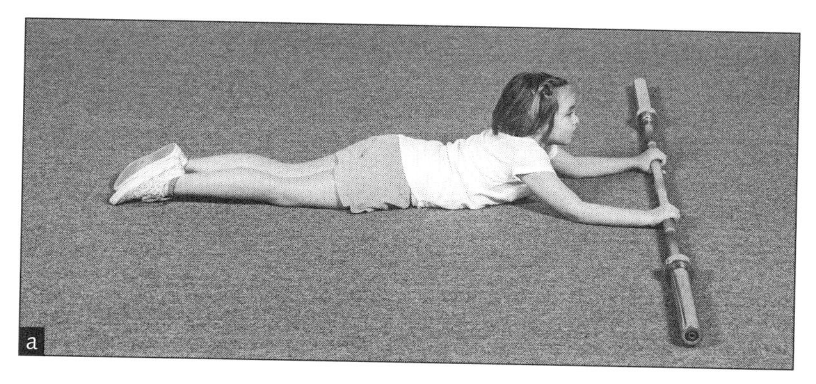

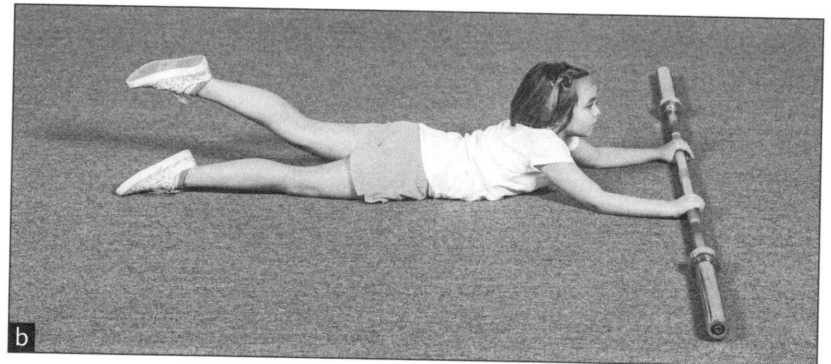

Chest Raise and Clap

Area worked: lower-back muscles

1. Lie on the stomach with the arms extended forward on the floor.
2. Raise the chest with the arms extended and perform two or three claps.
3. Relax the trunk and lower the arms to the floor.

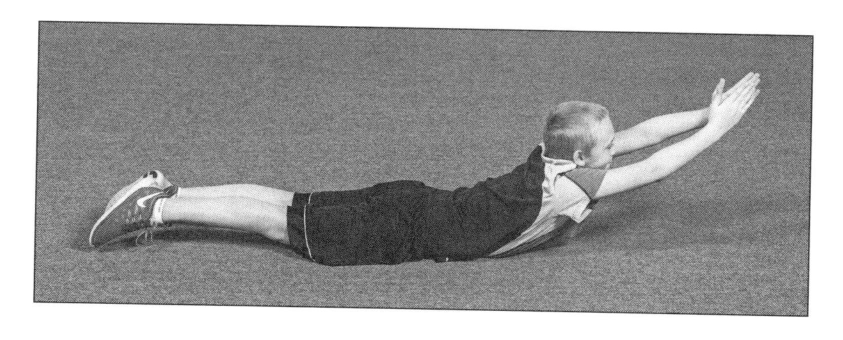

Double-Leg Skip

Areas worked: calf and knee extensor muscles

1. Two children hold the ends of a skipping rope; a third child stands ready to skip the rope.
2. The rope holders rotate the rope. The performer jumps up and down to avoid being hit by the rope.
3. Stop the action after 15 to 20 seconds and change roles.

Variations

- Single-leg skips in place
- Double-leg skips forward
- Single-leg skips forward
- Double-leg skips backward
- Single-leg skips backward
- Alternate single- and double-leg skips forward and backward

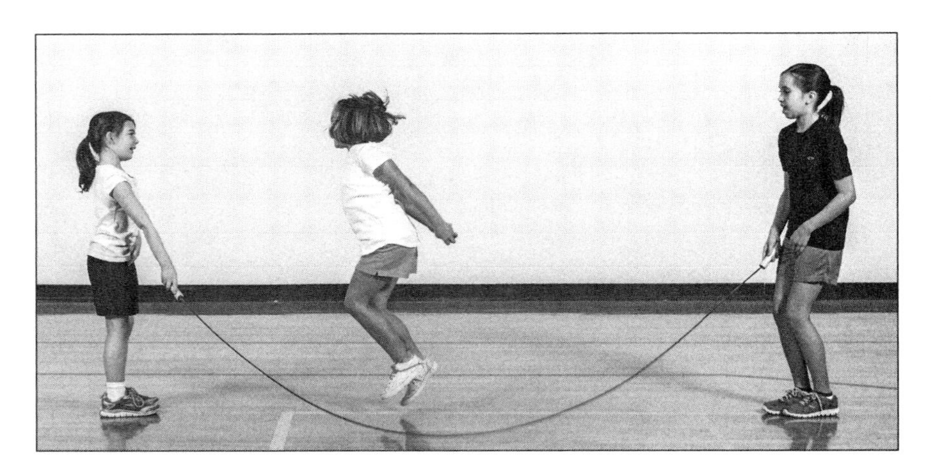

Loop Skip

Areas worked: calf and knee extensors

1. Two teams line up behind a starting line. Place a cone 15 meters or yards in front of each team.
2. At the signal, players skip a jump rope while moving forward as fast as possible, loop around the cone, and return to the starting line.
3. The rope goes to the next player, and the first performer goes to the end of the line.
4. The winning team is the one on which all players skip over the course and the finish line first.

Variation

Time individual performance (i.e., going over the course from start to finish).

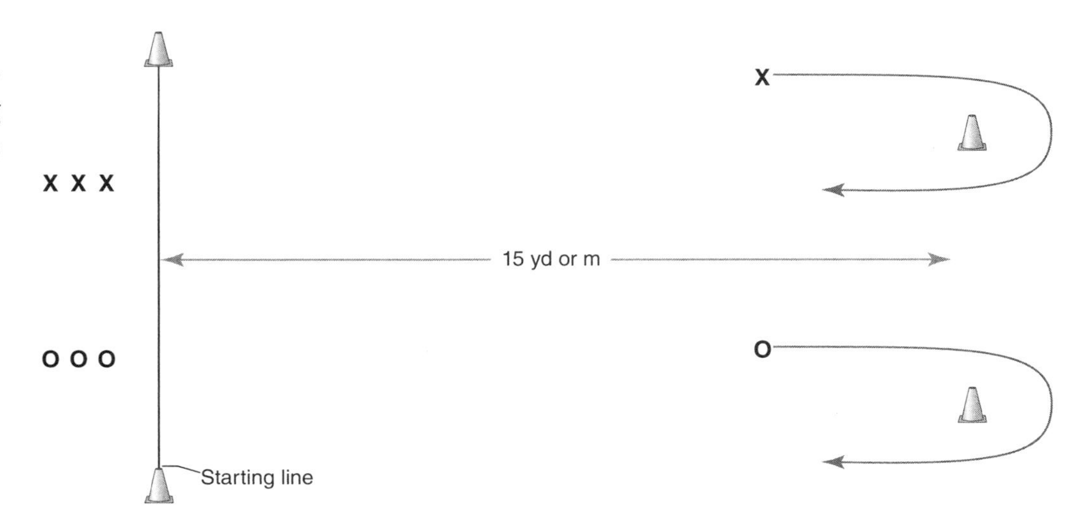

Dodge the Rope

Areas worked: calf and knee extensors

1. A group of players forms a circle. In the middle of the circle a player holds the end of a skipping rope. The distance from the middle player to the circle is equal to the length of the rope.
2. The player in the middle swings the rope in a circle at ankle height. Each player in the circle jumps over the rope as it approaches.
3. When the rope hits a player, that player goes to the middle of the circle and takes over swinging the rope.

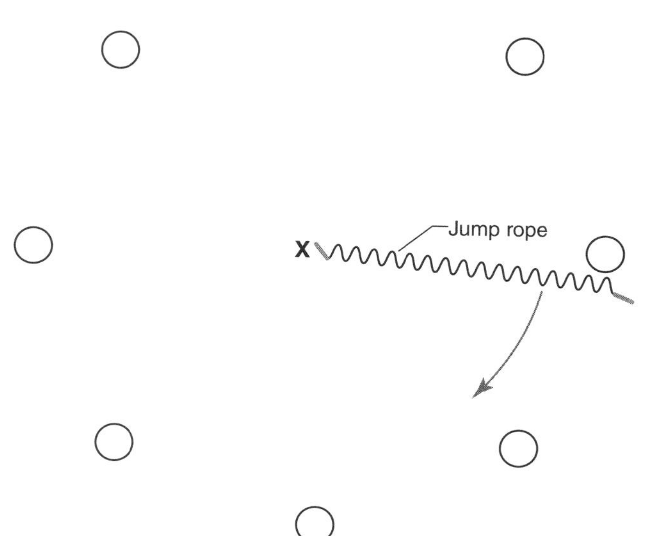

Abdominal Crunch

Areas worked: abdominal and hip flexor muscles

1. Lie on the floor with the arms crossed at chest level, feet flat on the floor, and knees slightly bent.
2. Raise the upper body up and forward, touching the elbows to the knees. The feet should remain on the floor during the movement.
3. Relax and bring the trunk slowly back to the starting position. Maintain proper form during all reps.

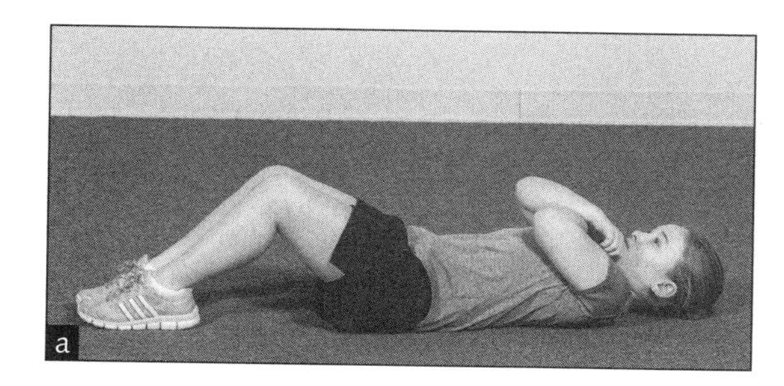

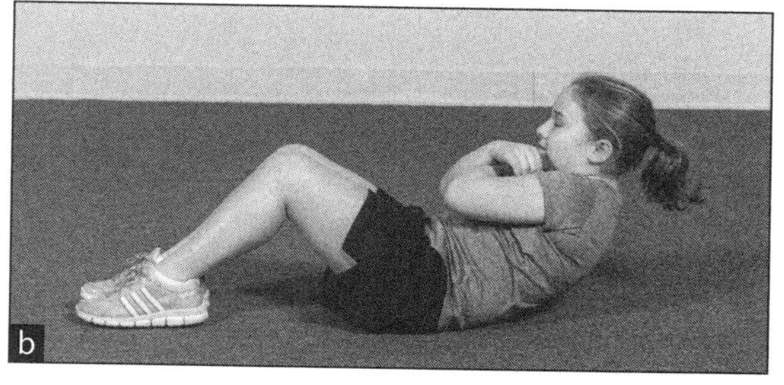

Exercises for Puberty

Exercises for puberty take the form of play or games in which children perform a basic strength exercise. The variety of movements performed helps children develop basic coordination, agility, and awareness of how muscles work in different positions.

Single-Leg Burpee

Areas worked: shoulders and back muscles

1. Begin in the push-up stance by placing hands flat on the floor and directly below the shoulders. The right leg is bent under the chest and the left leg extended back.
2. Exchange leg positions by bringing the left leg under the chest and extending the right leg back.
3. Repeat to fatigue.

Variation

Perform a double-leg burpee: while in a push-up position with legs extended, tuck both legs into the chest and return to the starting position.

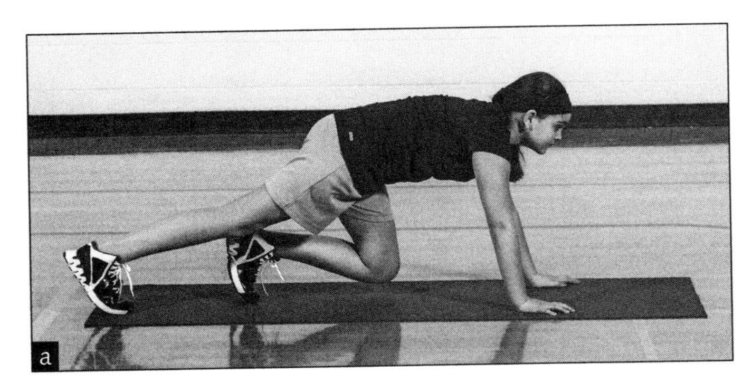
a

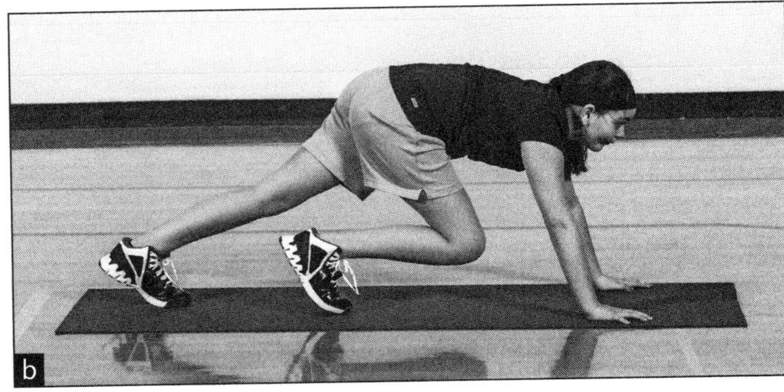
b

Push-Up

Areas worked: shoulders, triceps, and back muscles

1. Begin in the push-up stance with the elbows extended and legs extended back.
2. Bend the elbows and lower the body to the floor.
3. Extend the elbows and return to the starting position.

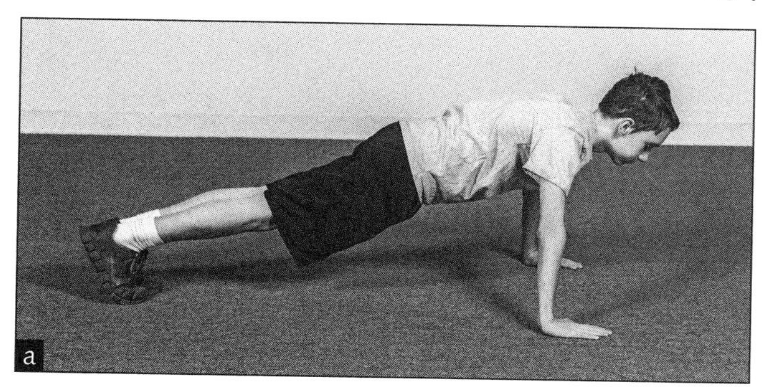
a

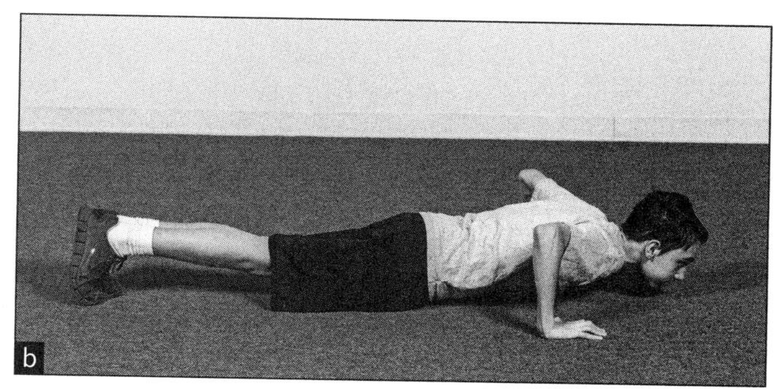
b

Clap Push-Up

Areas worked: shoulders, triceps, wrist extensors, and back muscles

1. Begin in the push-up stance with the elbows extended and legs extended back. Weight of the body should be on hands and toes.
2. Bend the elbows and lower the body to the floor.
3. Extend the elbows vigorously. When the body is at the highest level, push the palms off of the floor and quickly clap the hands together.
4. As the body descends toward the floor, place the palms back on the floor. Push up aggressively to continue the exercise.
5. Return to the starting position after performing the desired number of repetitions.

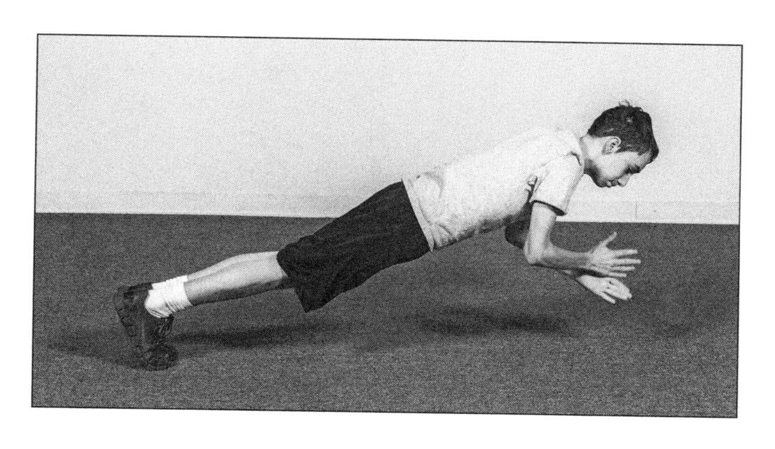

Medicine Ball Backward Overhead Throw

Areas worked: hip and knee extensors, back, and shoulder muscles

1. Stand with the feet apart, hands holding the medicine ball between the legs.
2. Extend the knees, hips, and upper body. Swing the arms backward and throw the medicine ball backward over the head.
3. Retrieve the ball and repeat the movement.

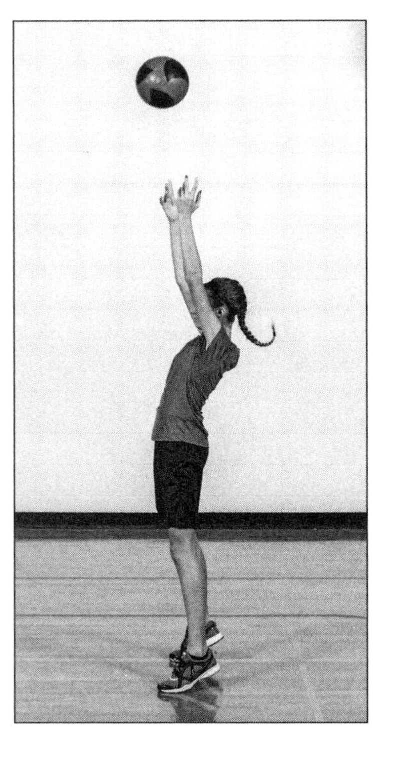

Medicine Ball Side Throw

Areas worked: abdominal obliques, leg extensors, and shoulder muscles

1. Partner A holds the medicine ball on the right side of the hips, with the back facing partner B.
2. Partner A rotates the trunk, hips, and shoulders dynamically, throwing the ball toward partner B.
3. Partner B catches the ball, turns to face partner A with the back, and repeats the movement.

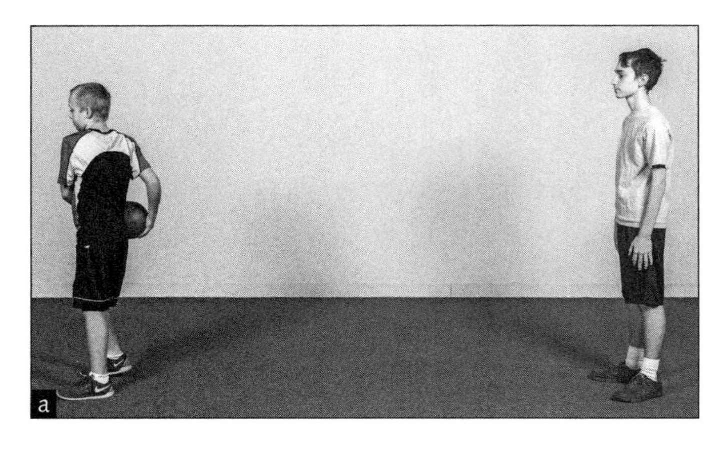
a

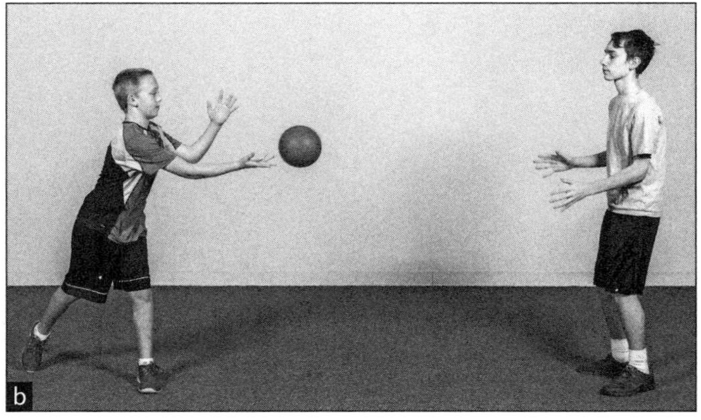
b

Medicine Ball or Shot Forward Throw

Areas worked: leg extensors, hips, back, and arm and shoulder muscles

1. Stand with the hips facing the direction of the throw, knees flexed and feet shoulder-width apart. Hold the medicine ball or shot in both palms with the arms fully extended.
2. Swing the arms back between the legs. Swing the upper body and arms forward, extending the knees and hips, and release the medicine ball or shot forward.
3. Fetch the shot and perform the movement again.

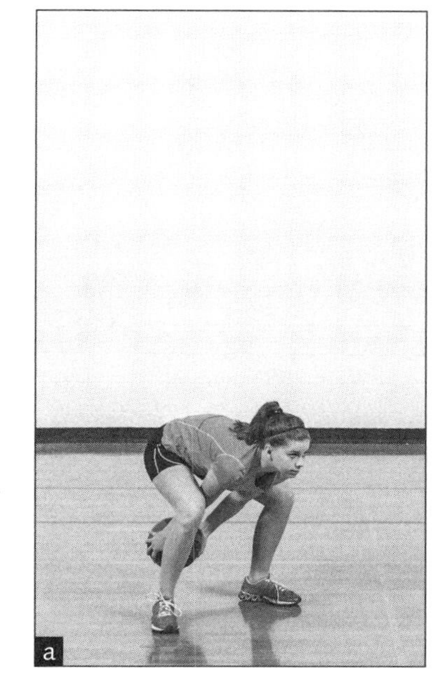

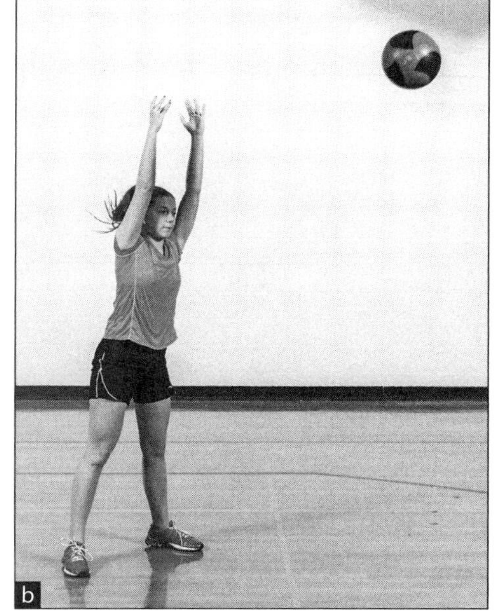

Variation

Perform the movement with a partner. Partners stand 15 feet (4.5 m) apart.

Hip Thrust

Areas worked: abdominals, hip flexors, and arm and shoulder muscles

1. Sit with the feet resting on a bench or any object 1 foot (.3 m) above the floor. Place the hands on the floor slightly behind the hips.
2. Thrust the hips up to horizontal (or higher) and fully extend the body.
3. Relax and lower the hips to the starting position.

Variation

Lie on the floor with the knees bent, feet on a bench, and arms extended at the sides of the body. Thrust the hips up and return to the starting position. For a greater challenge, place a medicine ball between the knees and thrust upward.

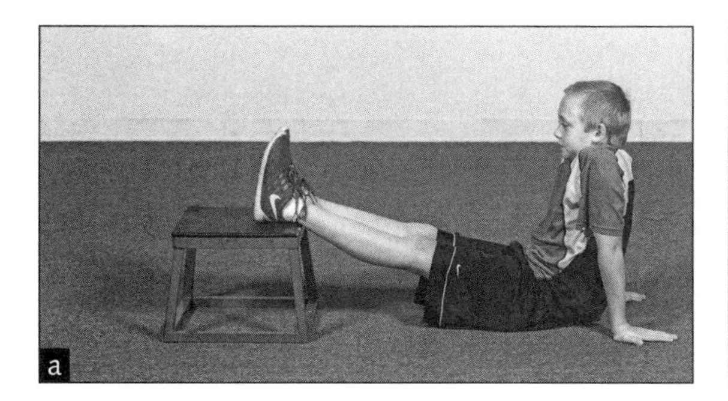

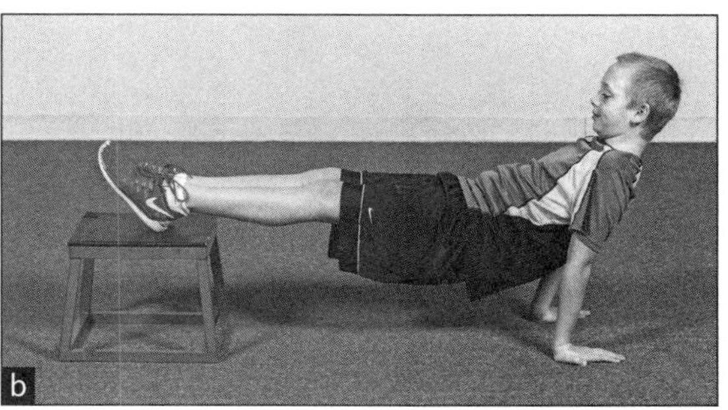

Hanging Hip Flexion

Areas worked: abdominals, hip flexors, and finger flexor muscles

1. Grip a high bar or rings, letting the body hang straight down.
2. Lift both knees up toward the stomach.
3. Relax and return the legs to the starting position.

Variations

- Lift one leg at a time.
- Lift the legs with the knees straight.

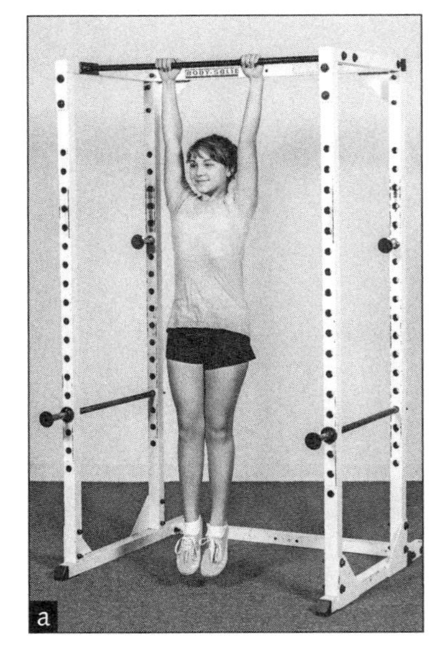

a

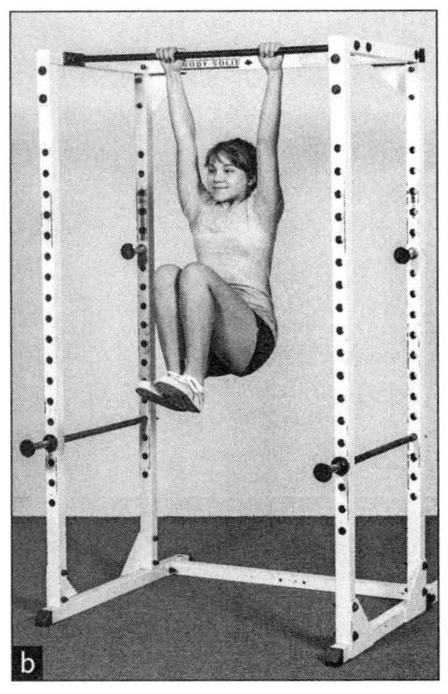

b

Medicine Ball Sit-Up Throw

Areas worked: abdominal and shoulder muscles

1. Partner A stands with the feet apart, holding the medicine ball. Partner B sits with the feet apart and knees slightly flexed.
2. Partner A tosses the ball toward the chest of partner B. As partner B catches the ball he rocks back toward the floor. Then, using the momentum of an upper-body forward thrust, partner B throws the ball back to partner A.
3. Players return to the starting position and then alternate roles.

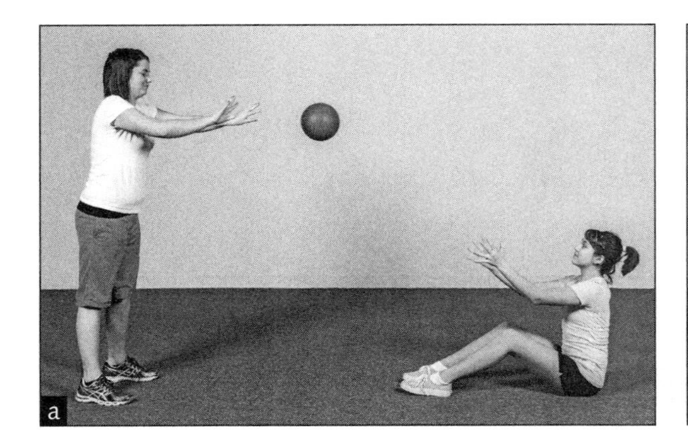

a

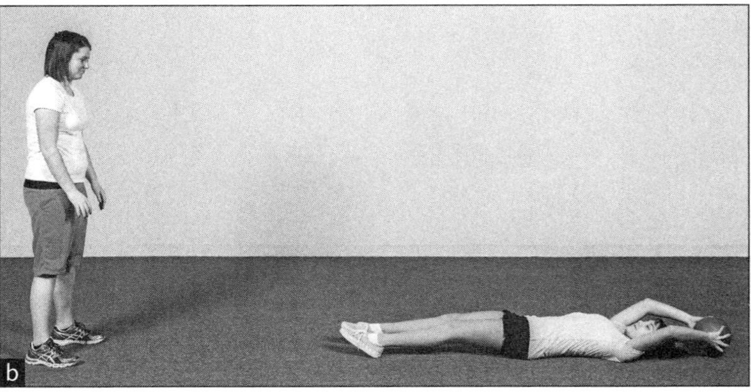

b

Medicine Ball Between-Legs Backward Throw

Areas worked: abdominal and shoulder muscles

1. Partner A stands with the feet apart, holding the medicine ball above the head. Partner B faces the back of partner A.
2. Partner A flexes the hips dynamically, brings the hands between the legs, and releases the medicine ball backward toward partner B.
3. Partner B catches the ball, turns around, and performs the same movement toward partner A.

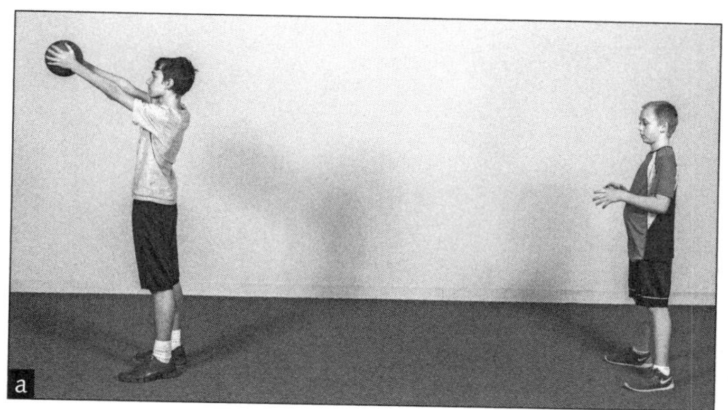
a

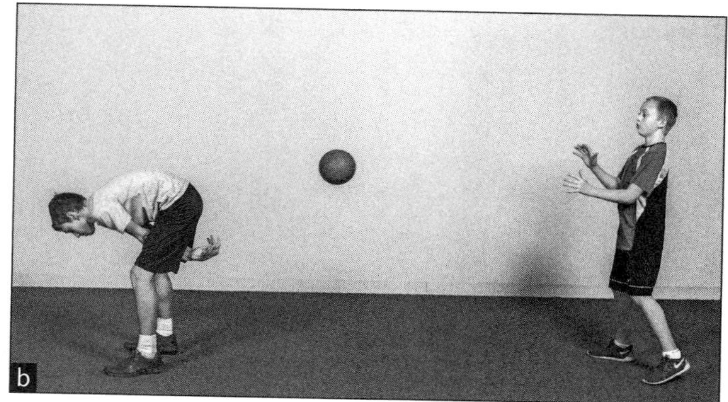
b

Double-Leg Side Lift

Area worked: abdominal obliques

1. Partner A stands with the feet apart. Partner B lies on the floor with the head near partner A's feet and grasps partner A's ankles.
2. Partner B lifts the legs up to vertical, lowers them on the floor to one side, lifts them up again to vertical, and lowers them down again to the other side.
3. Partner B returns the legs to the starting position. Players alternate roles.

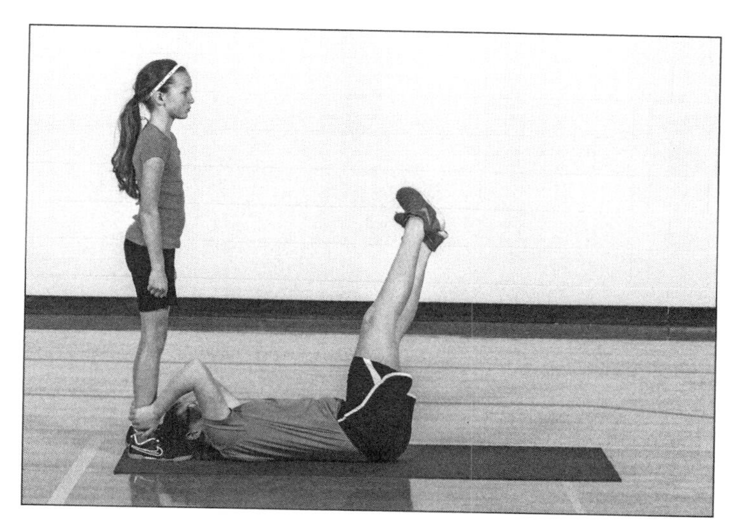

Medicine Ball Chest Pass Relay

Areas worked: arms, legs, core, and acceleration

1. Two or more teams line up facing their captain.
2. The captain passes the ball to the first player, who passes it back to the captain and runs to the back of the line.
3. The captain then passes the ball to the next player in line, who passes it back and goes to the end of the line, and sits down.
4. The team that finishes first because all the players have received the chest pass and sat down is the winner.

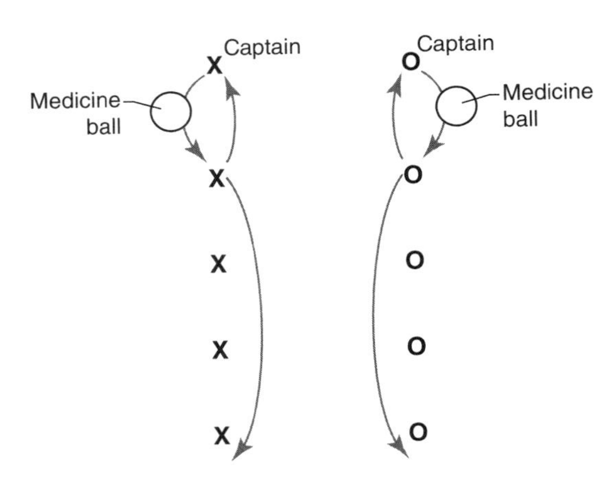

Over–Under Bridge Relay

Areas worked: knee extensors, abdominals, and trunk extensors

1. Teams line up and pass the medicine ball alternately over the head and between the legs.
2. The last player in line runs quickly with the ball to the front of the line and starts the sequence again.
3. When the last player of the team has taken the ball and ran to the start of the line and sat down, the game is over.

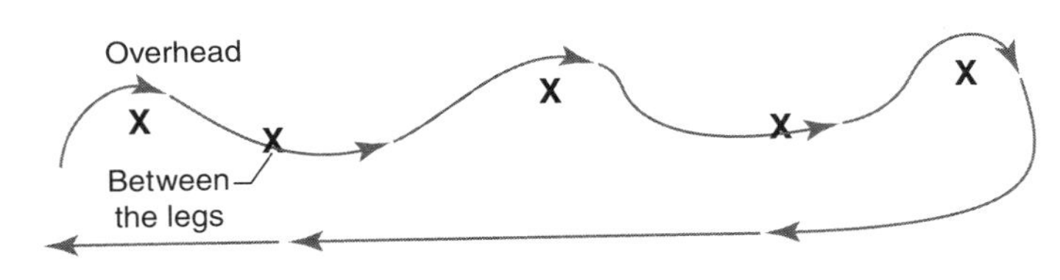

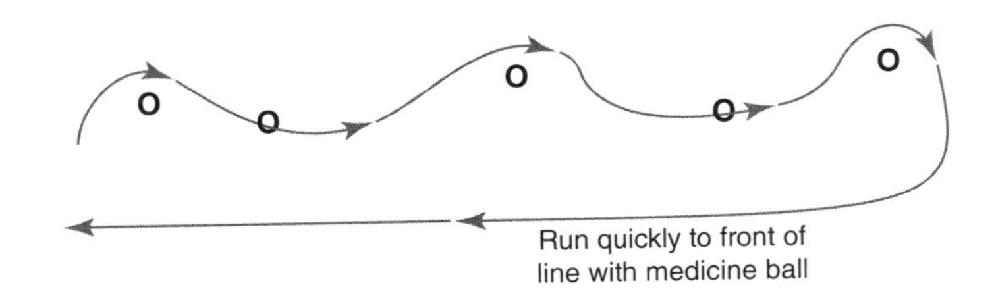

Medicine Ball Roll Under the Bridge

Areas worked: shoulders and legs

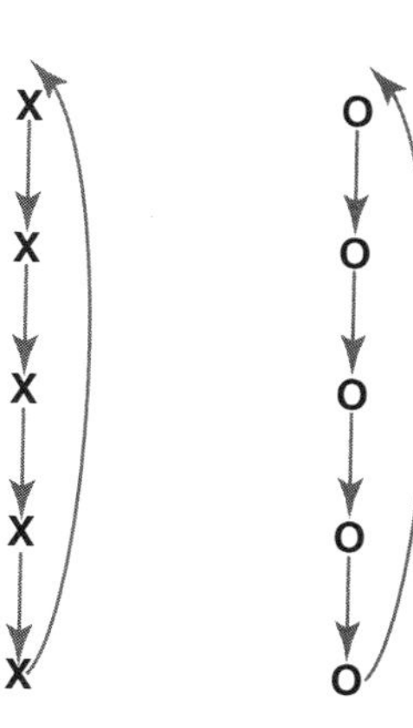

1. Teams stand in line with the feet apart. The first player in line rolls the ball between the legs to the last player in line.
2. The last player catches the ball and runs quickly to the front of the line to continue the task.
3. The team that finishes first, by having every player catch the ball and run to the head of the line, wins.

Obstacle Run Relay

Areas worked: balance, leg power (sprinting)

1. Create an obstacle course from available equipment and objects.
2. Mark the course so that each player has to perform the same tasks.
3. Time each athlete's performance to monitor individual improvement.

Variation

Hold a competition by creating equal teams and calculating each team's total time.

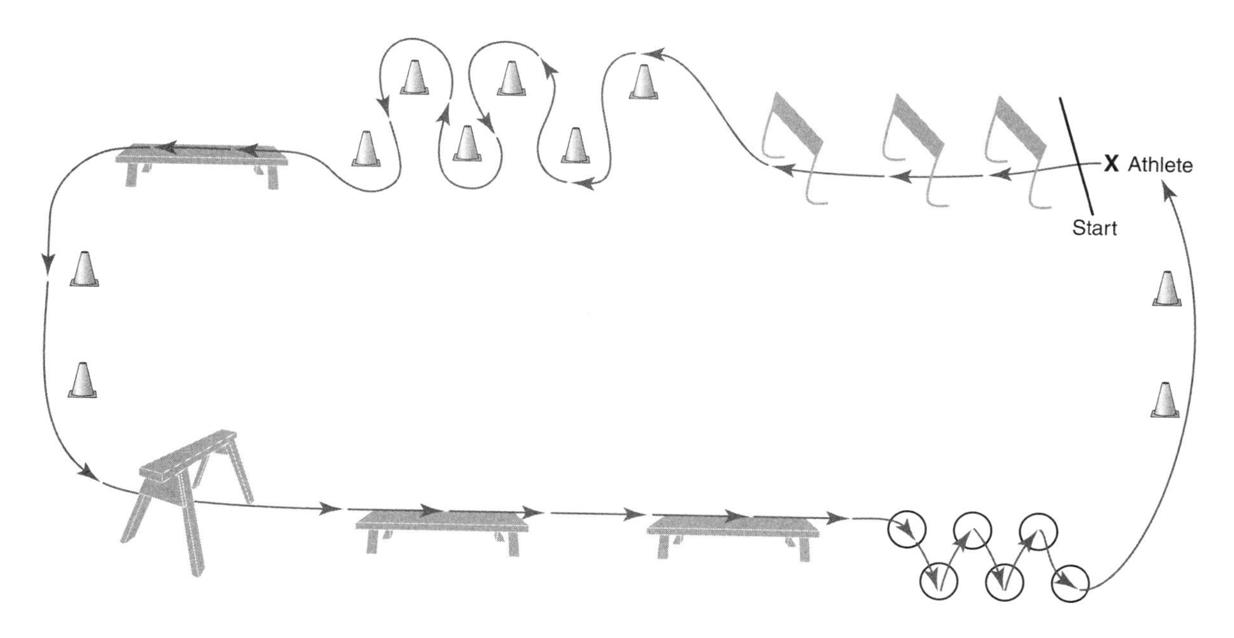

Exercises for Early Postpuberty

Most of the suggested exercises in this section don't require a lot of equipment and therefore can be performed at home or in a health club.

Push-Up Progression

Areas worked: shoulder and elbow extensors (triceps and trapezius)

1. Perform push-ups against a wall (stand with the feet away from the wall and push vigorously against the wall to bring the body to vertical).
2. Perform incline push-ups with the palms supported on a chair or box.
3. Perform push-ups on the ground (knees). Start with a push-up on the knees if regular push-ups are too difficult and progress to regular push-ups. Athletes may also choose to start a set with regular push-ups until they can no longer perform the exercise properly and then drop to the knees and complete a few more repetitions to total fatigue.
4. Perform regular push-ups (figures *a* and *b*).
5. Perform clap push-ups.
6. Perform incline push-ups with the feet on a chair or box and hands on the ground (figure *c*).
7. Perform clap push-ups from the same position as in 6.

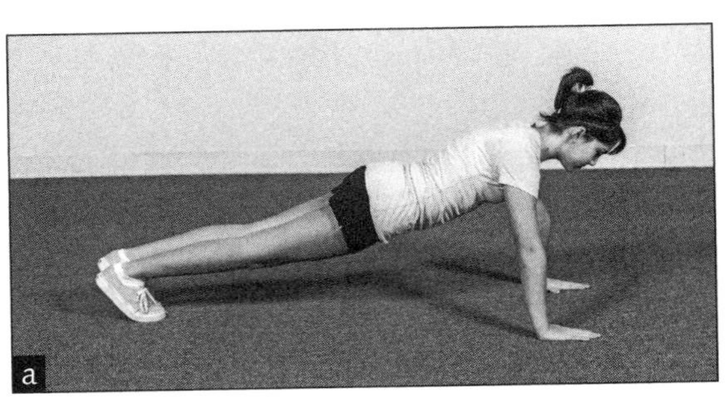
a

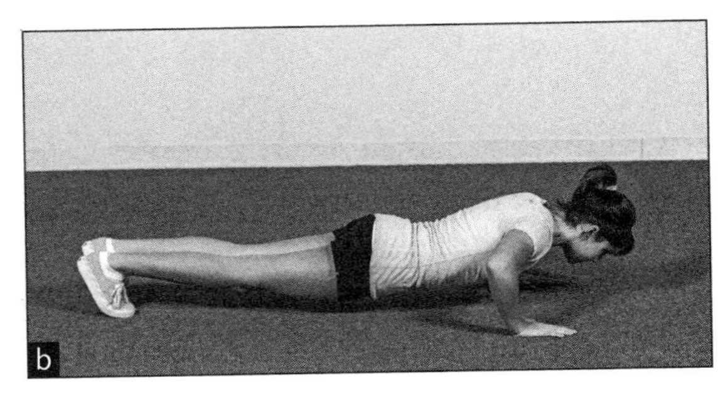
b

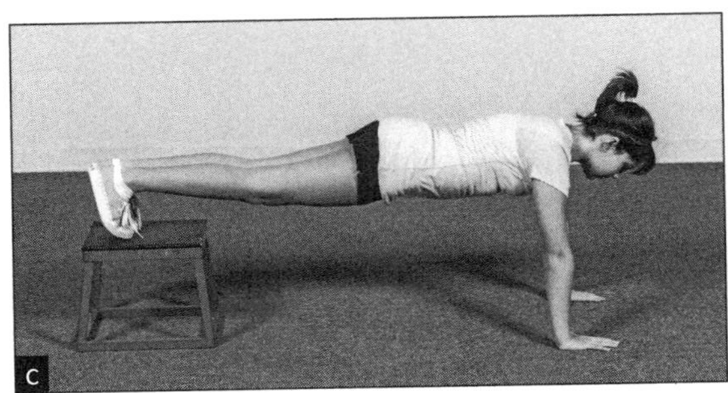
c

Dumbbell or Barbell Chest Press

Areas worked: elbow extensors (triceps), shoulders, and chest

1. Lying on the back, grasp the dumbbells, barbell, or chest press machine. Bend the knees and place them on a bench so your feet are on the bench, or place the feet on the floor. If feet are on the floor, make sure not to hyperextend the back.
2. Press the weight or handle up.
3. Slowly lower the weight or handle to the starting position.

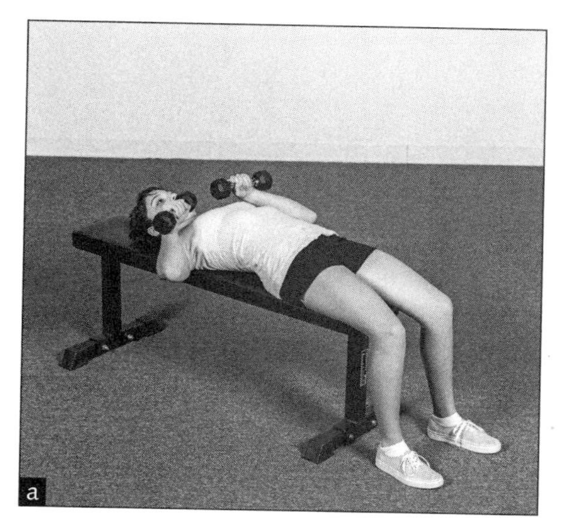

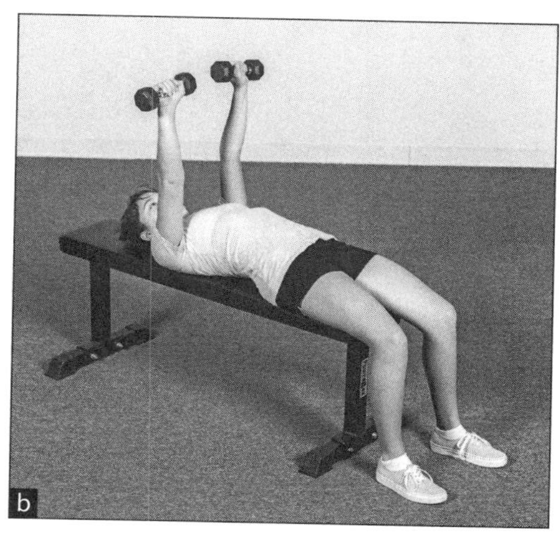

Cable Triceps Extension

Area worked: elbow extensors (triceps)

1. Stand facing the cable triceps bar with feet apart. Grasp the bar with the palms down, elbows bent, and hands at chest height.
2. Press the handle down to hip height.
3. Slowly return to the starting position.

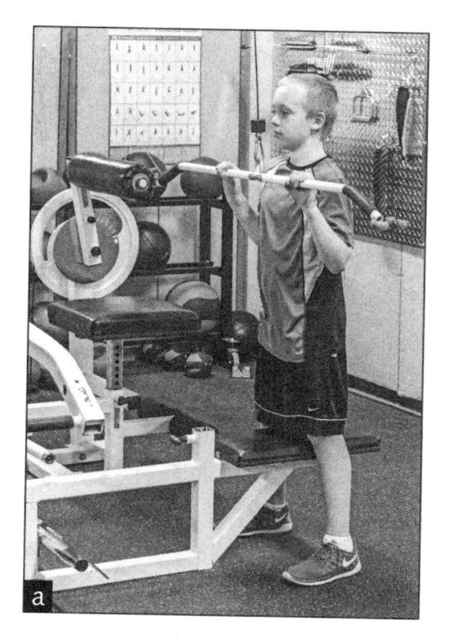

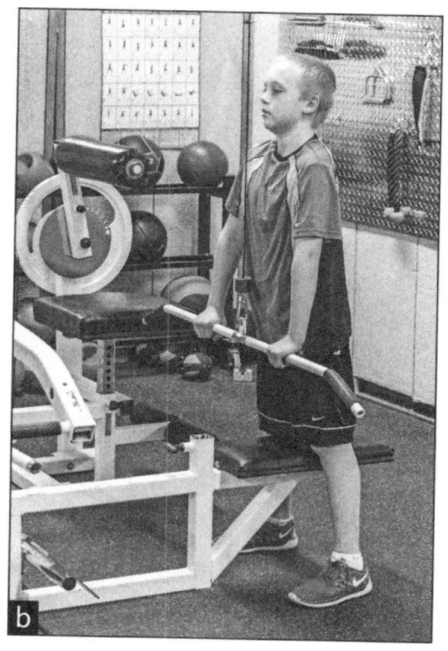

Dumbbell or Machine Shoulder Press

Areas worked: shoulder and elbow extensors (trapezius and triceps)

1. If using a machine, sit with the hands placed on the handle, palms up. If using dumbbells, hold the dumbbells at ear level, palms facing forward.
2. If using a machine, press the handle up vertically; do not lock the elbows. If using dumbbells, press the dumbbells up and slightly in so that they meet at the top of the movement. Imagine a triangle, with the base of the triangle at shoulder level and the apex at the top of the head.
3. Return slowly to the starting position.

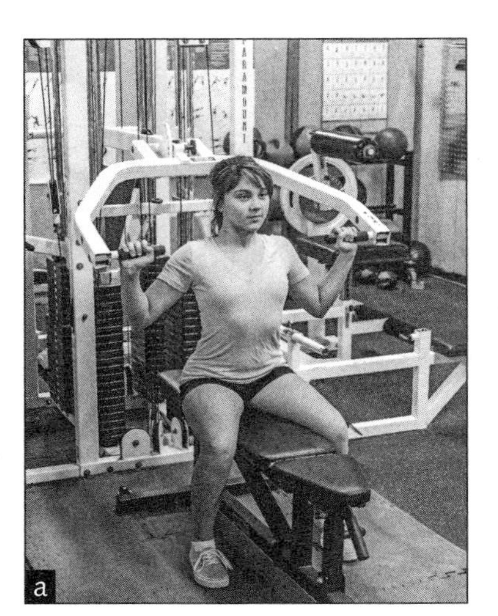
a

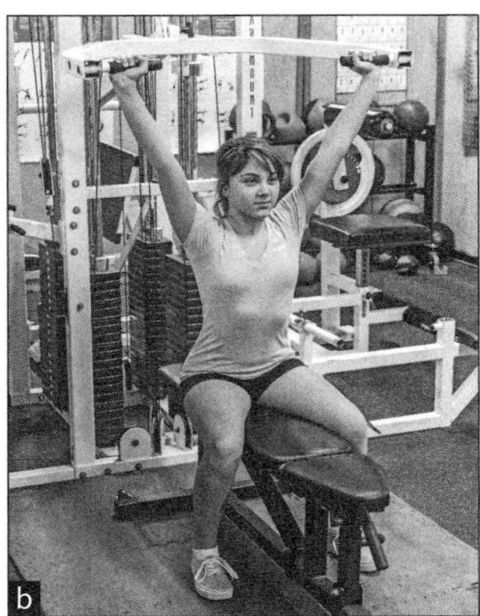
b

Lat Pull-Down

Areas worked: arm flexors and latissimus dorsi

1. Sit facing the lat pulldown machine. Grasp the handle with both hands.
2. Lean back slightly and pull the handle down to chest level.
3. Return to the starting position.

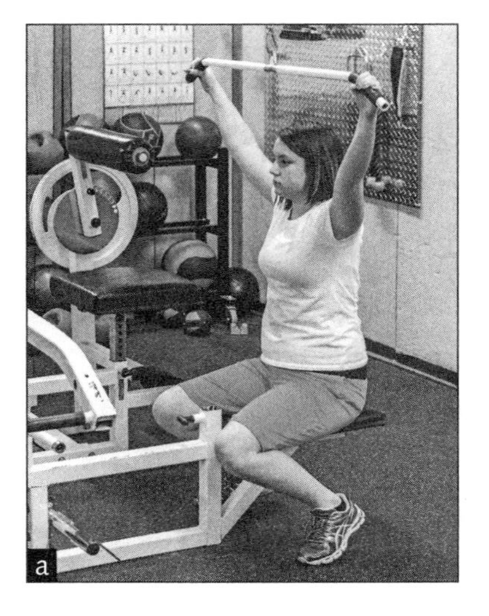
a

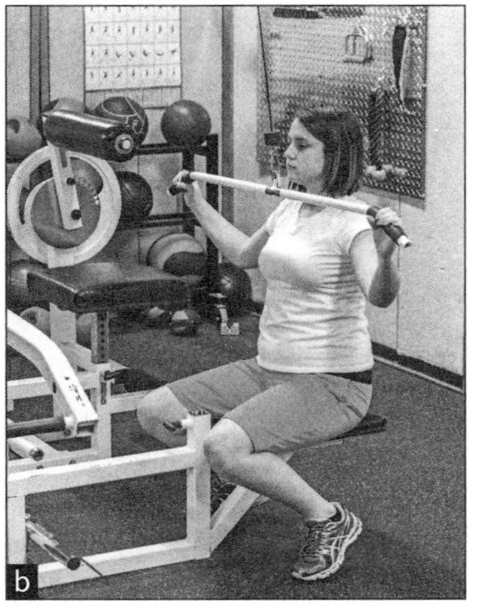
b

Dumbbell Preacher Curl

Area worked: elbow flexors (mostly biceps)

1. Sit with the arms extended and the elbows resting on the preacher curl pad. Hold a dumbbell in each hand with the palms facing up. The pad should be at chest level, and the body should stay close to the pad during the movement. You can also use a preacher curl machine.
2. Bend the elbows to bring the dumbbells or handle to chest level.
3. Return to the starting position.

V-Sit

Areas worked: abdominal and hip flexor muscles

1. Lie on the floor with the arms extended over the head.
2. Bring the arms and legs up into a V-sit position.
3. Return to the starting position.

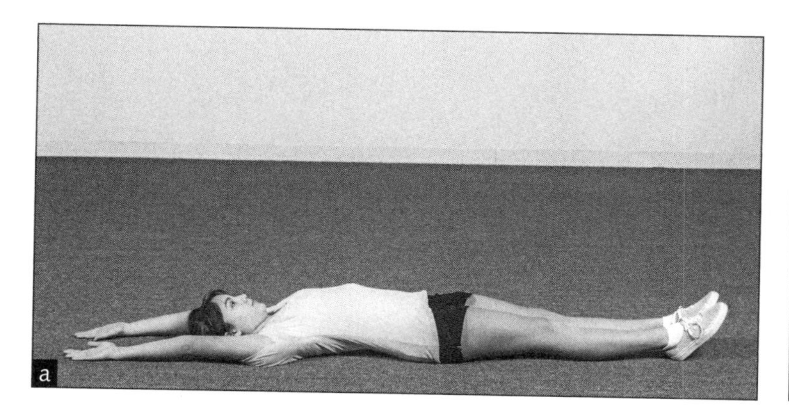
a

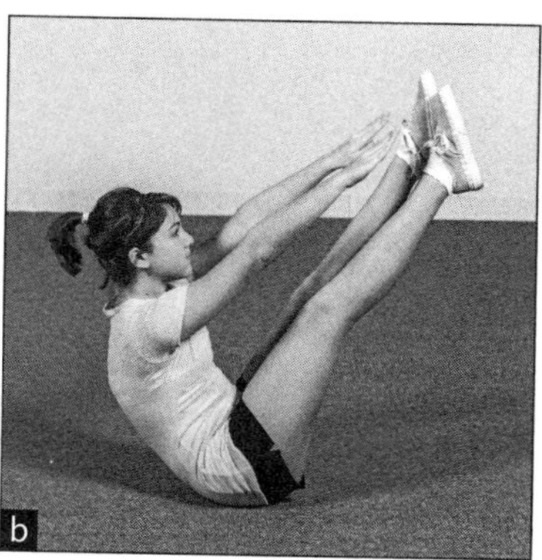
b

Abdominal Rainbow

Areas worked: oblique abdominals and hip muscles

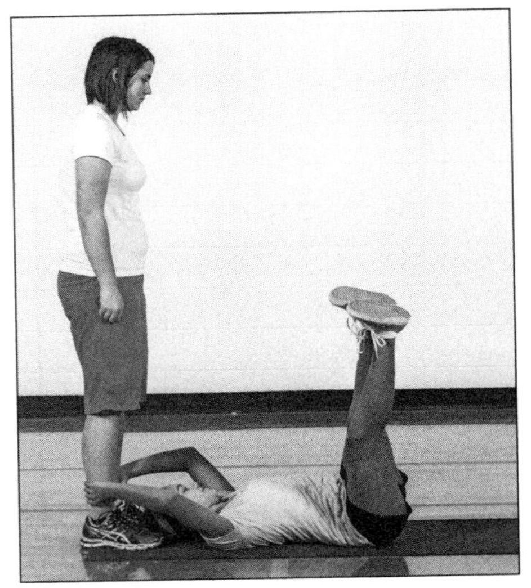

1. Lie with the head near the lowest rung of a stall bar. Grip the bar with the hand.
2. Lift the legs up and lower them to the right side. Lift them on the other side. Lift them again and lower them to the other side.
3. Rest the legs on the floor.

Variation

Instead of a bar, place the hands around the ankles of a partner to help stabilize the body, or simply place the arms out to the sides on the floor, creating a "T" shape. The arms should not leave the ground during the rotation.

Leg Press

Area worked: knee extensors (quadriceps)

1. Sit on a leg press chair and place the balls of the feet on the upper plate of the machine.
2. Press the feet into the plate, fully extending the legs.
3. Return to the starting position. Avoid bringing the knees into chest—stop the legs when they reach a 90-degree angle.

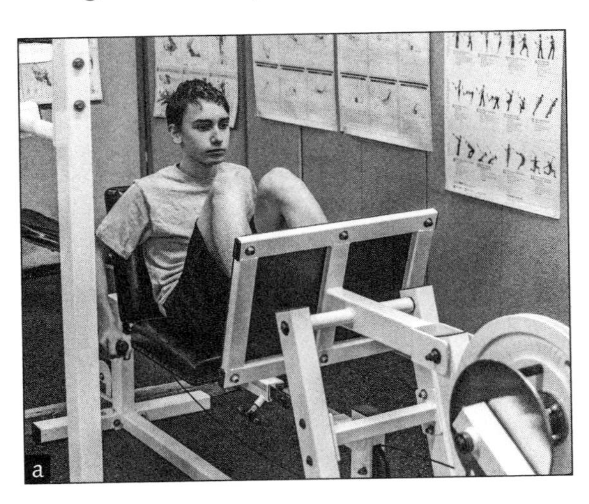

a

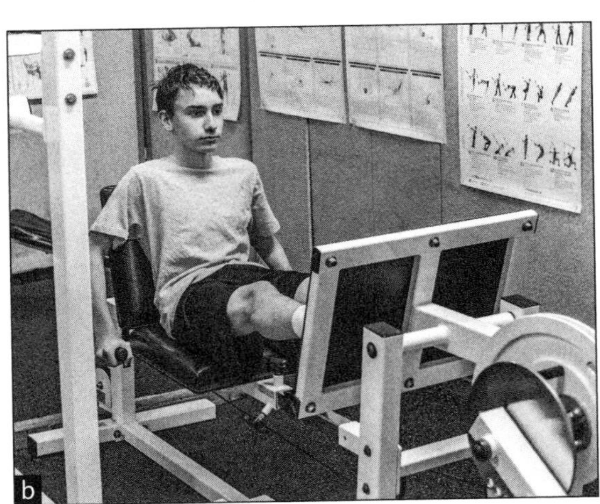

b

Leg Curl

Area worked: knee extensors (hamstrings)

1. Lying on the stomach, place the heels under the top padded roller of the hamstring machine and extend the knees.
2. Bend the knees, bringing the pad as close to the buttocks as possible.
3. Return to the starting position.

Variation

Perform this movement on a seated or standing leg curl machine.

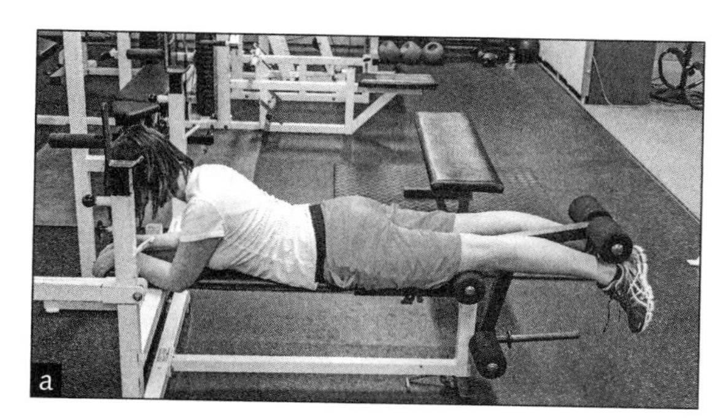

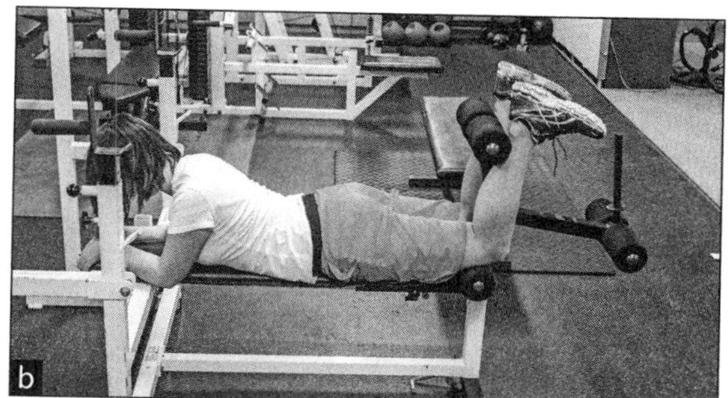

Barbell Half Squat

Areas worked: knee and hip extensors

1. Using a squat rack, place the shoulders squarely under the barbell and grasp the bar with the hands. Stand with the feet shoulder-width apart and knees bent, and hold the back straight.
2. Bend the knees and extend the hips back until the upper legs are parallel to the floor.
3. Return to the starting position.

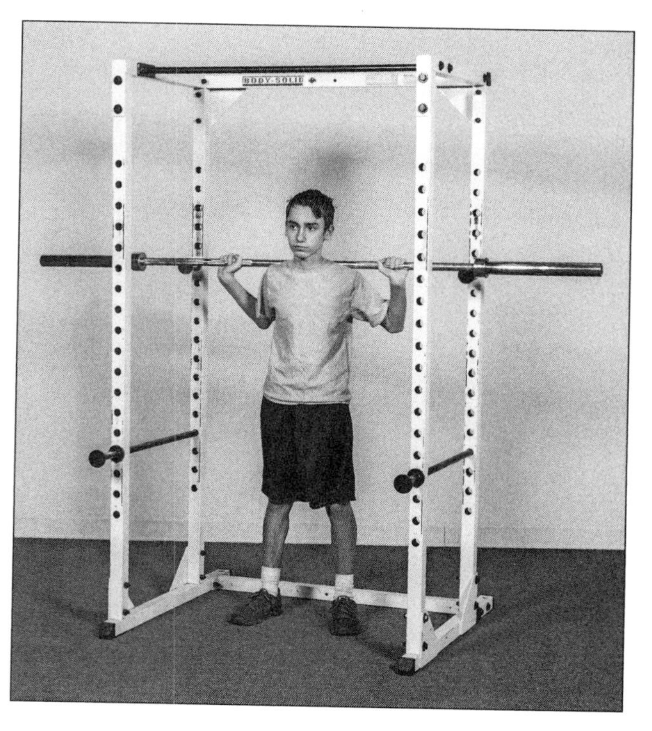

Variation

Perform this movement using a standardized weighted bar or dumbbells.

Slalom Jump

Areas worked: calf and knee extensors

1. Begin in a standing position.
2. Make continuous diagonal jumps on two feet, progressing forward in a slalom pattern.

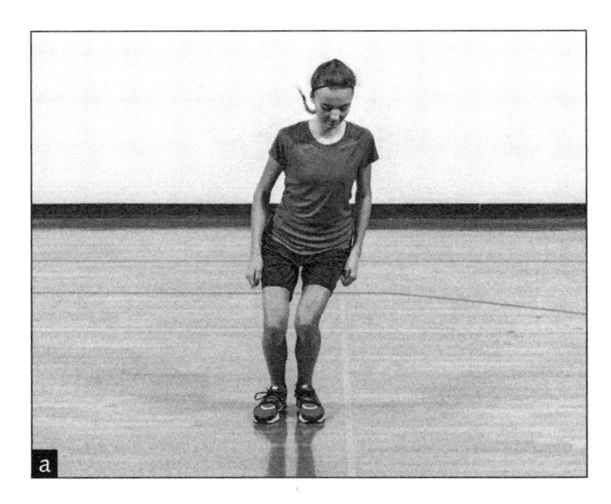
a

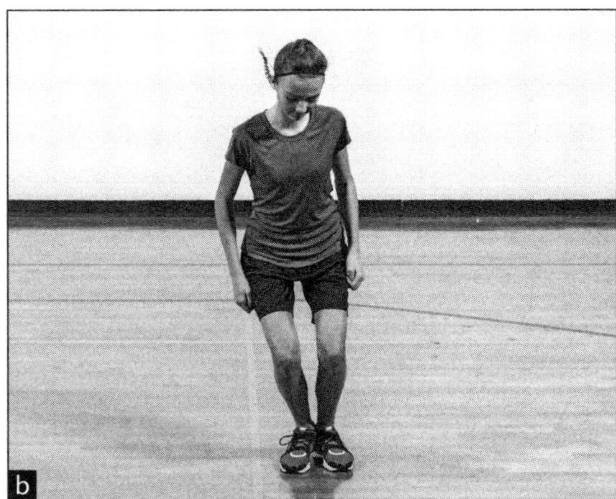
b

Scissors Splits

Areas worked: calf and knee extensors

1. Stand with one leg forward and the other leg behind.
2. Take off for a vertical jump and quickly switch the position of the legs in midair. Land and immediately jump, again switching the position of the legs in midair.
3. Perform continuous jumps.

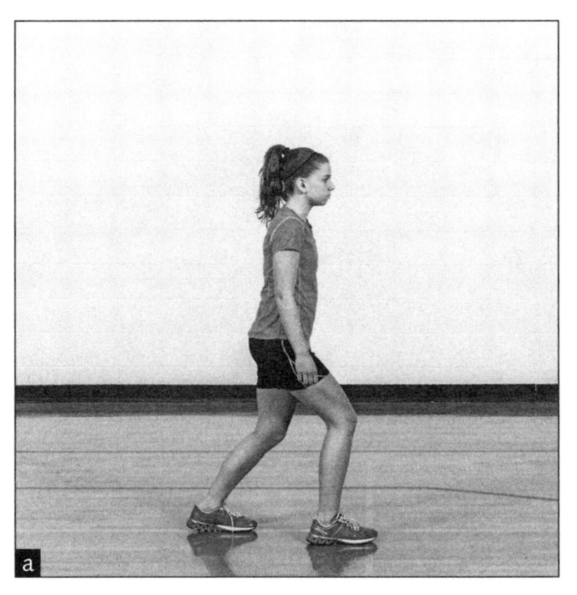
a

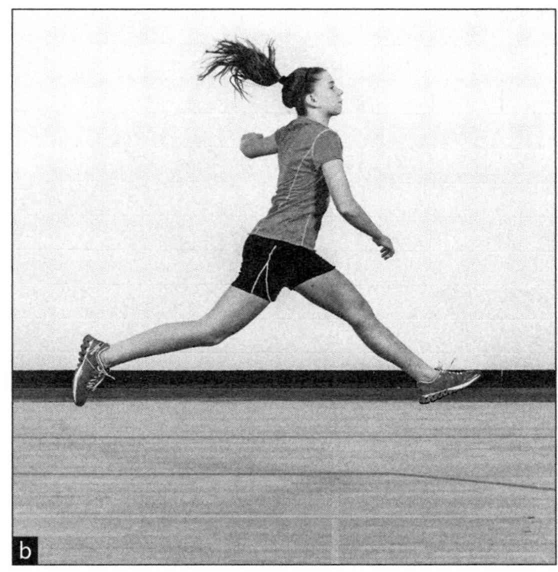
b

Vertical Hop

Areas worked: calf and knee extensors

1. Begin in a standing position.
2. Swing the arms upward and actively press the feet against the ground for a vertical spring.
3. Land, absorbing the shock, by bending the knees, tightening the core, and lowering the arms to hip level.
4. Repeat.

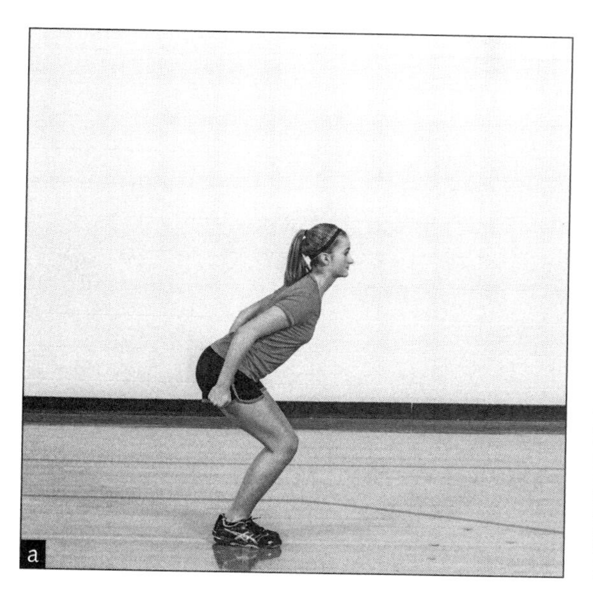

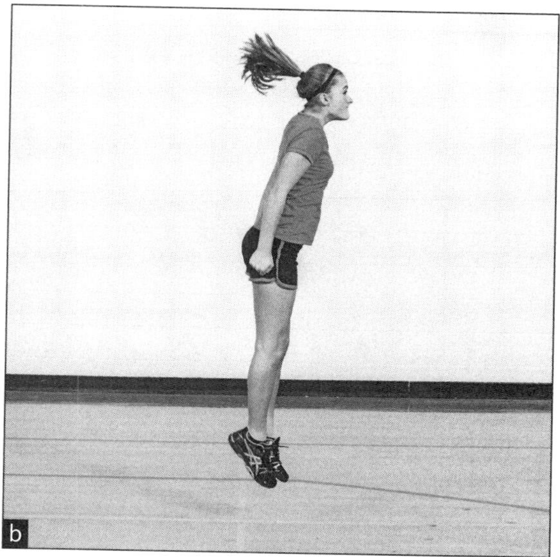

Cone Jump

Areas worked: calf, knee, and hip extensors

1. Begin standing in front of a row of 7 to 10 cones placed 2 meters or yards apart.
2. Run down the row, jumping over each cone.
3. Return to the starting line.

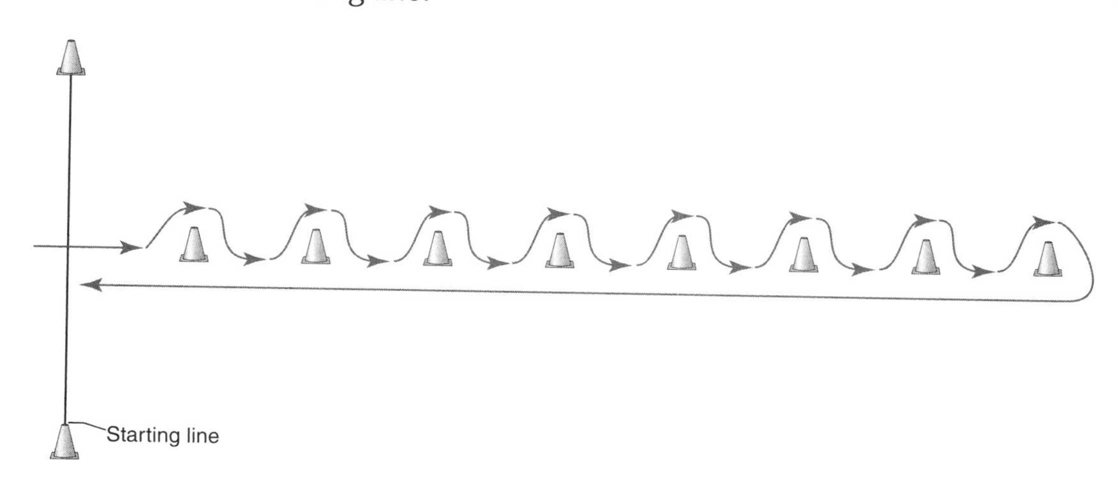

Continuous Squat Jump

Areas worked: calf, knee, and hip extensors

1. Stand with the feet apart and the hands placed behind the head.
2. Use explosive upward-forward movements, attempting to jump up as high as possible and upon landing explode upward again. Land on the toes, lower the heels, and slightly bend the knees to absorb the shock.
3. Repeat the movement.

Baseball or Tennis Ball Throw for Accuracy

Area worked: shoulders

1. Two teams stand 10 to 15 meters or yards apart on two lines. Both teams stand side-by-side facing the target that is placed 5 to 10 yards from the teams. In the middle of the gym or field place two balls, bowling pins, or upside-down cones which act as targets and that fall easily when hit by a ball.
2. Each team is given 3 to 4 tennis or baseballs for throwing. The first player throws at the target and then moves to the back of the line. An instructor or helper can stand beyond the target collecting the balls and resetting the target in place if successfully knocked over.
3. Each team or individual scores points for knocking over the cones.

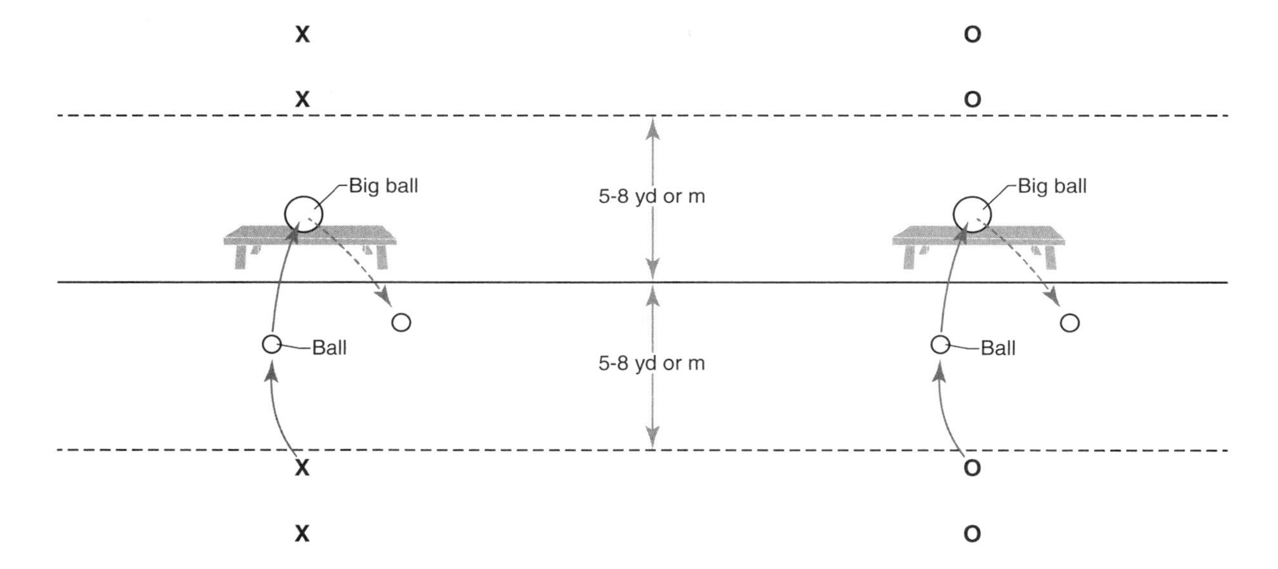

Exercises for Late Postpuberty

The training program and exercises for late postpuberty are closer to the programs for high performance than to those for early postpuberty. The exercises in this section are the most sport specific. In addition to the following exercises, use some exercises from early postpuberty, such as the chest press, cable triceps extension, shoulder press, lat pull-down, and dumbbell preacher curl.

Assisted Pull-Up

Areas worked: elbow flexors, chest, and lats

1. Grasp the handles of the bar with the feet resting on a bench or low box.
2. Pull the body up by flexing the arms.
3. Extend the arms to return to the starting position.

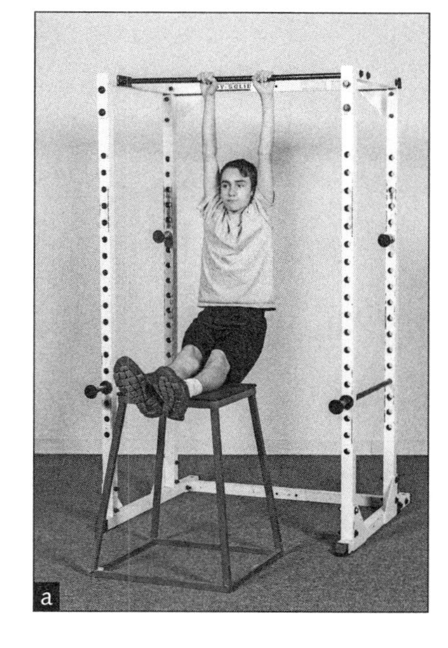

a

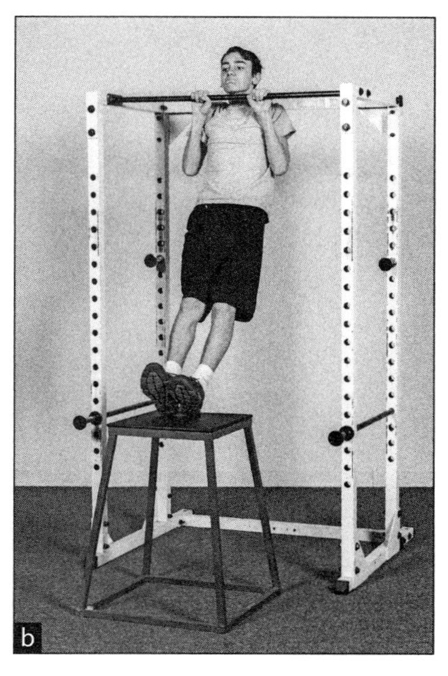

b

Pull-Up

Areas worked: elbow flexors, chest, and lats

1. Grasp the handles or bar with the palms facing inward, arms extended and body hanging.
2. Pull the body up by flexing the arms.
3. Extend the arms to return to the starting position.

Variation

Grasp the handles or bar with the palms facing away from the body or the palms facing the body—also called a reverse pull-up.

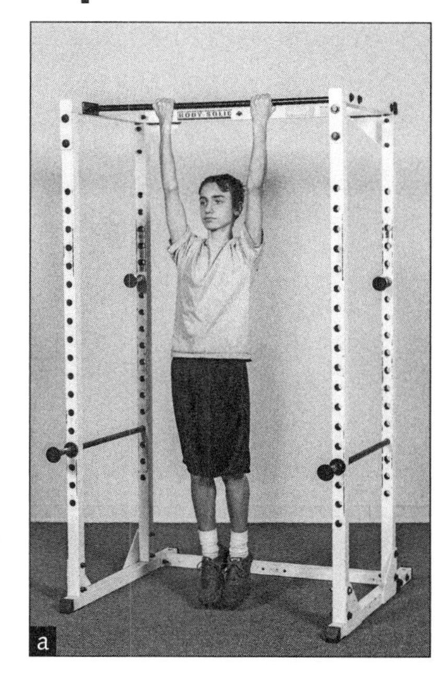

a

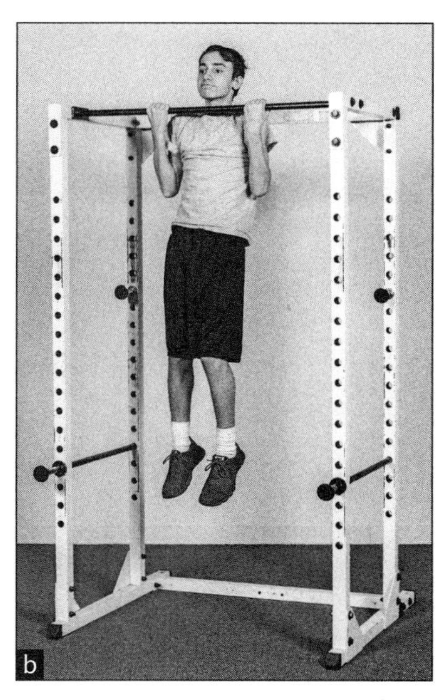

b

Caterpillar Push-Up

Areas worked: hands, elbow extensors, shoulders, and back muscles

1. Bend the hips. Place the feet on the floor, legs extended. Place the hands on the floor at shoulder width.
2. Bend the elbows and lower the shoulders toward the floor. Drive forward, lifting the head and extending the arms straight.
3. Bring the feet close to the hands (as in the starting position) and repeat the movement.

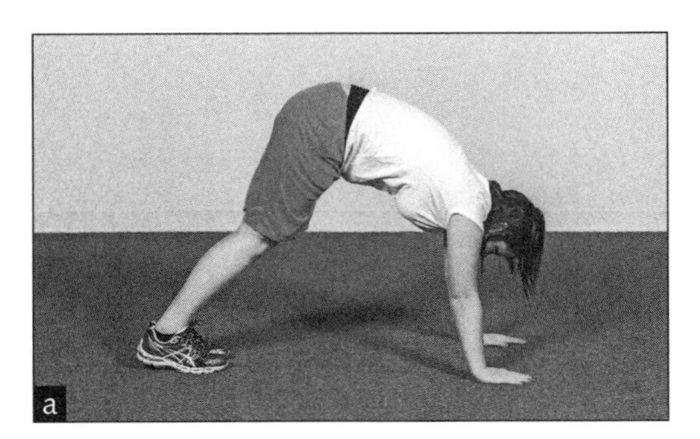
a

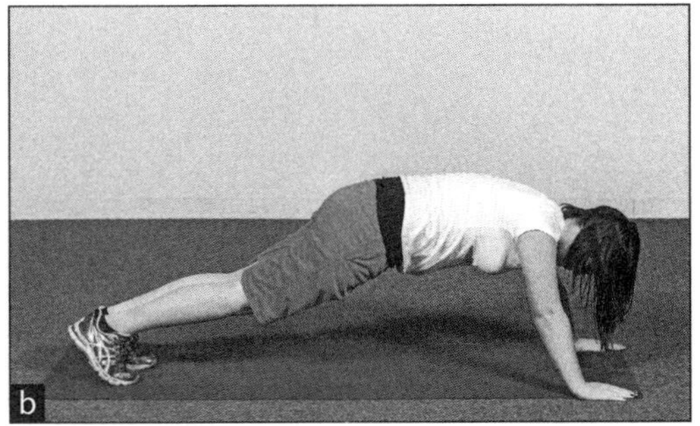
b

Dips

Areas worked: elbow extensors and chest

1. Grasp the handles of the dip machine with the palms facing in.
2. Bend the elbows and lower the chest toward the bar.
3. Return to the starting position.

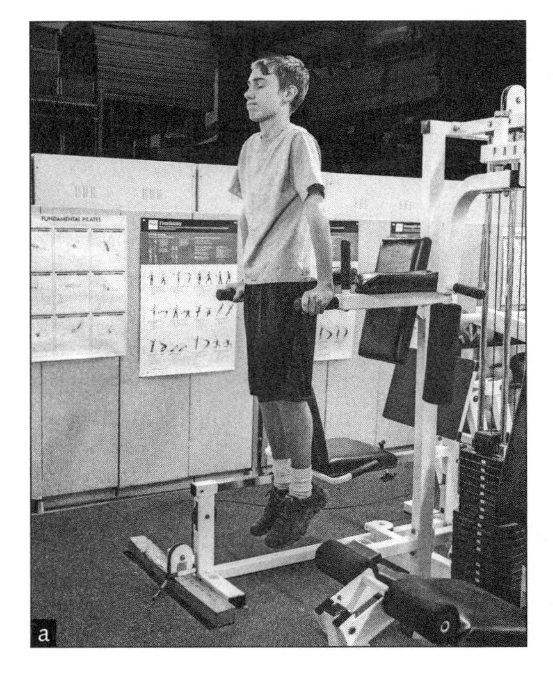
a

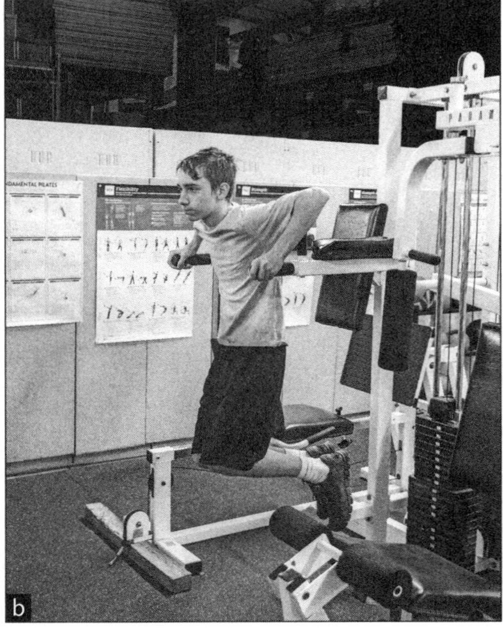
b

Wall Push-Up

Areas worked: elbow extensors, chest, and shoulders

1. Partner A stands about 3 feet (1 m) away from the wall. Partner B places the palms on partner A's upper back.
2. Partner B pushes partner A toward the wall. Partner A bends the elbows slightly to absorb the shock.
3. In a dynamic action, partner A immediately pushes against the wall to return to the starting position. The partners perform several push-ups without stopping.

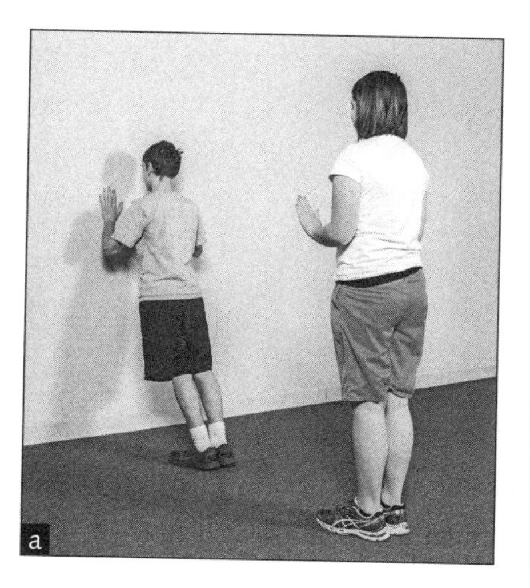

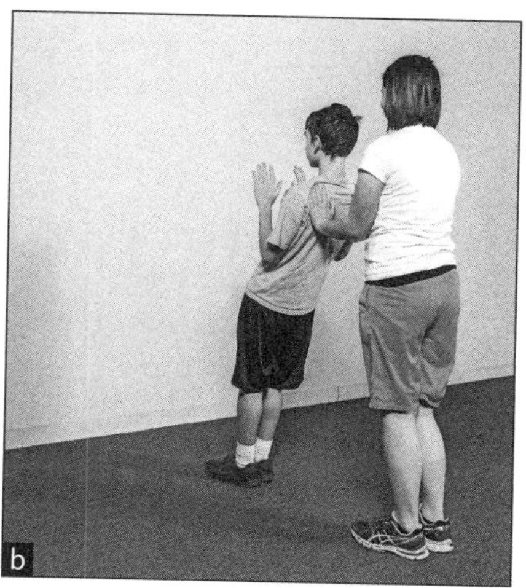

Drop Push-Up

Areas worked: arms flexors and extensors, chest, and back muscles

1. Kneel on the floor with the elbows bent 90 degrees.
2. Drop the body toward the floor in a free fall, keeping the elbows bent 90 degrees.
3. Perform a dynamic push-up to return to the starting position.

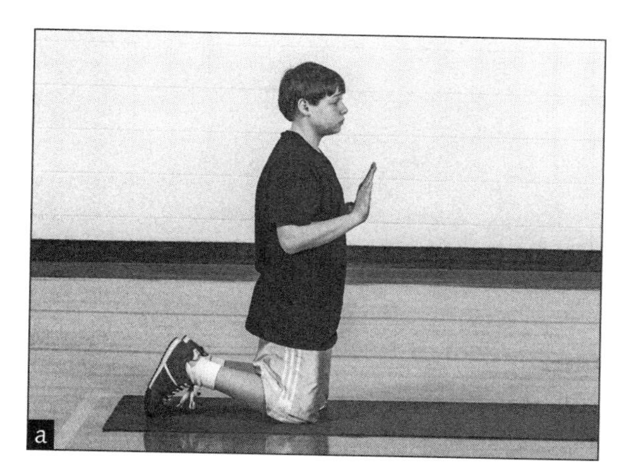

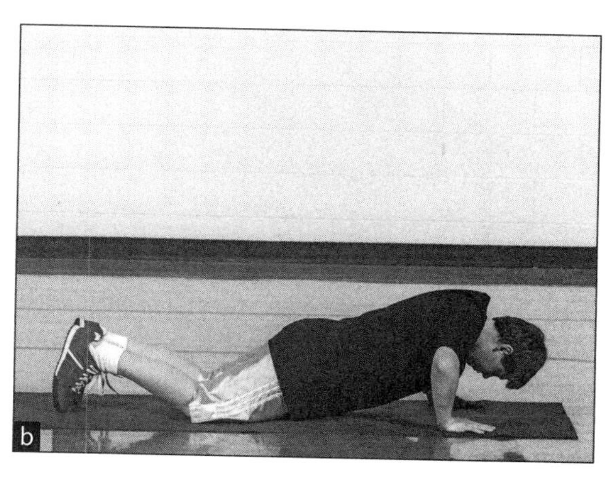

Dumbbell Squat to Press

Areas worked: legs, shoulders, and core muscles

1. Stand with the feet shoulder-width apart, holding a dumbbell in each hand at shoulder level.
2. Bend the knees until the thighs are parallel with the floor.
3. Pause, bring the hips forward to the starting position, and extend the dumbbells overhead.
4. Return the dumbbells to the starting position and repeat the entire movement, beginning with the squat.

Variation

Begin with the dumbbells to the side of the body and perform a squat followed by a biceps curl and a shoulder press, all in one movement. Return the dumbbells to the side of the body and repeat.

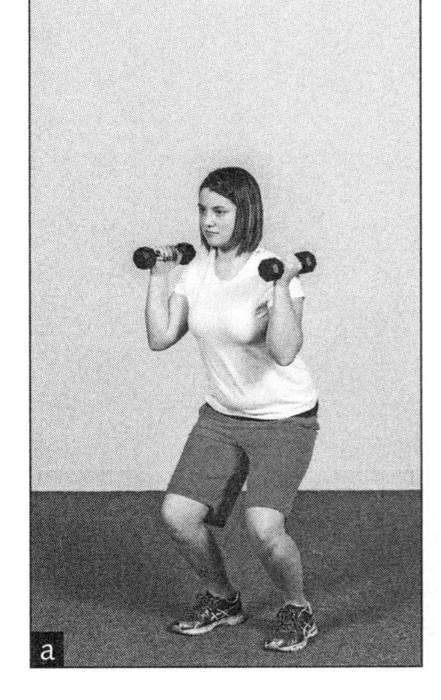
a

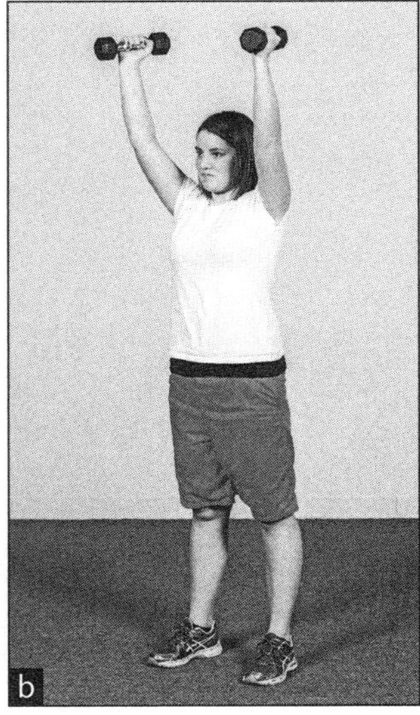
b

Abdominal Thrust

Areas worked: abdominals and obliques

1. Partner A lies on the back with the legs on the floor and holds partner B's ankles.
2. Partner A lifts the legs toward partner B's chest. Partner B pushes the legs down or to one side for a series of abdominal thrusts, creating high tension on the abdominal muscles.
3. Partner A lowers the legs to the starting position. Partners alternate roles.

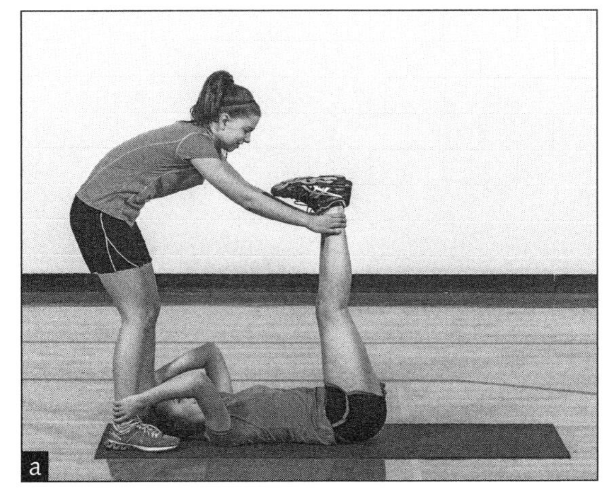
a

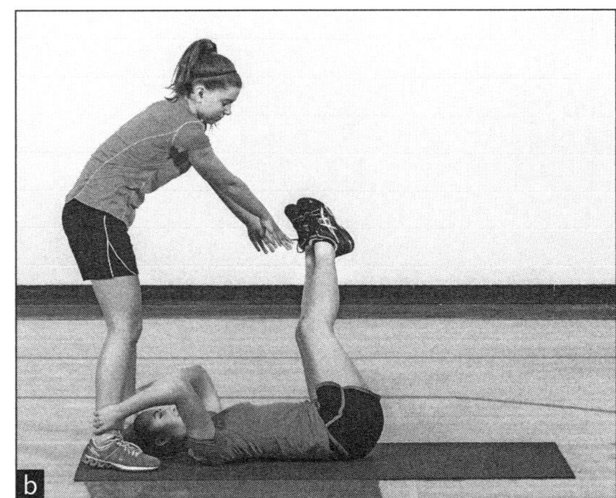
b

Push-Up Plank

Areas worked: arms, abdominals, and lower back

1. Assume a push-up position, with the palms on the floor at shoulder level and the feet together.
2. Hold the position for as long as possible.
3. For more intensity, place a weighted plate or medicine ball on the upper back.

Variation

Perform a regular plank by lowering the upper body onto the elbows.

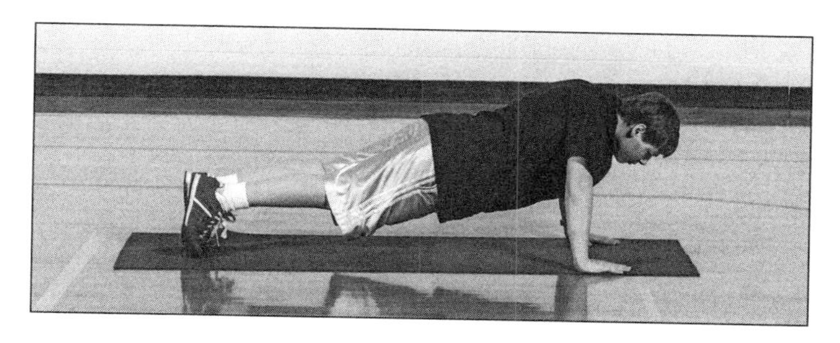

Medicine Ball Chops

Areas worked: abdominals, obliques, legs, and shoulders

1. Stand with the feet shoulder-width apart, holding the medicine ball at shoulder level.
2. Bring the medicine ball down toward the left knee by bending forward and transferring the body weight to left leg, lifting the right leg off the floor.
3. Transfer the weight to the right foot, lift the left foot off the floor, and drive the medicine ball up to the right shoulder.
4. Repeat for both sides of the body.

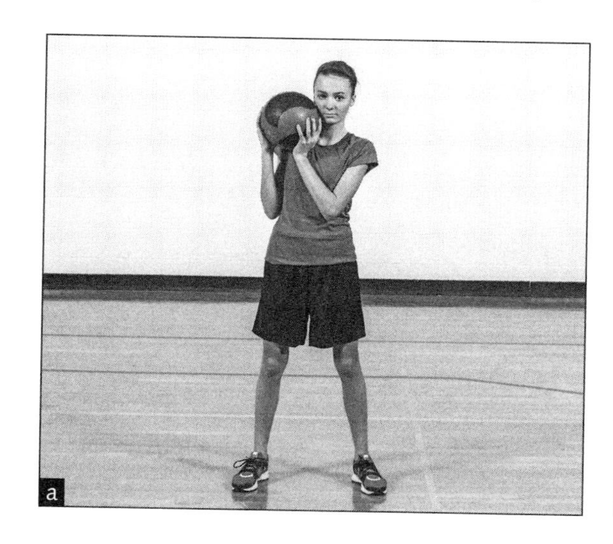
a

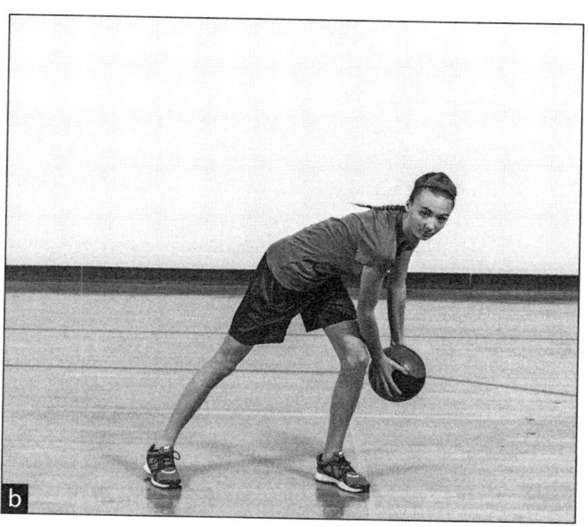
b

Medicine Ball Double-Leg Forward Toss

Areas worked: leg extensors and abdominal muscles

1. Two partners stand facing each other 10 feet (3 m) apart. Partner A grasps a medicine ball between the feet and toes (the toes are slightly under the ball).
2. Partner A performs a two-foot take-off. When approaching the highest point of the jump, partner A slightly arches the hips, brings the feet backward, forcefully contracts the abdominal muscles, brings the legs forward, and releases the ball toward partner B's chest.
3. Partner B catches the ball and performs the same action.

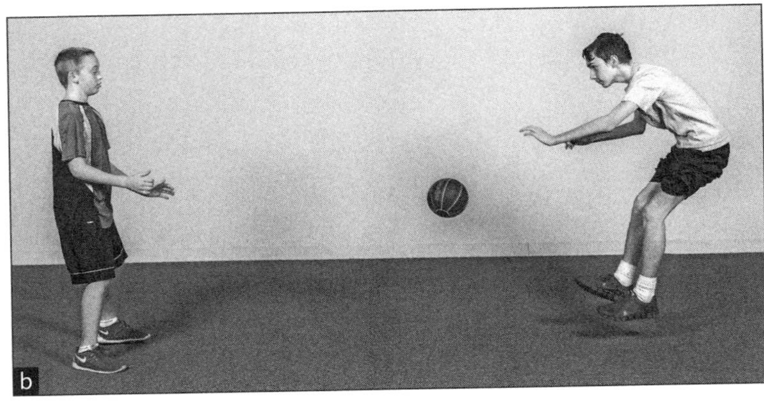

Superman

1. Lie on the stomach with the arms extended forward.
2. Simultaneously raise the upper body and lower body as high as possible.

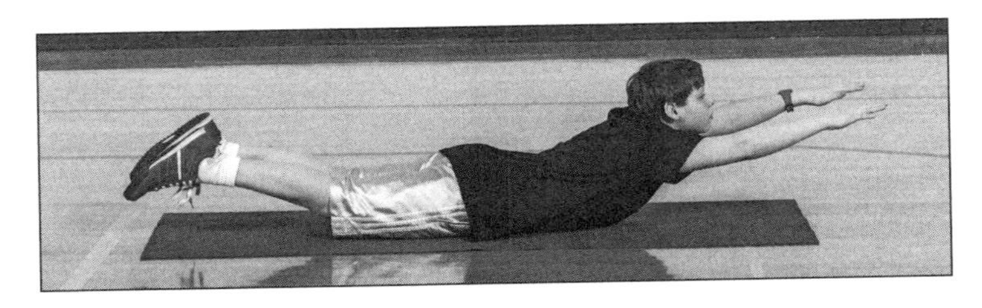

Reverse Hyperextension

Areas worked: back and hip extensors

1. Lie on the stomach, hips resting on a pad of the machine and arms holding the machine handle.
2. Thrust the legs upward.
3. Lower the legs to the starting position and repeat.

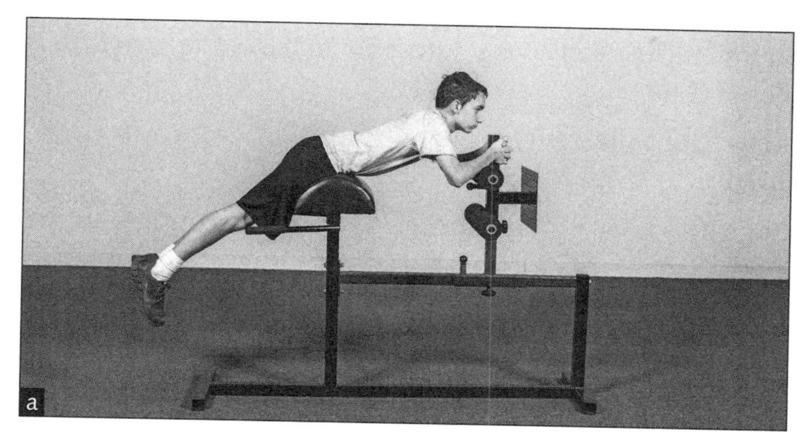

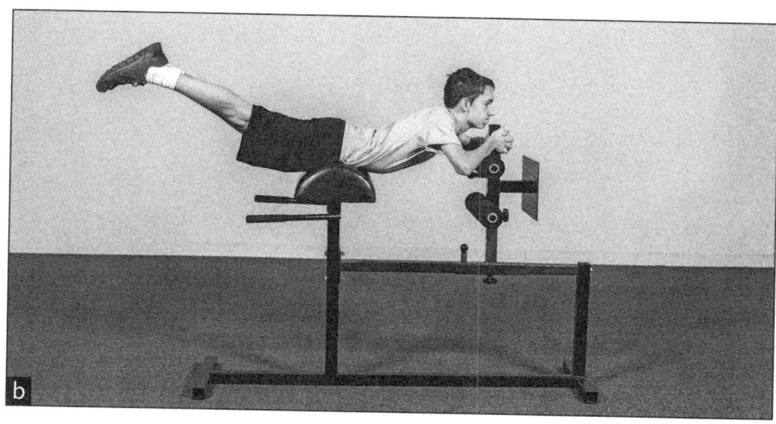

The following exercises focus mostly on leg power, which is often not well represented in athletic training. For leg strength, the instructor can also use exercises suggested for early postpuberty.

Knee-Tuck Jump

Areas worked: calves, knees, and hip extensors

1. Begin in a standing position.
2. Swing the arms upward and actively press the feet against the ground for a vertical tuck jump. Perform a tuck jump by jumping high and tucking your knees into your chest.
3. Land on the toes of both feet and lower the arms. Immediately drive the arms up and spring upward again.
4. Land by flexing the knees to absorb the shock and stop the jumps.

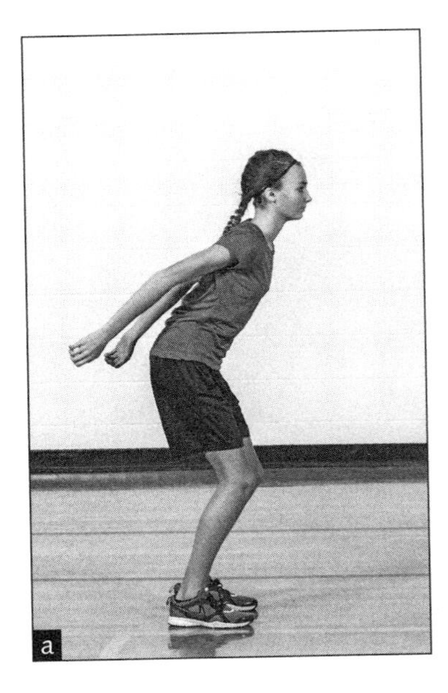
a

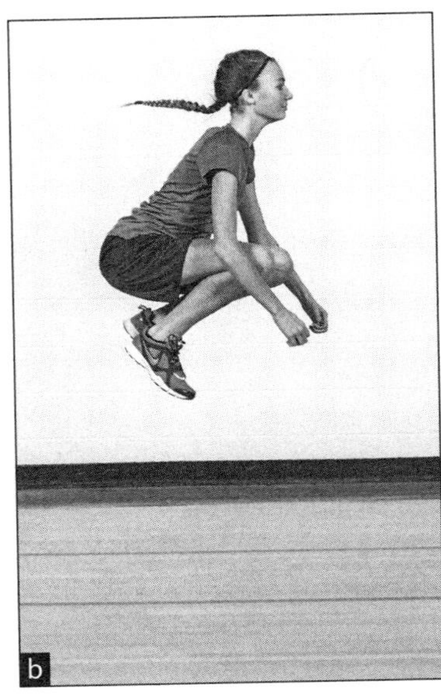
b

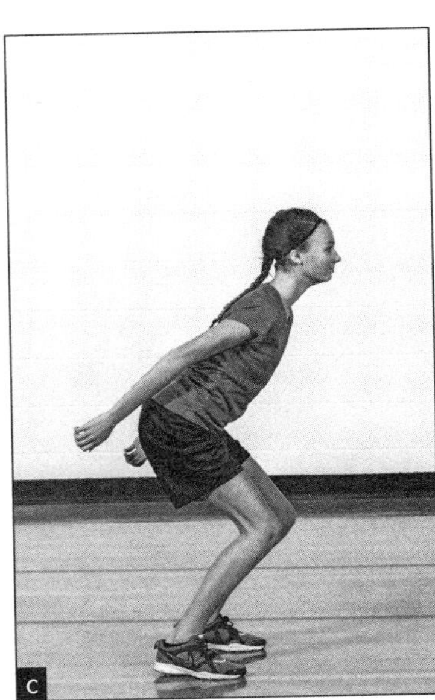
c

Back Kick

Areas worked: calves, knees, and hip extensors

1. Begin in a standing position.
2. Jump up vertically, bringing the heels to the buttocks.
3. Land on the toes to absorb the shock and then either continue or stop the jumps.

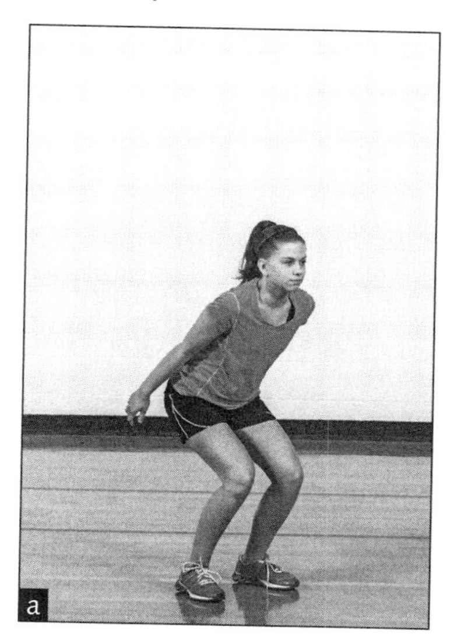
a

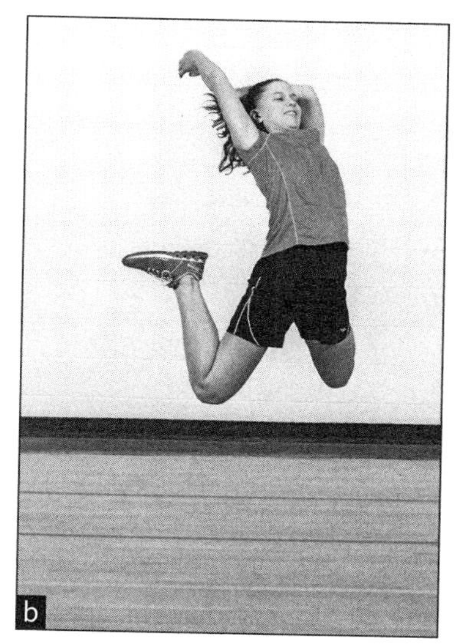
b

Forward Roll and Vertical Jump

Areas worked: calves, knees, hip extensors, shoulders, and arms

1. Begin in a low crouch position with the hands flexed at knee level.
2. Tuck the head under and roll over to a half-squat position. When the feet contact the floor, actively extend the legs to perform a vertical jump.
3. Land and repeat.

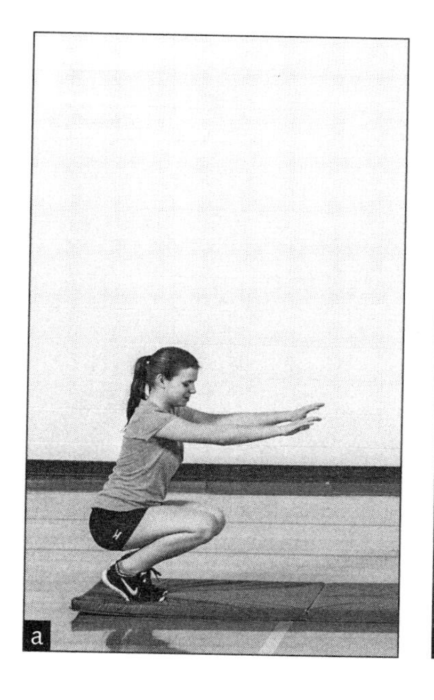
a

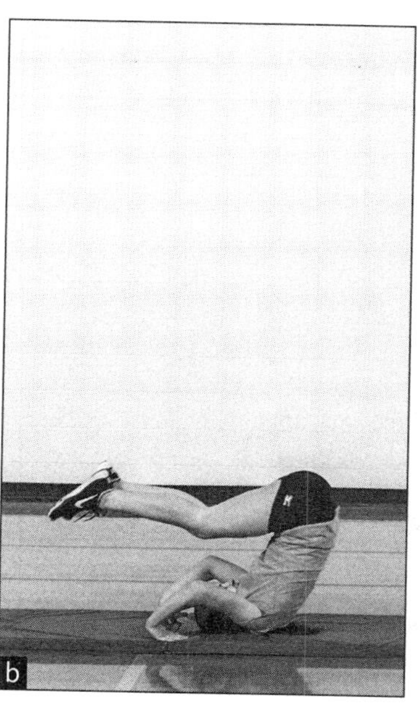
b

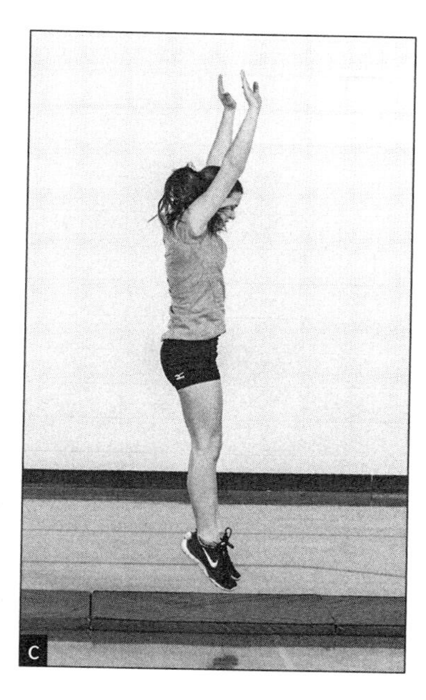
c

Dumbbell Side Swing

Area worked: core, shoulders and legs

1. Clasp the fingers of both hands around the long bar of the dumbbell.
2. Stand with feet shoulder-width apart, knees slightly bent, and dumbbell rested on the right side of the body at hips with your upper body slightly bent forward.
3. With arms extended (but not overextended at the elbow), swing the dumbbell up toward the left shoulder and slightly twist the body to the left, contracting the core throughout the entire movement. Slowly lower the dumbbell back to starting position and repeat.
4. Perform movement on both sides of the body. When starting with the dumbbell on left side of the body at hip level, swing the dumbbell upward toward the right shoulder.
5. Perform 12 to 15 repetitions per side with proper technique.

Medicine Ball Speed Throw

Areas worked: shoulders and elbow extensors and back muscles

1. Organize two rows of players. Partners (one from each row) stand facing each other 15 feet (4.5 m) apart. Each player in one row has a medicine ball.
2. Partners throw the ball back and forth using a technique determined by the coach. The aim is to perform the most throws in 30 (or 60, 90, or 120) seconds.

Note: For forward and backward throws between the legs, increase the distance to 35 to 40 feet (10-12 m).

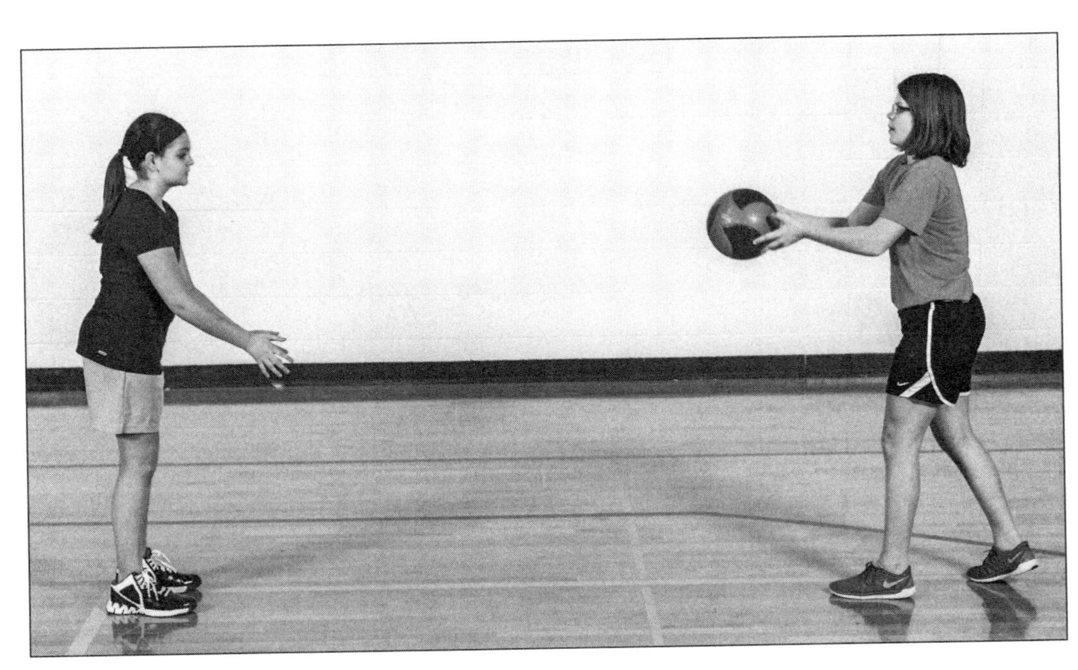

chapter 8

Endurance Training

The ability to sustain physical activity for long periods of time, often called endurance, is important for sports in which activity lasts longer than one minute. Endurance is not simply an ability of long-distance runners, swimmers, rowers, or cross-country skiers. A good endurance background is necessary for most athletes. Endurance helps athletes in any sport withstand the strain of training and competition. Furthermore, an athlete with a good endurance base will cope with the fatigue of training, schoolwork, and an active lifestyle more easily than an athlete without such a foundation.

For most athletes, fatigue is public enemy number one! Athletes who cannot effectively cope with fatigue have a high probability of performing poorly and losing the game, race, or match. Fatigue also affects the ability to concentrate on the task at hand, resulting in technical and tactical mistakes and inaccuracies in throwing or shooting. This explains why more mistakes are visible toward the end of a game or match. An athlete who wants to improve her game must develop her endurance capability.

Two types of endurance exist. In aerobic endurance, the athlete always performs the activity in the presence of oxygen. In anaerobic endurance, the activity is fast, dynamic, and of short duration, so the heart does not have time to pump oxygen to the working muscles to produce energy. Anaerobic endurance is more specific to team sports, tennis, and martial arts, whereas aerobic endurance is more specific to sports of longer duration such as cycling, swimming, triathlon, distance running, and cross-country skiing. Most athletes need a good aerobic base before they focus on sport-specific anaerobic endurance.

Endurance training also has tangible benefits for health. Individuals involved in endurance activities have stronger hearts and lower heart rates and blood pressure. Research shows a dose–response relationship between the volume and intensity of endurance training and health benefits. Moderate levels of endurance training improve heart rate, blood pressure, and other heart health indices. Further increases in both the volume and intensity of endurance training provided little benefit (Iwasaki et al., 2003). Interestingly, inability to maintain an adequate level of endurance, especially during the off-season, results in a decline in cardiovascular benefits, similar to what is observed in competitive athletes. Thus, athletes should make endurance training an important part of their training regimen to improve health and performance and must maintain an adequate level of endurance during the off-season. Compared with sedentary individuals, fewer regularly active individuals experience cardiorespiratory diseases, and incidents of death from cardiac disease are rare (Prasad and Das, 2009). Make endurance activities part of your lifestyle and a complement to a regular resistance-training program.

Like speed, endurance performance is strongly influenced by genetics, or an individual's biological makeup, because the proportion of slow-twitch muscle fibers to fast-twitch muscle fibers largely determines an athlete's endurance potential. Genetics may affect as much as 70 percent of final performance in a sport or event in which endurance is the dominant motor quality (Bouchard et al. 1984; Matsui, 1983). Most people are born with a 50:50 ratio of fast-twitch to slow-twitch muscle fibers. Gifted endurance athletes most likely have a higher proportion of slow-twitch muscle fibers, whereas gifted sprinters have a higher proportion of fast-twitch muscle fibers. Slow-twitch muscle fibers, also known as Type I fibers, are used for endurance-type sports such as long-distance running, cross-country skiing, and other aerobic activities. Type II muscle fibers are divided into two subcategories: Type IIA and Type IIX. These muscle fibers are used for short-duration anaerobic activities that require fast, explosive movements such as sprinting and discus throw. Many team sports require a combination of both fiber types for maximal performance. For example, in a soccer game the athletes must sprint back and forth between plays (which requires the use of fast-twitch muscle fibers) and at the same time maintain an adequate level of recovery and aerobic output for the duration of the match (which relies on slow-twitch muscle fibers).

The question on researchers' minds is whether athletes can convert muscle fiber types with training. In other words, if an athlete was born with a 50–50 split between slow-twitch and fast-twitch muscle fibers, can training shift the muscle fiber types to match the level and type of training? Can endurance training convert Type II fibers to Type I, and can explosive training convert Type I fibers to Type II? Although some research illustrates the potential to shift fiber types within groups (e.g., convert Type IIA to Type IIX), at this point little evidence illustrates the conversion from Type II to Type I or vice versa. Nonetheless, scientists continue to address the question of fiber type conversion and still hold to the belief that various forms of training, such as a long-duration, high-endurance type of training, can possibly convert Type II fibers to Type I fibers, which would benefit the endurance athlete (Wilson et al., 2012). While we wait for science to catch up, as coaches we continue to advocate for a style of training that provides the safest and most effective way to improve the athlete's endurance and that utilizes methods that complement and focus on the desired adaptations.

However, the fact that an athlete is naturally gifted for endurance activities does not mean that he will always be the best performer. Psychological factors, such as motivation, willpower, and competitiveness, also influence endurance performance. Training ethics, determination, and motivation to work hard often can make up for a lack of talent. Irrespective of talent, all athletes can improve their endurance capacity from childhood to maturation. In early childhood, endurance can improve as much as 10 percent to 20 percent per year. As athletes reach athletic maturation, improvement may decrease to 5 percent to 10 percent per year, although Olympic-class athletes are expected to improve their endurance potential by between 3 percent and 7 percent each year.

Performance ability in endurance-dominant sports improves constantly from early prepuberty to postpuberty and into late adolescence. Athletes reach high performance during maturation. Female athletes may peak at a slightly earlier age than their male counterparts, perhaps because girls tend to mature earlier than boys. Throughout these phases of development, boys perform better overall than girls (Baxter-Jones and Maffulli, 2003; Hughson, 1986).

With the exception of swimming, most endurance-dominant sports (e.g., running, cycling, triathlon, rowing, cross-country skiing, and canoeing) are not as popular as team sports among children. Yet the medical community and fitness specialists often associate these activities with the health benefits of physical activity, therefore implying that more people should engage in endurance activities. Unlike team sports, children can perform endurance activities individually or in small groups and at their own pace. Involvement in such activities can mean the beginning of a lifetime of fitness enjoyment and health benefits. It is not mandatory to train for three or four hours per day to enjoy these sports. Exertion of a shorter duration can also improve endurance, especially in early childhood (Baxter-Jones and Maffulli, 2003).

The adaptation of children's organs and systems to endurance training improves pulmonary (lung) and cardiac (heart) function and increases the number of red blood cells that transport oxygen to the working muscles. Only in the presence of oxygen do glycogen and fatty acids burn to produce the energy necessary for endurance activities. As athletes train, they also become more economical in using energy, which results in improved performance.

Endurance-Training Model for Initiation

Prepubescence can be the beginning of long-lasting athletic activity for many. Children's skills are poor in the early years because they have low economy of locomotion and poor tolerance for heat stress. Prepubescent children also have inferior cardiac output (i.e., the amount of blood the heart pumps in one minute), low blood oxygen–carrying capacity, and low maximal oxygen uptake or $\dot{V}O_2$max. However, athletes score consistently better than nonathletes, which demonstrates that adaptation to training does occur (Rowland and Boyajian, 1995).

The average prepubescent boy has greater endurance than the average prepubescent girl, partly because toward the end of prepuberty the $\dot{V}O_2$max of girls is about 10 percent to 15 percent lower than that of boys. $\dot{V}O_2$max is closely related to lean body mass, increased muscular system, and low body fat, which are greater in boys. On average, boys perform 10 percent to 20 percent better than girls in endurance activities. Before puberty, however, $\dot{V}O_2$max and endurance performance improve for both boys and girls due to training and the increase in the size of the lungs, heart, and muscular system (Baxter-Jones and Maffulli, 2003; Hughson, 1986; Roberts et al., 1987).

Lung function is a strong element in the oxygen delivery system. However, because of improper breathing techniques, breathing economy and the amount of air being ventilated do not increase correspondingly as lung work increases. Children hyperventilate (i.e., they take high and superficial breaths) compared with adult athletes, whose breaths are longer and deeper. For example, maximum ventilation in a five-year-old can be 40 liters per minute compared with 110 liters per minute for an adult (Kenney et al., 2011). Respiratory frequency decreases with age. The respiratory frequency at rest for prepubescent children is around 18 to 20 breaths per minute; by the time children reach postpubescence it decreases by approximately 3 to 4 breaths per minute. The cardiovascular system (heart, arteries, and veins) of children differs from that of adults. The heart rate (number of beats per minute) during both rest and activity is higher in prepubescence (about 200-215 beats per minute) and decreases progressively during the other developmental stages (Young et al., 1995). As children grow, heart rate frequency decreases while efficiency increases; the lungs' vital capacity (the amount of air brought into the lungs that the body can use) also increases (Hebbelinck, 1989; Shephard, 1982).

As a result of exercise, red blood cells and hemoglobin (a complex molecule in red blood cells that contains iron and enriches the capability of red blood cells to transport oxygen) increase. This elevates oxygen delivery and, consequently, increases the efficiency of aerobic endurance. During prepubescence, hemoglobin concentration is approximately equal for boys and girls; the differences in endurance proficiency are due to the other factors mentioned previously.

Scope of Endurance Training

The main scope of training for prepubescence is to progressively make children able to perform an increased duration of physical activity before experiencing fatigue. Anaerobic or aerobic endurance training can take the form of activity (e.g., play), games, or endurance-related sports (e.g., track and field, swimming, cycling, cross-country skiing). Organized drills consisting of a prolonged duration or several repetitions can have positive results in endurance development.

Endurance for prepubescence doesn't have to be developed in a regimented fashion, such as running laps for a given distance or speed. This would in fact be a gross disservice to children. Children have a limited attention span and should not be considered young adults (Reider, 2011). Traditional endurance training such as running laps or paced cycling or dribbling will not work for children. They will easily get bored and prematurely complain of fatigue. If it is not fun, they are more likely to want to stop the exercise or to associate the exercise with fatigue. The earlier children feel pain, the faster they will be hurt, burned out, and even willing to quit sport. Playing fun games and activities and promoting friendly competition makes kids willing to run faster, jump higher, and have a great time pushing their potential. We have seen this time and time again. Ask children to run three laps around the field and they will walk, complain, and want to stop due to fatigue. Alternatively, set up two lines and create an activity that requires sprinting, changes in directions, jumping, and rolling to the finish line and kids will run the equivalent of 30 laps at a higher intensity without a whisper of fatigue. With kids, structured exercise should always take a backseat to fun and intense play.

Endurance activity should be part of multilateral development at this stage of development, and often children can perform endurance training as part of or in addition to technical training. Endurance-related activities should be enjoyable, fun, and interesting for children so they can get cardiorespiratory development as well as varied, pleasant training.

Program Design

Prepubescent children seem to cope better with activities that are either short and fast or longer than two minutes and performed at a slow pace. Competition distances between 200 and 800 meters or yards are unsuitable for prepubescent and pubescent children. These distances should not be part of any track and field program for young athletes because children are unable to tolerate the lactic acid build-up specific to this type of high-intensity activity. Only in late adolescence should athletes incorporate these distances into a competitive program. At this stage of development children have had the time to build strong aerobic and anaerobic backgrounds, improve the power and efficiency of the cardiorespiratory system, and, as a result, improve their lactic acid tolerance.

Prepubescence is the time for early anatomical adaptation of the heart, lungs, joints, and muscles to prolonged physical activity. This should be the base on which athletes build demanding aerobic and anaerobic endurance for specialization and high performance.

Training programs that boys and girls perform together (i.e. coed programs) should be carefully planned and progressively increased over at least two or three years, depending on the age of entry into the sport. Organizing such programs requires carefully applying the principles of individualization with the knowledge that children have their own levels of tolerance to work and fatigue and different degrees of motivation.

Prepubescence is the time to introduce different forms of play and games and to involve children in team sports with simplified rules and the least rigidity possible. In addition, to facilitate restrictions and scheduling, children should play for as long as it is fun and not stressful.

Table 8.1 Periodization Model for Endurance Training for Prepuberty

Form of interval training	Distance or duration	Speed of activity	Reps	Rest interval (min)
Play and games	—	Medium to fast (for short play)	2-4	Variable
Continuous relays	40-200 m/yd	Medium	2-4	2-3
Nonstressful aerobic activity (e.g., running, swimming, rowing, cross-country skiing)	20-60 min	Low and steady	1-2 (depending on the distance)	—

Children can also develop basic endurance by running on varied terrain using the least-boring methods. The instructor should use his imagination to organize running in small groups with various tasks and games of tag. The emphasis should be not only on running but also on performing various tasks while completing the course. This is a great way to integrate multilateral development, which requires children to perform movements at varying levels of intensity and at different angles and to utilize all muscle groups in the activity.

Children can develop basic endurance through individual activities such as swimming, running, cycling, or cross-country skiing. Do not make such activities into traditional competitions; rather, simply ignite the competitive spirit so that the children enjoy the activities and training.

Use table 8.1 as a guideline for planning endurance activities for prepubescent athletes. The first form of training considers play and games, which children could perform at a fast pace for a short duration or slower pace for a prolonged duration. The number of repetitions (how many games performed or how many times children do a game in a session) is two to four. The rest interval is as long as necessary so children are fully rested before starting again.

If children perform relays of longer distance (up to 200 meters or yards), the speed cannot be higher than medium. At this age children cannot run 200 meters or yards with high velocity. Children can repeat relays two to four times, always taking a break of two or three minutes before doing it again.

Children can easily perform longer-duration activities (e.g., running, swimming, cross-country skiing) for 20 to 60 minutes if the speed of activity is low. Do not push children while they are performing such activities. Let them find their own activity speed and allow the real challenge to be the distance. It is better for them to perform an activity for a long distance at slow pace than to do a short distance at a fast pace.

Endurance-Training Model for Athletic Formation

As athletes reach puberty, their endurance improves. If pubescence represents the beginning of organized training, then young athletes can expect fast improvements in endurance capacity simply because their pretraining endurance level was low.

Children can improve $\dot{V}O_2max$ during puberty; the highest gains occur during the growth spurts. Although $\dot{V}O_2max$ increases at approximately the same rate for boys and girls during prepubescence, puberty accelerates endurance gains for boys. This is mostly because boys tend to increase in muscle mass, whereas girls tend to gain body fat. As a result, boys have a higher aerobic capacity and larger cardiac and pulmonary capacity (Hughson, 1986; Kenney et al., 2011; Shephard, 1982).

Most changes pubescent athletes experience are genetically determined. Some of the dramatic changes that occur during puberty manifest in aerobic endurance. Young athletes experience visible phases of stagnation of endurance development. At times, coaches notice a temporary plateau or even a decline in aerobic endurance despite the continuity of training.

Temporary changes in trainability also occur during pubescence. Endurance-training potential can noticeably decrease about half a year before a leap in growth. Before and after a growth spurt, however, gains in endurance capacity appear at a faster rate. We can conclude, therefore, that the improvements in aerobic capacity depends on a child's change in growth and physiological maturity.

For girls, pubescence is the stage of the fastest and probably best gains in endurance, although, as already mentioned, males accelerate faster. It is possible that girls will never reproduce the performance they reach during pubescence unless they participate in organized training. The main reason for performance depreciation in girls is postpubescent gains in total body fat.

The size of the heart and lungs directly affects the oxygen delivery (cardiorespiratory) system. Boys' organs are better developed due to the size of the lungs and to increased involvement in physical activities. The respiratory frequency at rest is approximately 18 breaths per minute for both sexes; however, compared with adults, children's respiratory pattern is more superficial and rapid. This makes children hyperventilate during exercise, which results in higher breathing frequency and lower efficiency in oxygen use. Other sex differences also exist during puberty. Boys have significantly greater red blood cell counts and hemoglobin concentration due to increased physical activity levels.

Beginning with puberty and continuing to maturation, boys have slightly lower heart rates because they have larger and more powerful hearts. At puberty the highest rates begin to decrease at approximately one or two beats per year. The highest heart rate during exercise is recorded before or during puberty and ranges from 195 to 215 beats per minute (Kenney et al., 2011; Malina, 1984). Factors such as poor fitness levels, obesity, anxiety, and heat stress also influence heart rate, especially in untrained individuals.

During growth spurts, children may be vulnerable to muscle injuries resulting from long-distance activities, and, if the young athlete continues to train and ignore the injury, the overuse syndrome may be visible. This can be even more likely when running long distances on hard surfaces. Therefore, consider the benefits of regular aerobic training against the potential negative results. Parents and coaches should be careful in applying regimented training that may result in pain or even health risks. Long-distance activities require an extended training time, which may stop children from doing enjoyable social activities such as playing and learning other skills.

Scope of Endurance Training

Any endurance-training program for pubescent athletes should attempt to increase the foundation for aerobic and anaerobic endurance and take any endurance gains made during prepuberty to a higher level. An equally important goal is to continue developing and strengthening the cardiorespiratory system, thus increasing the power of the heart to pump blood to the working muscles more effectively. Such power manifests as a progressive decrease in heart rate and an increase in cardiac output (the amount of blood pumped per minute).

From puberty, the endurance capacity of girls and boys clearly differs. Therefore, training programs have to address their specific conditions.

View pubescence as the beginning of effectively organized endurance training. The development of endurance benefits overall fitness and buffers fatigue. The better the endurance level, the easier an athlete will cope with an increased number of training hours per week and the total demand in training, which increases during puberty and postpuberty. Improved endurance also results in faster recovery between training sessions, making athletes better conditioned to tolerate a progressively increasing training load.

Program Design

Endurance training for pubescence should progress toward specialization, in which training specificity becomes dominant. As table 8.2 shows, the program can expand to include middle-distance events in track and field and can increase to longer distances (800-2000 meters). Because running is an important activity for most sports, now is the time to teach children correct running technique. To accomplish this, the athlete should perform the distance or the number of repetitions only as long as the skill is correct. When fatigue sets in, technique starts to fall apart, and continuing to work under these conditions will be counterproductive.

Continue to develop endurance mostly during the technical and tactical work (i.e., conditioning). However, also consider performing endurance training apart from conditioning. In such situations, when endurance training is trained both as a technical skill and also in following a specific endurance training program (conditioning), the instructor must remember that each segment of training is fatiguing and should consider total fatigue when calculating the training load (including conditioning).

Consider the following steps when progressively increasing the load in endurance-related training.

1. Increase the duration of a training session from 45 minutes to 60 minutes, from 60 minutes to 75 minutes, and then from 75 minutes to 90 minutes.
2. Increase the number of training sessions per week from two or three to four or five (or more in some sports, such as running or cross-country skiing).
3. When both the duration of a session and the number of workouts per week reach the limit, increase the number of drills or repetitions per training session. This makes training demand higher, and endurance benefits increase as a result.
4. Increase the duration of each repetition. If in the past a drill or repetition has lasted 45 seconds, extend the duration to 60 or 70 seconds or more.

As the duration of training increases, children start perspiring more and therefore should take fluids before, during, and after training. Parents and coaches must allow for

Table 8.2 Periodization Model for Endurance Training for Puberty

Form of training	Distance	Speed of activity	Reps	Rest interval (min)
Play and relays	40-200 m/yd	Fast to medium	3-5	Variable
Interval training runs	200-400 m/yd	Medium	3-5 (low numbers for 400 m/yd)	2-3
Aerobic activity (long repetition)	800-2000 m (.5-1.25 miles)	Medium and steady, with slight discomfort at times	1-3	3-5

frequent water breaks, especially in hot and humid conditions, so that children maintain body heat balance and avoid losing too much fluid.

Training Program

A training program for pubescent athletes should still include different forms of play and games in addition to elements of more formal training aimed at developing endurance. As much as possible, the coach should incorporate variety and enjoyment in the activities she is planning. Although training for endurance often means perseverance in repeating the same kind of work over and over, avoid regimentation.

Repeating certain types of endurance training does not necessarily mean performing boring laps. Coaches can make training enjoyable by varying the distance and terrain and arranging a fun course. For team sports, coaches should set the duration of technical and tactical drills with endurance development in mind. A drill that lasts 60 seconds has technical and tactical merit and develops sport-specific endurance.

An endurance-training program should include different distances or durations because each may develop a component of endurance. For instance, an activity performed at a long, steady pace will develop the pumping power of the heart and the stroke volume (the amount of blood pumped per beat) and, in the long run, will decrease the resting heart rate. Some types of work, mainly aerobic training, develop the capillary network (the branching out of veins and arteries), allowing oxygen to travel to every part of the body.

Interval training—a method of repeating a distance or time several times with a prescribed intensity, duration, and rest interval—strengthens the heart and lungs. If the duration of work is between two and three minutes, the athlete develops $\dot{V}O_2$max. By performing shorter repetitions, the athlete will progressively adjust to anaerobic endurance. Because such a training program produces lactic acid, a fatiguing by-product of anaerobic training, you must apply it carefully and progressively. Interval training is used the most during postpuberty and mostly during training for high performance. Given this, the latter part of pubescence is the time to introduce interval training.

Training for anatomical adaptation, rather than training for physiological improvement and performance increases, is the type of interval training most appropriate for puberty. This means medium distance and time, medium intensity, and a rest interval that allows for full regeneration. Such a program should give children the time (two to four years) to adjust anatomically before training physiologically. Children can achieve the anatomical adaptation phase of interval training without the typical strain of high-intensity interval training of shorter duration, which results in a high heart rate (close to or even more than 200 beats per minute). Such a heart rate has a low stroke volume and decreases the ability to effectively pump oxygen and the glucose needed for producing energy. The idea that interval training is short and must hurt is a misconception.

The main law for endurance training for puberty is "before training physiologically, train anatomically." That is, train the anatomy of the cardiorespiratory system before training the physiology of the cardiovascular system. Before the body of a pubescent athlete can be pushed with high-intensity exercise and benefit from physiological adaptations, the heart, lungs, and vessels need to be strong enough to withstand the pressures of a high-intensity workload.

Considerations for Specialization

Endurance and endurance performance improve steadily throughout the growing years. During adolescence, a slight improvement occurs for males but not as much for females. As athletes better adapt to training, energy expenditure becomes more effective and economical and performance may constantly improve. The biological differences, as well as performance differences, continue to grow during postpuberty. In addition, females are less likely to reach their full physical potential because of social factors, not necessarily because of biological handicaps. Society is accustomed to males dominating sport participation. Despite society's acceptance of equal opportunities for males and females in sport participation and the increase in media coverage of female sports (Berstein, 2002), men's sports are still more visible. However, powerful female athletes such as tennis players Maria Sharapova and Serena Williams and LPGA golfers Michelle Wie and Stacey Lewis have inspired thousands of young girls to participate in sport. Furthermore, the popularity of soccer continues to grow among young girls because of the positive influence of many female soccer stars, including American Amy Wambach and Canadian Christine Sinclair. In fact, at the 2012 London Olympic Games, U.S. female athletes outnumbered U.S. male athletes (269 to 261) for the first time in Olympic history. The tides are changing.

Scope of Endurance Training

On the foundation of endurance built during prepubescence and pubescence, training now becomes more specific to meet the needs of the selected sport. Diverse training is progressively narrowed during this stage of development, especially as the athlete approaches high performance. For endurance training, diversity in training is achieved by varying the total training time devoted to aerobic and anaerobic training.

The long-term approach to endurance training pursued during prepuberty and puberty reaches a peak during postpuberty as more emphasis is given to anaerobic training and sessions of high-intensity aerobic and anaerobic training postpuberty. A postpubescent athlete who was given adequate time to mature and prepare the cardiorespiratory system for higher workloads is physiologically prepared to develop a more specific long-term training program. From postpuberty on, the coach has to develop annual plans that include aerobic and anaerobic training as well as introduce ergogenesis training.

Ergogenesis is a term of Greek origin. *Ergon* means work, and *genesis* refers to beginning or creation. In sport, ergogenesis implies creating work that combines the elements of endurance as the specifics of the sport require. As such, ergogenesis refers to the total contribution of anaerobic and aerobic endurance to performance, expressed as a percentage. For instance, the ergogenesis of rowing is 83 percent aerobic and 17 percent anaerobic. In 800-meter running, the ergogenesis is 51 percent aerobic and 49 percent anaerobic. In 200-meter swimming it is 70 percent aerobic and 30 percent anaerobic. In basketball it is 40 percent aerobic and 60 percent anaerobic. Consequently, an annual plan must include phases in which ergogenesis, or the right combination of aerobic and anaerobic endurance, dominates. Such a program results in the progressive improvement of performance.

Program Design

Because postpuberty is the stage when athletes start to specialize in an event, sport, and position (in team sport), training specificity gets high visibility. However, coaches should not exclude multilateral training in this stage. The athlete must continue to work on the foundation of aerobic capacity—the ability to produce energy under aerobic conditions. Anatomical adaptation of the cardiorespiratory system—that is, strengthening the heart and improving the oxygen transport system—must be a constant objective of aerobic training. A training program for postpubescence should continually develop aerobic capacity to effectively produce and efficiently consume the oxygen this system provides.

During the first two or three years of postpubescence, developing aerobic capacity becomes the major training objective for individual-sport and team-sport athletes. In the last part of postpubescence, endurance training becomes more specialized according to the needs of the selected sport. As mentioned previously, from this stage on athletes should use anaerobic endurance and ergogenesis to build a strong aerobic base.

Constantly improving aerobic capacity to the highest possible level has certain benefits:

- It develops the oxygen transport system, in which a powerful heart plays an important role.
- Athletes can prevent hyperventilating by focusing on active exhalation—filling the lungs with fresh, oxygen-rich air—and taking deep, steady breaths.
- High aerobic capacity positively influences anaerobic capacity because it lengthens the athlete's ability to function before reaching fatigue. An athlete with a high aerobic capacity can tolerate anaerobic work and the accompanying highly fatiguing lactic acid buildup.
- An athlete with high aerobic capacity can recover quickly from fatiguing training sessions or after repeating work or drills. Consequently, the athlete can slightly reduce the rest interval between repetitions and thus perform more work. More work usually translates to improved performance.

A training program designed for postpubescence, especially the second part of this stage, also has to develop anaerobic capacity. This refers to an athlete's ability to produce energy in the absence of oxygen and to progressively tolerate the buildup of lactic acid, which is the by-product of anaerobic training.

Developing aerobic or anaerobic capacity depends on the selected training method. Long-distance training methods, including long-distance uniform (steady state) training, alternate interval training of long repetitions and specific racing endurance to develop aerobic capacity. Particularly for team sports, however, the instructor should remember that athletes also can develop these capacities through specific drills, especially tactical drills. Drills of longer duration (more than three minutes) improve the aerobic component, whereas drills of 30 to 60 seconds improve anaerobic capacity. Both methods should be used in training to improve the foundational qualities of endurance.

The training methods we suggest in table 8.3 do not exhaust what is available in sport training. However, it is critical during this stage of development, especially the early postpuberty years, to constantly emphasize aerobic training—both uniform long-distance runs and long repetitions of interval training. A solid aerobic base developed at this age without strain and stress guarantees improved performance during maturation. After all, athletes reach high performance at maturation and not at early postpuberty! Pushing young athletes often burns them out. As a result, young athletes quit sport and miss out on many benefits—both long term and short term—of sport participation that can positively affect a teenager in the formative years leading to adulthood. Not every child will become a champion on the field, ice, or court, but all children can become champions in life through the lessons learned in sport.

Table 8.3 suggests the duration of rest intervals. These are just guidelines. To calculate the rest interval between repetitions, use the heart rate method.

1. Take the heart rate immediately after a repetition of an activity.
2. Continue to monitor the heart rate. When it decreases to 120 beats per minute, start another repetition.

Table 8.3 Periodization Model for Endurance Training for Postpuberty

Form of training	Distance or duration	Speed of activity	Reps	Rest interval (min)
Uniform training (long distance)	2000-5000 m (1.25-3.1 miles)	Low to medium	1	—
Interval training (long repetitions)	800-1500 m (0.5-1 mile)	Medium	2-4 (up to 6)	2-3
Interval training (short repetitions)	200-400 m/yd	Medium	4-6	3-5
Tactical drills for team sports (long)	2-5 min	Medium	3-6	2-3
Tactical drills for team sports (short)	30-60 sec	Fast	4-6 (up to 8)	3-5

Predicting Maximum Heart Rate

The variability in heart rates for pre- and postpubescence makes it difficult to accurately predict maximum heart rate (HRmax) without conducting an individual heart rate test. Given the time required to test each athlete's HRmax and the potential for inaccurately measuring HRmax, coaches often opt to use rate of perceived exertion, in which the athlete rates his level of training intensity as easy, difficult, hard, or extremely hard. Furthermore, the "220 minus age" formula for predicting HRmax in adults aged 19 to 65 years does not appear to accurately predict the mean average HRmax of younger athletes.

Recently, an updated HRmax formula was accepted as a plausible way to predict HRmax in children. This formula helps coaches more accurately assess the level of intensity used in training and technical or tactical drills. The following formula has been touted as the best formula to date for predicting HRmax in children aged 7 to 17 years:

$$208 - (.7 \times \text{age})$$

One study illustrated the efficacy of using this method to predict HRmax in children aged 7 to 17 years (Mahon et al., 2010), and a similar study validated the formula for children aged 10 to 16 years (Machado and Denadai, 2011). Both studies acknowledge that the formula is not perfect but that it is a good indicator of HRmax for both pre- and postpubescent athletes.

Using a 16-year-old soccer player as an example, HRmax would be calculated as follows:

$$208 - (.7 \times \text{age})$$

$$208 - (.7 \times 16) = 208 - (11.2) = 196.8 \text{ (predicted HRmax)}$$

If the prescribed level of intensity for specific aerobic-training drills (e.g., 90 seconds to 3 minutes) was between 85 percent and 90 percent of HRmax, the heart rate training zone would be calculated as follows:

$$196.8 \times .85 = 167 \text{ beats per minute}$$

$$196.8 \times .90 = 177 \text{ beats per minute}$$

Coaches can use this formula as a general basis for planning intensity levels and can modify the heart rate range or percentage of HRmax to better suit the individual athlete.

Exercises for Prepuberty

The following four exercises are appropriate for prepubertal athletes.

Controlled Speed Exercise

Focus: general endurance

1. Create a triangular shape with rounded end points (or ask the athletes to), and divide it into three sections. Each rounded end is a section. Divide the participants into small groups. One group stands at each section's start point.
2. Maximum running time is 15 seconds in any one section. Choose the running route around the triangle – either clockwise or counterclockwise. Have every group start to run from their section at the same time.
3. Include a variety of speed movement (e.g., jog for 40 meters or yards [section one], run for 60 meters or yards [section two], walk for 20 meters or yards [section three] to recover, and repeat).

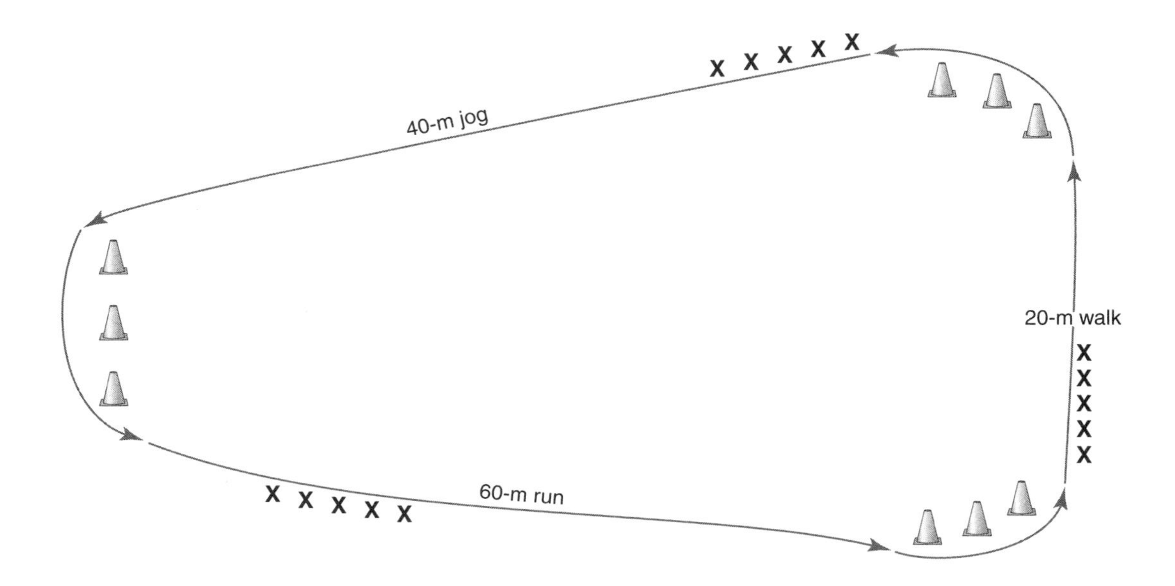

Square

Focus: general endurance

1. Mark a square that is 50 meters or yards by 50 meters or yards. The corners of the square are rounded. Each team begins at a corner.
2. The athletes walk the first side of the square (40-50 seconds), jog the next side (18-20 seconds), walk the next side (40-50 seconds), and jog the last side (18-20 seconds). They can also run backward for variety and to improve spatial orientation.

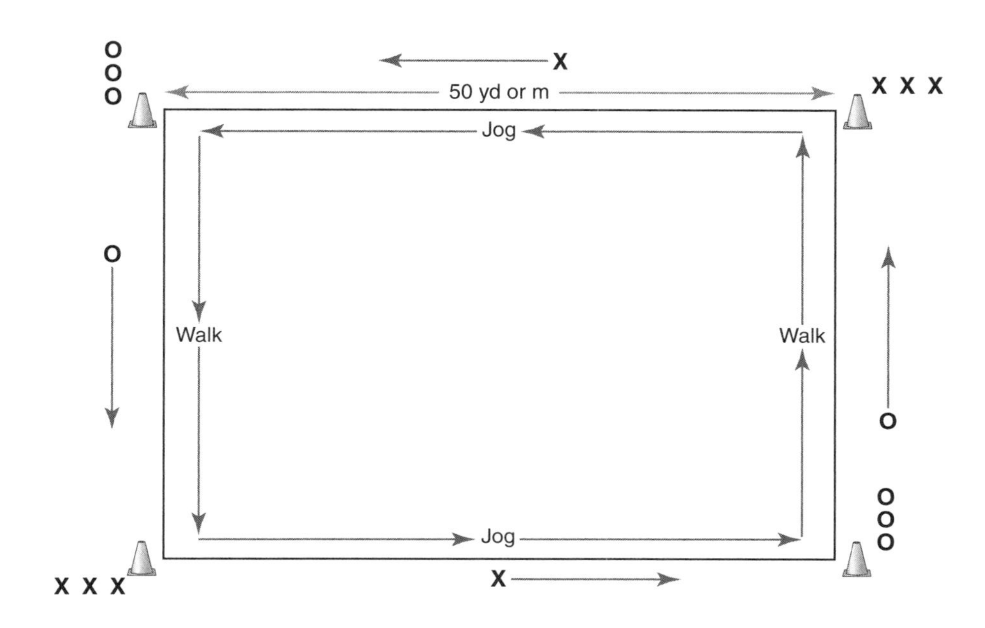

Quad

Focus: general endurance

1. Divide athletes into four groups and place them at the four corners of a square. The length of each line of the square is 50 meters.
2. The athletes walk, briskly walk, jog, or run the square at their own pace.
3. The athletes complete two to four nonstop loops.

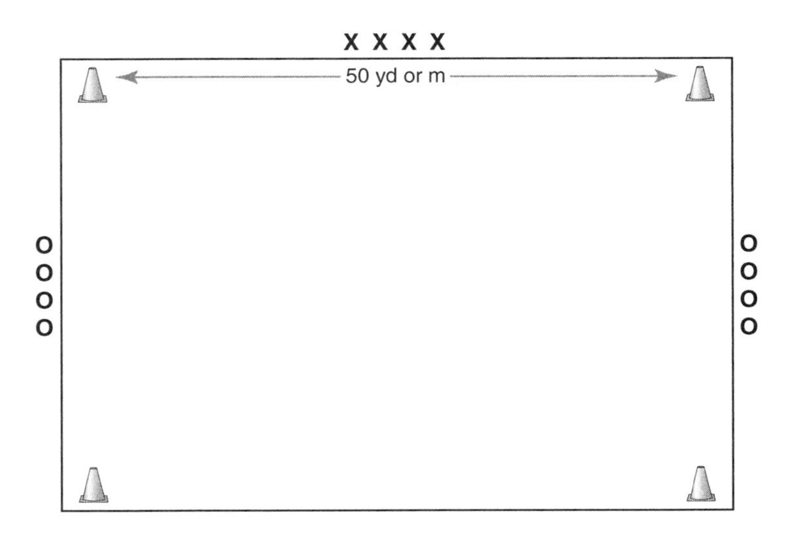

Outdoor Course

Focus: general endurance

1. Mark a running course of 300 to 500 meters in a natural setting on varying terrain.
2. Divide the course alternately into 100-meter and 50-meter sections using natural landmarks.
3. Athletes walk the 50-meter sections and jog the 100-meter sections. Each athlete completes the course two to four times.

Variation

More advanced athletes run the whole course but vary the speed of the sections.

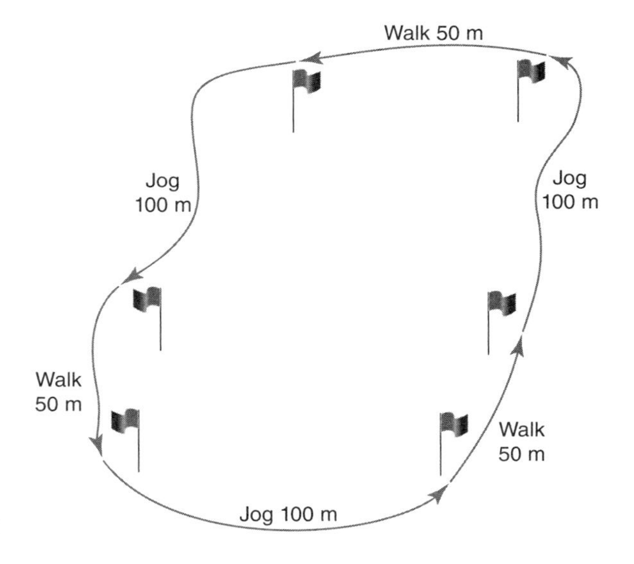

Exercises for Puberty

The following five exercises for endurance training are appropriate for pubertal athletes.

Aerobic Technical Run

Focus: running technique

1. In distance running, the athlete runs tall with the head up, the shoulders down and relaxed, and the arms swinging back and forth in coordination with the leg actions.
2. The knee drive and leg recovery are lower than in sprinting. The athlete lands on the heel and rolls over the toe for a new propulsion phase.
3. Steadiness of running and pace judgment are always important in endurance running.

Long Repetitions for Pace Judgment

Focus: aerobic endurance and pace judgment

1. Athletes run distances of 800 to 2000 meters in a steady rhythm and at an even pace.
2. To ensure pace judgment, time each repetition and give feedback to each athlete individually. This will help athletes get in touch with their pace and will improve awareness of pace and changes in heart and breathing rates. Make sure that timing the athletes does not create a competitive environment.

Interval Training Runs

Focus: aerobic and anaerobic endurance

1. Athletes run repetitions of 200 to 400 meters at a medium, even pace on a track or open field. They should concentrate on good form and maintain a relaxed, steady pace.
2. Athletes perform each repetition at the same pace.
3. Athletes should run with medium (60 percent) velocity and should not push themselves.

10-Minute Triangle Run

Focus: aerobic endurance

1. Divide the athletes into three groups. Each group starts at a corner of a triangle. One side of the triangle is a 50-meter run, a second side is a 40-meter jog, and the third side a 30-meter walk.
2. The athletes walk, jog, and run the sides of the triangle according to their ability.
3. Each athlete should be encouraged to complete two to four full rounds of the triangle at their level of comfort and pace. Athletes with higher levels of aerobic fitness may finish the four rounds faster than athletes who are less fit.
4. Recording an athlete's time to complete the course (either one time around or a predetermined number of rounds) can be used to assess improvements in aerobic capacity on a retest basis. Athletes walk for 2 or 3 minutes between repetitions or full rounds (i.e., one full completion around the triangle constitutes a full round or one repetition).

Variations

- Make the triangle larger.
- Decide on a number of loops to perform for jogging, running, and walking. For instance, at first when making the loop larger, the coach may choose to dedicate two sides of the triangle to walking and one to jogging. Progressively, one side can be dedicated to walking, one to jogging, and one to running. Eventually, one side can be dedicated to running and one side to walking or jogging. The goal is to progressively increase the distance between lines, intensity, and time devoted to aerobic movement (i.e. total time to perform the exercise.
- Progressively increase the duration to 12, 15, 20, or 30 minutes.

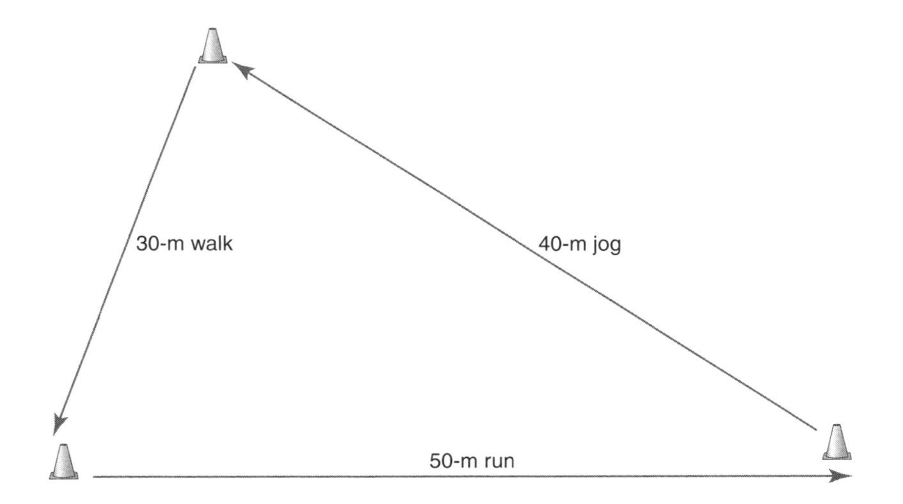

Passing on the Right

Focus: anaerobic and aerobic endurance

1. Runners line up in single-file lines. Each team starts at a marked point in the oval of a stadium.
2. The teams run single file. Every 10 steps, the last person in the line moves to the front of the line, passing on the right.
3. Every time the runners pass the point where they started, the instructor blows a whistle to signify the beginning of a sprint.
4. When the instructor blows the whistle again, the runners revert to the initial pace.
5. Continue for a predetermined number of laps.

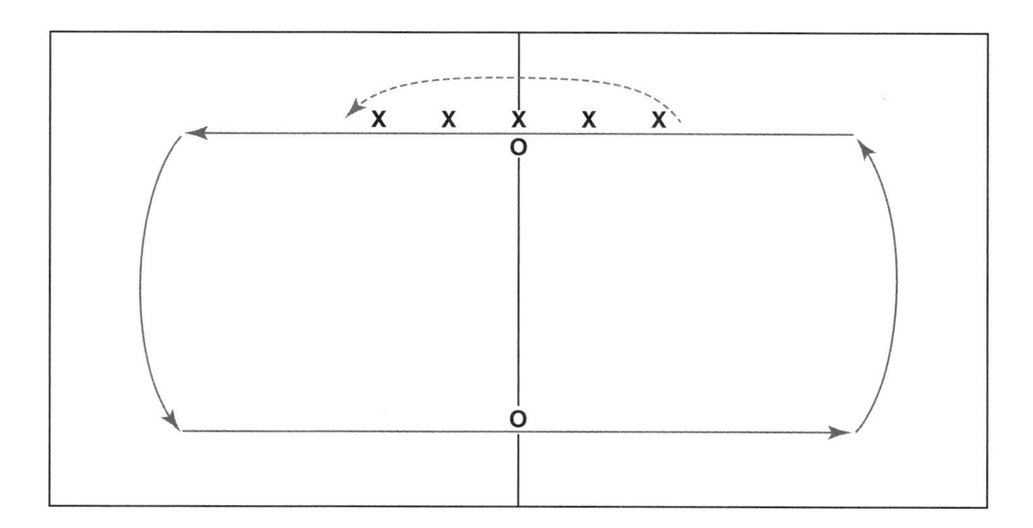

Exercises for Postpuberty

Building on the base of the aerobic and anaerobic training of prepuberty and puberty, the scope of endurance training for postpuberty is sport specific. Athletes perform most forms of training with the implement (e.g., ball) they use in the chosen sport. Figures 8.1 and 8.2 exemplify the periodization of endurance training for postpuberty. The training program performed in the suggested phases progresses from aerobic (October and November) to mixed training, in which half of the program is interval training, to develop anaerobic endurance while aerobic training continues. During the competitive phase, endurance training is clearly sport specific: Ergogenesis is at least 50 percent.

During the competitive phase, the specific training for aerobic and anaerobic endurance using technical and tactical drills can follow these examples.

- Aerobic training
    - Specific drills for 90 seconds to 3 minutes or longer
    - Rest interval of 1 or 2 minutes
    - Target heart rate of 166 to 174 beats per minute (approximately 85 percent to 90 percent of predicted HRmax)

- Anaerobic training
  - Specific high-intensity drills for 20 to 60 seconds
  - Rest interval of 2 or 3 minutes
  - Target heart rate of 176 to 186 beats per minute (approximately 90 percent to 95 percent of predicted HRmax)

The coach decides the number of repetitions for each type of drill depending on athletes' potential and the schedule of games and competitions.

Figure 8.1 Periodization for an Annual Plan for Early Postpuberty

Month	Oct	Nov	Dec	Jan	Feb	Mar	Apr	May	Jun	Jul	Aug	Sep
Training phase		Preparatory							Competitive		Transition	
Type of training		Aerobic endurance			Aerobic long intervals		Mixed aerobic and anaerobic		Mixed specific endurance, introduce ergogenesis		Aerobic	

Notes: Note the progression regarding the type of training and training content. Types of training change according to the objectives of training phases.

T = Transition

Figure 8.2 Periodization for an Annual Plan for Late Postpuberty

Month	Oct	Nov	Dec	Jan	Feb	Mar	Apr	May	Jun	Jul	Aug	Sep
Training phase	Preparatory			Competitive		T	Preparatory		Competitive			T
Type of training	Aerobic		Mixed ergo.	Specific endurance ergo.		A	Aerobic	Mixed ergo	Specific endurance ergo.			A

Notes: A = Aerobic; Ergo. = Ergogenesis; T = Transition

chapter 9

Excelling in Competition

Competition or an opportunity for children to play with peers and feel part of a team is essential to build character traits such as perseverance, team play, good sportsmanship, and physical maturity, and to develop children in the sport environment. Properly guided competitions can benefit overall development and play an active role in children's growth and social interrelationships. Competitions give children the opportunity to apply the technical and tactical skills learned in practice to an organized game, experience winning and losing, and develop skills and values that will serve them later in life. However, many competitive sport programs place excessive physical and psychological demands on children. The adverse effects of these early stresses can be detrimental to growth and may lead young participants to lose interest and drop out before fully developing their talents. Therefore, coaches and parents should treat competitions as a way to foster better sporting skills and social skills that help kids interact and communicate with other children, not as a way to immediately produce a champion. A positive experience in sport and competition can lead to an active lifestyle for many years to come, and this is more important than being a champion athlete.

Why Do Children Drop Out of Sport?

In the United States alone, more than 45 million kids participate in some form of competitive sport. Unfortunately, by age 15 years, 70 to 80 percent of these kids quit playing sport altogether (Merkel, 2013). Considering the societal, psychological, and physical benefits of play, it is in our best interest to keep kids interested and active in sport for as long as possible in the hope that they will carry their love for exercise into adulthood.

Of course, some kids play sport out of interest and for exercise and have no intention of taking their skills to a higher level. There needs to be room for these kids to compete and feel safe and adequate in a sporting environment. There also needs to be programs and opportunities for the kids who want to reach a higher level of play and competition. One inherent problem is that we push kids too fast and foster an environment in which fun is prematurely replaced with winning. In this scenario, many "would be" competitive athletes are lost in the shuffle because they are unable to handle the stress and pressure of competition and choose to drop out of sport early. Furthermore, kids who need play and exercise as an outlet from life stress or problems at home or simply for better health and fitness are let down and geared toward living a sedentary lifestyle—and all the negative health effects that follow.

Competition is important. Winning is important. However, prematurely stressing either competition or winning in lieu of fun will result in losing many kids, and we will continue to experience a 70 percent dropout rate.

Given the opportunity, kids will discuss many reasons for dropping out of sport, including the following:

Lost interest. It is normal for kids to lose interest in a sport, especially if they didn't join for themselves but rather because their parents signed them up. Some kids are inclined to exercise and play but dislike organized sport. That is understandable. However, once kids are enrolled and on a team, it is up to the coach to make practice and competition fun by offering variety in training and, most importantly, not overly stressing winning. Building team cohesion, cheering for all players, and taking the time to say "Great run," "Good play," or "Wow, great effort" can go a long way in making the experience more about fun and teamwork than about winning the game. It is easy to lose interest in something that is one-dimensional. It is more difficult to lose interest when building team spirit.

No longer fun. There is only one way that playing a sport can go from fun to "I'm done!" That is when fun is replaced with competition, pressure, and feelings of inadequacy. This should not happen in the early years of sporting competition. Even with the need for competition and the thrill of winning, sport for 8- to 13-year-olds should always be about fun. It is up to the coach and the parents to make the sporting experience fun and to provide an environment in which less-skilled players feel like part of the team and believe that their contribution not only matters but is vital for team success.

Takes too much time. This is a complaint we often see, especially in higher levels of play. Once an athlete joins a team—a team that she will mature with both on and off the field—she must adhere to certain rules and guidelines and a vigorous schedule. It is not uncommon for a 10-year-old hockey player to play two games per week, practice on ice two days per week, and complete one off-ice conditioning program per week. For a 10-year-old who is in school and in essence still a kid, five days of hockey per week is a demanding schedule—but this is standard for these kids. For younger kids or for kids who are not playing at a higher level, one game and one practice can suffice. In some cases, especially for 5- to 7-year-olds, they can practice for 30 minutes before a game. Parents must understand what is important to the child and place him in the appropriate program while allowing room for kids to be kids.

Too much emphasis on winning. Too often winning is seen as being everything, even to the detriment of proper technique and team play. Especially in the early years of play, the player who scores the goal or gets the basket is rewarded with cheers and high fives while the athlete who passed the ball or defended the play is ignored. We tend to overemphasize winning and scoring. As parents, we can all swear truth to this one fact: We want our kids to be the ones who score the goals! But, too much emphasis on getting the goal or winning the game undermines the important skills and techniques that are necessary for higher-level play. Yes, scoring is important, but no goal can occur without a much-needed assist! Because winning will always be on the forefront of each parent's and coach's mind, we recommend that coaches take a few minutes at the end of the game or at the start of practice to discuss the good and bad points of the game and some of the plays that helped the team open up scoring chances. This is a good way for the coach to emphasize technique, tactical drills, and the importance of teamwork—all under the guise of winning the game! Winning is important, but so is the road that gets a team there. It is in the journey that kids become champions, both on and off the field.

We were recently chatting with a set of parents whose boys were invited to try out for a higher-level hockey team. The boys were intimidated, having heard that the coaches are demanding and have high expectations. One coach in particular was known as a "tough guy," benching players who did not perform to standard. When we asked the parents how the tryout went, they both smiled with joy. The boys, who were longtime friends, both made the team, and the parents were pleasantly surprised by how inspiring and welcoming the coaches were. They spoke to the players, helped them on the ice, and didn't push too hard. The parents had two concerns. First, the boys would have to practice two days per week, play two games per week, and attend weekend tournaments—some out of town—once or twice per month. Second, they hoped that their boys wouldn't be discouraged by the high level of competition and pressure. As one parent put it, "I would hate for my son to drop out of hockey. He loves it so much, but I know that he feels a bit inadequate since he is smaller than the other boys on the team." You would think we were talking about teenage boys, but both boys had just turned 10 years old!

Some controversial issues surround highly organized competitive sport for children. The next sections discuss how coaches and parents can use competition to develop a child's love for the sport, fitness, social skills, friendship, and life skills, such as winning, losing, dedication, respect, and good sportsmanship.

Problems With Competition

Children love to compete, but parents love it even more! In an attempt to satisfy their own thirst for competition, parents and coaches may expose children to programs that are too aggressive or too advanced. Even if children are able to tolerate the physical component of the program, they may have difficulty coping mentally with the excessive emotional demands of training and competition. Pushing children into overly demanding training and competition schedules too early and keeping the competition-to-training ratio too large are two common ways in which coaches and parents create stress and burnout in young athletes.

Competing Too Early

Most children have their first sporting experience in organized competition. Often children as young as four years are participating in structured leagues with formal rules, referees, and official team uniforms, and winning is the primary objective.

In the United States, children aged three to five years participate in competitions in swimming and gymnastics, and those aged five to six years compete in track and field, wrestling, baseball, and soccer! In Brazil, children aged six years compete in soccer and swimming, and in Canada, children aged six to eight years already compete at the provincial (state) level (Passer, 1988; Passer and Wilson, 2002).

Some horror stories exist. In the late 1980s, a 9-year-old girl ran a marathon in Phoenix, Arizona. A few years later, a 12-year-old girl ran a similar distance in San Francisco. Did the organizers and, especially, the parents pay any attention to the medical concerns, such as excessive early training, burnout, heat injury risks, cardiac damage, reproductive changes, and impaired nutrition? In another case, we spoke to a father whose son was cut from a hockey team. The team began to practice in August for games that began in mid-September and ended in mid-March. In December the coach told the young boy that he should be looking for a new team because he would be cut from the team the following year. The coach saw this move as an act of compassion because it offered the kid time and an opportunity to look for another team. Such an act would in fact be deemed responsible if the kid wasn't 11 years old! He ultimately decided to quit competitive hockey and unfortunately, according to his father, began to struggle with confidence issues. This type of treatment and behavior is quite common in sport (Bigelow, 2000).

Early participation in competitions is one way in which children are pushed. From the first or second year of their training, parents or coaches enter children in important state, provincial, or national competitions. Demanding training and challenging competitions force coaches to artificially push young athletes to adapt to highly intensive work. In many cases, this approach causes children to peak at an early age, and they can indeed achieve incredible performances. The downside is that they burn out well before they have the opportunity to excel in competitions at the proper time of physiological and psychological maturation. By this time, some have given up sport and others rarely duplicate the performance they achieved in their midteens. Even worse, they can experience soft-tissue injuries in both the upper and lower body due to repetitive strain on their maturing physical systems. Practicing vigorously and playing multiple intense sports throughout the year while devoting little or no time to rest and regeneration can predispose young athletes to numerous soft-tissue injuries (Mariscalco and Salvan, 2011). Also, numerous studies have shown that children find activities such as sport more enjoyable when they are not pushed to compete or win and are encouraged by their parents to have fun (MacPhail et al., 2003; Mulvihill et al., 2000).

In track and field, children enter such events as the 400 meters, 800 meters, and 1500 meters, which are physiologically and psychologically taxing. These events require a good training background because speed, speed endurance, anaerobic endurance, and aerobic endurance are in high demand. Similar negative conditions can occur when children prematurely enter the triple jump, which involves a series of repetitive shocks. These shocks are not absorbed by sand and the motion of bending the knees to land, as they are in the long jump; rather, they are directed straight to the spine. The ground reaction forces can be too great for the immature muscular and ligament-stabilizing systems to handle, thus causing back pain (MacDonald and D'Hemecourt, 2007). Approximately 30 percent of adolescents have experienced some form of back pain due to intense activity or sport (Cupisti et al., 2004). Children aged eight years and up enter the triple jump, which requires the force of take-off and the shock of landing. In many countries in Europe, children are banned from competing in the 400 meters and the triple jump before the age of 16 years, when they have established enough background training.

The culprits of such mistreatment are coaches, parents, and competition organizers. To demonstrate their competency, coaches often keep win and loss records and, for some, children become just statistics! Children should not pay the price for the ambitions of coaches. Ambitious parents who want to see their children become successful in sport and become champions are impatient and do not want to wait four to six years—they want it now. Competition organizers and boards of education can be positive elements in children's athletics if they organize competitions according to children's potential and impose age limits based on the proper age for children to participate in high-level competitions.

Competing Too Often

Coaches and instructors often try to duplicate the number of games professional athletes play. Take, for instance, ice hockey in Canada or soccer in the United States. In ice hockey, children aged 8 to 10 years play anywhere from 60 to 80 games per season. The logic goes like this: Professional players play 80 games per season, so if you want to become a professional player you have to do what professional athletes do! We have even heard of parents planning their child's week based on the hours of work they put into their sport because they read that some professional athlete practiced the same number of hours in a week! Even worse, we once heard a father tell his son, "You can go to the party if you want, but just know that while you are relaxing with your buddies, someone out there is practicing his slap shot."

By contrast, when the Soviet system of training was in full swing (1950s-1980s), team sports had a four-to-one ratio of training sessions to games. This means that for every game, children had four training sessions to work on skills and developing motor abilities. In North America, in some team sports children are lucky if they get a one-to-one ratio of training to games. In ice hockey, the ratio is outrageous at three games to one practice! When do these children have time to work on their skills and fitness? Often, in team sports such as ice hockey, baseball, soccer, or basketball, children attend weekend tournaments. In these circumstances the ratio of training sessions to games may be even worse than one to one. Is it any wonder that the improvement rate in technical skill, physical fitness, and recovery from a game is slow and that children are emotionally taxed far beyond their tolerance level?

In individual sports such as track and field, gymnastics, and skiing (although not necessarily swimming), the situation is far better. The ratio in these sports is often 8 or 10 to 1.

We must be aware that early success offers no promise of the same later on and does not guarantee future stardom. Success during childhood means more competition, which leads to psychological stress and failure in skill proficiency. The higher the number of games children play, the lower the number of practices, which means decreased skill proficiency and weaker performances. It is essential that children practice more and compete less. That is the secret to success—not always professional success, but athletic success!

Emphasizing Winning

If our prime interest is to develop talented athletes, then it is essential for us to emphasize skill development and de-emphasize winning in sport programs for children. Emphasis on winning creates stressful situations in which children cannot adequately develop skill. Instead, they often reinforce and further develop skills that are technically incorrect.

The best way for children to develop skills is to practice them in a fun, nonstressful, nonthreatening environment. Such an environment seldom exists in competitive sport programs. In many cases, children are competing too frequently and have little time available to practice the necessary skills that will help them become better athletes.

In some leagues, such as hockey, in which young children have to compete in as many as 80 games a season, little time is devoted to skill development. During games children are applying, not developing, their skills. If children do not properly develop their skills before application, they will be reinforcing poor techniques and unquestionably developing bad habits. Once developed, bad technical habits are difficult to correct. They may be suitable for success at a lower stage of development but are not suitable for higher levels of competition.

For example, assume that a coach wants to develop a top-notch 10-year-old amateur wrestler. The coach may encourage the child to learn some fancy throws, which will provide the young wrestler with terrific opportunities for success as a 10-year-old. At 14 years of age, however, the child will likely have a poor throwing technique because at the earlier age he did not have sufficient strength and power to learn the technique properly. Instead of developing a strong fundamental technical base, the young wrestler spent too much time practicing throws. As a result, he may become discouraged when, at 14 years of age, other children are much better at performing the fundamental techniques necessary for wrestling success, such as leg attacks.

Discriminating Against Late-Maturing Children

Coaches who want to win usually play their best players. Often, the best players are those who have matured early because they are bigger, stronger, faster, and have more endurance. In such cases, early-maturing children occupy starting positions on the sport teams while late-maturing children sit on the bench.

Early-maturing children are undoubtedly better athletes during childhood. However, much research indicates that late-maturing children may have greater potential to reach international standards in a specific sport during adulthood. In fact, in the 1980s, in their quest to dominate the athletic world, the former communist countries of Eastern Europe switched their selection of talented children from early-maturing children to late-maturing children. Experience had shown that early-maturing children had only sometimes met their expectations. The late-maturing children, however, displayed more consistency and, in most cases, achieved higher performance levels. This has also been demonstrated in soccer, with late-maturing children experiencing greater success at higher levels of play (Ostojic et al., 2014).

In late-maturing children, the adolescent growth spurt starts at a later stage of development and lasts longer than it does in early-maturing children. As a result, when late-maturing children reach adulthood, their athletic development is usually better than that of early-maturing children. Unfortunately, in many sport programs for children, late-maturing children do not get equal opportunities to participate because of the overemphasis on winning. These children are discriminated against in many situations.

Risking Injury

Although the stress of intensive training that is physically demanding and psychologically taxing may result in burnout, it also often results in injuries. In many instances, children are not exposed to training programs that have a long-term perspective. On the contrary, parents and coaches want quick results. To achieve such results, coaches may not pay much attention to strengthening the anatomy of the children. When a coach ignores the condition of ligaments, tendons, cartilage, and muscle tissue, the injury-prevention portion of a program is missing. This shortcoming, when added to high-intensity training, can only result in injuries. We cannot emphasize enough the need for multilateral development, especially during the initiation and athletic stages of development. This is the point in an athlete's life when the anatomy is primed to adapt to various carefully applied forces and stressors. Taking the time to strengthen the ligaments, tendons, joints, and cartilage and following a moderate program that works all muscle groups in the body will build a solid foundation of strength that will serve as the building block for future speed, endurance, power, and, yes, higher levels of strength!

Take the time to teach athletes to properly warm up and the importance of preparing the body for competition. Exercises that can be overlooked as simple and nonconstructive are what are needed to properly strengthen anatomical structures and prevent injury. In one study (Wingfield, 2013), researchers worked with clubs from eight regional districts of the Swedish Football Association and tested the efficacy of performing 15 minutes of neuromuscular exercises, including simple jumping exercises, in adolescent female soccer players. The exercises were done twice per week. During 278,298 hours of play the teams recorded 21 anterior cruciate ligament injuries; 7 injuries occurred in the intervention group (those that completed the exercises) and 14 occurred in the control group. A few simple exercises resulted in 50 percent fewer severe injuries. Take the time to do what is necessary for greater performance and longevity in sport!

Start by doing what is necessary and eventually the young athlete will be able to handle the new stressors and will have a stable base on which to prevent injury and, if need be, properly and effectively recover from injury. Injuries are part of sport, especially contact sports. However, a strong and nurtured base that was not rushed into high-intensity training will be better able to withstand the vigor and intensity of competition and training.

When Are Children Ready for Competition?

In most cases, it is not the children who ask to enter competitions but rather the parents and coaches. Those who make decisions for children to participate in competitions should keep the following guidelines in mind.

- Enter children in competitions only when they are ready. This includes motivational readiness (i.e., they want to compete), demonstration of an appropriate skill level, and the motor abilities needed to be competitive.
- Ensure that the primary goals are to have fun; learn skills; and reach certain skill, tactical, or physical objectives, such as making five good passes during the game.
- For individual sports (e.g., running, swimming, rowing, or skiing), organize skills competitions in which whoever has the nicest skill wins. Emphasizing skills will benefit the athletes later, and it takes away the physiological stress of competitions and the need to train hard.
- Discourage children younger than seven or eight years of age from participating in organized competitions. They can test their skills in a noncompetitive environment. If they do participate in organized competition, stress having fun!
- Only at age 12 to 13 years do children understand the role of competition and what skills and abilities it takes to experience success or failure. Therefore, participation in organized competition should begin at age 11 or 12 years.

Table 9.1 illustrates some guidelines for the age of entering competitions and offers suggestions about the number of competitions per year in which athletes should participate. Note the difference between team and individual sports. For individual sports, the number refers to the number of starts (i.e., heats) and not the number of competitions. For example, in the 100-meter sprint there may be three heats per competition: heats, semifinals, and finals.

Preventing Stress and Burnout

Stress is usually perceived as an unpleasant emotional reaction to threatening situations or failure to meet performance expectations. Competitions expose young athletes to stress, especially for individual sports, in which teammates cannot share the stress. Regardless of the level of competition, excessive stress has negative consequences such as insomnia, loss of appetite, and sickness before competitions.

The pressure of winning, which comes from both parents and coaches, aggravates the degree of stress children experience. The stress level children experience is higher if the love and approval of parents is contingent on performing well. This pressure, coming from parents, coaches, and peers, is in most cases too much to cope with, especially for young children. Although training specialists and researchers often refer to the negative effects of competition stress, they do not often discuss the strain and pain children experience in the training sessions preceding important competitions. These workouts often produce negative effects similar to those of competitions. Moderate levels of stress, however, can provide a setting that enhances children's motivation and performance.

Table 9.1 Suggested Types and Number of Competitions

Age (yr)	Type of competitions	Organized competitions/yr
4-7	No formal competition—just for fun	—
8-11	Informal competitions—stress skill form rather than winning; participate in other sports just for fun	Team sports: 5-10
12-13	Organized competitions in which the goal is to achieve certain physical, technical, or tactical goals rather than winning	Team sports: 10-15 Individual sports: 5-8
14-16	Participate in competitions without pushing to reach the best performance possible	Team sports: 15-20 Individual sports: 8-10
17-19	Participate in junior competitions to qualify for state and national championships; get ready to reach peak performance at the senior competitions	Team sports: 20-35 Individual sports: short duration, 20-30; long duration, 6-8

Competition-related stress manifests before, during, and after competition.

- Precompetitive stress manifests in fears about not doing well, fear that one's contribution to the team's performance will not meet the expectations of teammates, sleeping disorders, restlessness, frequent urination, and diarrhea.
- During competition, stress manifests in fear of making mistakes, failure to take chances, poor performance due to high anxiety, sensitivity to coaches' or teammates' criticism, lack of energy, paleness, and trembling.
- Postcompetitive stress, which can occur after losing a game or after a poor performance, manifests in lethargy, depression, moodiness, irritability, isolating one's self from family and peers, lack of appetite, sleeping disorders, and lack of willingness to train or to show up for the next workout.

Burnout is the result of chronic stress induced by training and competitions. Symptoms of burnout include lack of energy, exhaustion, sleeplessness, irritability, physical ailments, headaches, anger, loss of confidence, depression, and a decrease in performance achievement. Some victims of burnout drop out from further participation in sport.

Athletes can prevent both stress and burnout to a high degree by using the following techniques (Rotella et al., 1991):

- Have a good time in training and competitions. Enjoy being with your friends and improving your skills. Set goals for yourself that are not directly related to the outcome of competition.
- Separate overall self-esteem from performance (especially for specific tasks). Failure to win the game does not rest strictly on you. Set goals for yourself that you can achieve. As long as you have achieved your own goals, be satisfied.

- Develop interests other than the chosen sport. Your life and satisfaction with life must not depend strictly on the performance you achieve in your sport. Have hobbies. Listen to music, paint, socialize, and find other reasons to be happy.
- Play a sport recreationally—just for the fun of it!
- Take time to relax and to enjoy family and friends.
- Remember that the sport is just a game.
- Learn to laugh at yourself, accept and learn from your errors and failures, and enjoy your successes. Sport is just one of many environments in which you are involved. A loss of a game can easily be offset by the satisfaction you have in other areas.

Coaches can help athletes avoid burnout by doing the following:

- Watch for the signs of staleness (i.e., lack of enthusiasm, irritability, decrease in performance).
- Provide variety and fun in training.
- Help the athletes have balance in their lives.
- Encourage athletes to have nonsport interests.
- Keep sport in perspective (for the athletes and yourself).
- Most importantly, emphasize the goal of doing certain skills well rather than performance.

Coaches can also help prevent stress and burnout by alternating training with other activities. Use tables 9.2 and 9.3 as guidelines for planning children's weekly activities.

Table 9.2 Weekly Schedule With Three Training Sessions

Monday	Tuesday	Wednesday	Thursday	Friday	Saturday	Sunday
Training	Free for socializing with friends	Training	Free for play and games	Training	Recreational sports or hobbies	Off

Table 9.3 Weekly Schedule With Four Training Sessions

Monday	Tuesday	Wednesday	Thursday	Friday	Saturday	Sunday
Training	Training	Free for socializing with friends	Training	Training	Recreational sports or hobbies	Off

chapter 10

Fueling the Young Athlete

Proper and progressive training starting at an early age is vital to performance and to the development of sport-specific strength, power, speed, endurance, and other motor abilities. Along with training, sound nutrition—a combination of foods we decide to feed our children and inevitably the foods they choose to eat—affects children's overall health on and off the field and helps shape their relationship with food as they mature into young adults. The young athlete's diet differs from that of adults. A young athlete's growing body needs an adequate amount of wholesome carbohydrate, a generous amount of lean protein, and a good source of fats. A young athlete's daily consumption of food should include 50 percent to 55 percent carbohydrate, 10 percent to 15 percent protein, and approximately 20 percent to 25 percent fat. A diet high in nutritious carbohydrate such as brown rice, pasta, whole-grain breads, vegetables, and legumes such as chickpeas and lentils is required for optimal energy and sport performance.

Furthermore, athletes must eat an adequate amount of lean protein from animal and plant sources in order to help the muscles recover from training and competition and to build stronger muscles and bones. Children should also consume good sources of fat such as fish; plants, such as avocados and coconut oil; nuts; and seeds to help develop the skin and hair and strengthen the immune system. Good sources of fat provide fuel for the athlete, insulate the organs, and move the important vitamins A, D, E, and K throughout the body. The bottom line: Young athletes need to eat real food and a variety of foods in adequate amounts. A balanced diet that is void of many processed foods will allow the athlete's body to train, perform, and recover well.

Performance relies on good nutrition. Athletes who eat poorly can feel fatigued, have insufficient fuel for training or competing, suffer from nutritional deficiencies, and jeopardize bone and muscle growth; this all inevitably affects performance. Parents and coaches can help shape the way kids eat and ultimately influence the foods that make up the majority of their diet. The proof is in the pudding (no pun intended). Kids who balance their diet with nutrient-dense foods report feeling better, stronger, and more energetic. It is up to the adult to provide the proper path to healthy eating. This chapter discusses five nutritional habits that can help shape young athletes who fully enjoy and appreciate the value of nutritious food, training, and sport.

Fueling Habit 1: Avoid Processed Foods

Is it possible to eat plenty of food and still not get the nutrients the body needs? The answer is an astounding *yes*. According to the American Heart Association, children in the United States eat seven times the recommended amount of extra sugar (i.e., sugar other than that naturally present in carbohydrate-rich foods such as fruits, oatmeal, bread, and so on) per day. This extra sugar provides no nutritional value, yet it fills the belly and prevents the child from wanting to eat foods that provide the nutritional support the body needs (Kavey et al., 2003; Gidding et al., 2005).

Many processed foods, such as snack bars, luncheon meats, white bread, convenience foods, and other "junk" foods, are filled with calories and are nutritionally poor. Most of these foods taste great and fill an athlete's belly but provide little vitamins and minerals (which help the body function optimally), protein, carbohydrate, and healthy fats (which aid in muscle growth, bone development, and recovery). Even some supposedly healthy food choices such as fruit juice, milk, yogurt, and cereals can be filled with added sugar, which outweighs the "nutritional" benefits of regularly eating these foods.

Many processed foods and junk food are also filled with sodium, sugar, and other chemicals that satisfy the palate and leave us wanting more. Unfortunately, convenience and lack of time have made junk and processed foods a staple of the American household. Avoiding processed foods is a challenge for both adults and children. It is much easier to toss a fruit-on-the-bottom yogurt in your lunch bag than to buy plain Greek yogurt, wash and cut some fruit, and place the fruit in a container to add to the yogurt later. To complicate things further, nutritionists often suggest adding healthy fats such as walnuts, almonds, or various seeds to your yogurt to add more nutrients. You would need to take a second container! The fruit-on-the-bottom yogurt with granola included in the container is much more appealing. Unfortunately, it comes with approximately three times the amount of sugar!

We once heard someone say that kids don't really like yogurt and that the entire "Don't eat yogurt with fruit on the bottom" argument isn't really an issue because kids aren't choosing this type of snack. The processed-food kings must have caught wind of that because it is no longer suggested that kids eat fruit-on-the-bottom yogurt. Instead, because kids are always on the run, why not give them the opportunity to run and eat at the same time? Hence, dairy shelves are filled with liquid yogurts that taste great and that kids can swallow directly from the cup—no mess, no fuss. Besides the extra calories from added sugar, fat, corn syrup, and other chemicals, the kids get some calcium and a bit of protein. What a deal!

As much as we would like to discuss the processed-food industry, childhood obesity, and how sugar is negatively affecting children both physically and mentally, the scope of this book is to help you train your athletes from early adolescence to the late teens. Part of the plan or training regimen includes adhering to a diet that promotes muscle and bone growth and provides a stable delivery of energy to help the athletes participate in numerous activities, recover well, and maintain a healthy body weight and body image as they mature to adulthood. Athletes need to eat, and they need to eat well. An average teenager can consume 2500 calories a day and maintain a healthy body weight, whereas an active teenager who plays two games and practices four times per week may require in excess of 5000 calories a day. Although the caloric requirements of these two teenagers may differ, their nutritional blueprint remains the same: They must eat foods that adequately provide the vital vitamins and minerals along with protein, carbohydrate, and fats that the body needs to function optimally. If they achieve their caloric needs by eating processed foods void of any nutritional value, they will feel low on energy, find it difficult to concentrate, and, for athletes, find both practice and competition fatiguing. Their diets must consist of whole foods—natural fruits, vegetables, oats, whole grains, and lean proteins—and meal plans that begin at home and can be consistently adapted to their life at school and extracurricular activities. Kids can't always eat at home, but they can bring the food values that were taught at home on the road with them.

Everything in Moderation?

We have all heard the saying that we should eat everything in moderation. Doing so can help us sustain a healthy body weight and prevent cravings or binging episodes that are created when we attempt to abstain from a particular food item. In other words, if you like ice cream, have it occasionally. Moderation may work for some adults, but it doesn't work for kids. Kids do not understand the concept of moderation because they are not hardwired to remember every morsel of food that they eat. Kids do not keep track of how many sodas, fruit juices, or cookies they have consumed. In addition, some kids don't handle sugar well and can develop allergies, get sick, or continue to crave unnatural sugary treats.

Parents need to decide what foods they will allow in their homes and what foods to avoid or eliminate altogether. Meals should always include real food choices, carbohydrate, protein, and vegetables. Processed food items such as ice cream, cookies, or other desserts are best consumed occasionally rather than in moderation. To some, the term *moderation* can mean chocolate chip cookies for breakfast, a double-chocolate granola bar for an afternoon snack, a bag of chips after school, and a soda with dinner. This is not moderation, but it is unfortunately part of the daily North American diet. It is best to choose a specific day of the week for kids to enjoy a dessert or treat, be it ice cream, cake, or other pleasure. Make it an event for the entire family to enjoy. Better to have a specific day that everyone can look forward to than to leave it up to chance—or, better yet, to moderation. During the rest of the week choose low-sugar alternatives for snacks. Make your own healthy cookies or cakes (with hidden goodies such as beets or avocado) or trail mix that includes dry fruit. Turn moderation into occasion to help the young athlete build a strong and healthy body.

A Word on Sodas

Soda is a processed food that provides absolutely no nutritional value and floods the body with a surge of sugar. Approximately one in five children consume excess calories from soda and other sugar-sweetened drinks (Rader et al., 2014). Males between the ages of 12 and 19 years consume approximately 12 percent of their total calories per day from sugar-sweetened beverages such as soda and juices (Miller et al., 2013). Soda should not be part of an athlete`s diet, either in moderation or on occasion. Studies have shown that soda consumption is linked to childhood obesity (Lim et al., 2009) and diabetes (Miller et al., 2013; Morgan, 2013) and that it can suppress the appetite of a growing child, thus preventing the child from eating vitamin- and protein-rich foods that the body needs. A can of soda can contain more than 50 milligrams of caffeine, a stimulant that can negatively affect a maturing brain (Miller et al., 2013). Furthermore, the acidic nature of soda and its lack of any nutritional quality can affect the alkaline balance of the body, causing inflammation and abdominal upset (Morgan, 2013). All of these consequences of drinking soda will prevent the young athlete from functioning at optimal levels and in fact can harm the athlete's long-term health. Although palatable and ingrained in the North America diet, soda is a health concern that should be eliminated from the young athlete's diet. Substitute soda with low-sugar sport drinks and flavored water to promote drinking and hydration.

Fueling Habit 2: Parents Control the Food Supply

Good nutrition begins at home. Most of us know and believe this, but the busyness of life has made food preparation and family meals very difficult to adhere to. It is not uncommon for most families to eat separately most days of the week. In today's fast-paced life, meal preparation is often reduced to takeout or simply defrosting some form of prepackaged meal.

Here is a typical scenario. Mom leaves work early to pick up the kid. The kid is starving—not because he hasn't eaten in hours or because he has been running around all afternoon but simply because he hasn't consumed the proper foods that satisfy his body's needs. Breakfast was fast and apparently healthy: a pack of instant honey-maple oatmeal and a glass of orange juice. By 10 a.m. the kid was hungry, so he opened his lunch bag and was happy to see a fruit granola bar, a small apple, and bag filled with jujubes. He wolfed down the bar, grabbed a handful of jujubes, and tossed the apple back in the bag for afternoon recess. At lunchtime the kid made his way to the cafeteria. It was pizza day, so he got a break from chicken fingers and fries. Two small slices of pepperoni pizza, a juice box, and a small chocolate chip cookie and the kid was satisfied. At recess the kid grabbed the apple and headed outside. He took a few barbeque potato chips from his friend's bag, kicked the ball around, and took a bite from his apple. When the bell rang and it was time to line up, the kid noticed that the apple was still in his hand, starting to turn brown and barely eaten. He tossed it in the garbage can as he walked inside the school. At 3:30 p.m. the kid waddles over to Mom's car and is starving. By this point in the day the kid has consumed approximately 1200 calories and 80 grams of added sugar. Amount of fiber, protein, whole-grain carbohydrate, and energy-fueling nutrients? Minimal. (Well, he did take a bite of the apple.)

We share this story not to make fun but rather to highlight a very important trend occurring in North America. Approximately one-third of children and adolescents in America eat fast food every single day. These foods, which include foods from hamburger, pizza and fried chicken establishments, are packed with fillers and inadequate and sometimes harmful foodstuffs that are robbing our children of the nutrients that are vital for growth and performance (Bowman et al., 2004). Between 1970 and 1990 the amount of high fructose corn syrup ingested went up 1000 percent (Bray et al., 2004)! The consumption of sugar and high fructose corn syrup continued to increase from 1990 to 2000, and use decreased slightly from 2000 to 2004 (Duffey and Popkin, 2008). By 2004 high fructose corn syrup provided approximately 8 percent of total daily energy intake, and total added sugar provided 17 percent of total daily energy intake (Duffey and Popkin, 2008). High fructose corn syrup is the primary ingredient in many processed foods and is used as an additive in many soft drinks. In fact, fast food and processed foods make up 16 percent to 17 percent of the total calorie intake for many teenage boys and girls (Sebastian et al., 2009). This number is alarming, especially as we battle childhood obesity and an increased risk of chronic disease. To make matters worse, dark-green and orange vegetables and legumes make up a very small portion of adolescents' vegetable intake (Kimmons et al., 2009).

Parents have a challenge. Not only do we have to sift through the marketing information bombarding television and the Internet, we also have to take the time to prepare and properly assess what we are feeding our families. We cannot take the word of food producers and advertisers about what we should be feeding our children. For example, a product that is gluten free may be loaded with additional sugar and other foodstuffs. Simply put, as parents we need to take charge and control the food supply. The best approach is to introduce whole foods for the entire family.

According to the United States Department of Agriculture (2015), kids between the ages of 6 and 18 years who eat foods away from home tend to eat at more fast-food outlets, restaurants, and schools compared to kids who eat at home. Furthermore, when dining out, kids are drinking greater amounts of soda, which is increasing the consumption of unnecessary and unhealthy sugar.

Back to our example from earlier, after Mom and the kid get home from school, the entire family can be out at various commitments within a few hours. Mom may drive Joey to soccer practice while Dad takes Lucy to her soccer game. Once again, the busyness of life makes proper meal preparation and planning extremely difficult, and parents succumb to the temptation of ordering out or simply defrosting a prepackaged frozen entree filled with sodium, sugar, and other unhealthy additives. As professionals in the field of athletic development, we see this all the time. Parents don't know how to overcome such a challenge and look to supplements and other nutritional products to help improve their children's nutrition. Although many products on the market—including multivitamins, low-sugar protein bars, and whey protein powder—can be useful for kids, these products should not be introduced until the kids are given an opportunity to eat healthier and truly taste and feel the difference of eating whole foods.

Building Your Food Supply

We have talked a lot about whole foods. In essence, whole foods are foods that are unprocessed and unrefined or have been processed very little—foods that nature has given us. Such foods are filled with protein, carbohydrate, and fats that our body tissues need in order to grow and regenerate. Many of these foods, especially an array of fruits, vegetables, and legumes, are filled with hundreds of vitamins and minerals that work together to sustain life and keep every cell healthy and nourished. If we take a look at a typical floor plan of a grocery store, the peripheral walls of the grocery are filled with whole foods—fruits, vegetables, lean protein, whole grains (e.g., rice, pasta, whole-grain breads), legumes (e.g., lentils, chickpeas), and nuts and seeds. As we look at the middle aisles of the store, we see an unending supply of refined and processed foods.

When building the food supply for your home, try to follow the 90–10 rule: Fill your cart with 90 percent whole foods and 10 percent processed foods (of course, you can go much lower than 10 percent)! We are also parents and grandparents, so we know and understand that going 100 percent whole food is impossible. Kids want to have some lunch meats, ice cream, and the occasional chocolate croissant, waffle, apple pie, chicken fingers, and, of course, fast-food treat! In addition, items such as wraps, various styles of whole-grain breads, and energy bars are not considered whole foods but can be part of a kid's diet—especially an active child whose energy intake needs to match his energy expenditure. We are not looking for perfection here, just the pursuit of perfection so that kids and parents alike can experience the energy that comes from eating right.

However, because whole foods are unprocessed and unrefined, it means that you have to take the time to prepare the foods! Grilled chicken with Greek salad is a wonderful meal, but someone needs to cut, clean, and cook the chicken; wash and dice the salad; and prepare the salad dressing. Similarly, a dish of pasta with lean meatballs and fresh tomato sauce is a wonderful Sunday lunch, but once again preparation is required. It is much easier to buy bottled tomato sauce and meatballs and simply boil the pasta, but with the convenience comes a significant price tag of more sodium, sugar, and chemical additives that increase shelf life. Besides that, you lose the opportunities to add your own vegetable blend and spices and to teach your kids the value of healthy home cooking. Kids are also able to enjoy a greater quantity of food when consuming whole foods because most whole foods are packed with fiber and protein, which satiate the appetite and prevent cravings for unhealthy snacks and beverages.

Table 10.1 lists whole foods from the different food groups. This list is not exhaustive; however, the important point is that all these foods are given to us by nature. Organic is arguably better when choosing many of these foods, but simply beginning to include a majority of these items in both meals and snacks is a great way to optimize your young athlete's health, energy, and recovery.

Planning Your Meals

We have all heard the saying "An ounce of prevention is worth a pound of cure." Although this statement is intended to emphasize the importance of maintaining a healthy lifestyle and preventing disease, it is also applicable to planning your meals. Eating is important—we need fuel on a daily basis—so meal preparation rightfully deserves the time and effort it requires. Without proper planning, we must resort to less healthy and sometimes harmful alternatives—harmful to the waistline, energy, digestion, and overall health. Because we cannot make more time, we must adequately plan to take more time, sometimes from other things, to make meal planning a priority. The following are some useful tips for properly planning and delivering high-quality meals for young athletes.

Make a list of items you need for the week, including all fruits, vegetables, legumes, whole grains, snack items, and lean proteins. If possible, include the kids in the shopping experience so they can understand the difference between a real food item and its prepackaged alternative.

Table 10.1 Whole Foods

Vegetables	Fruits	Nuts and seeds*	Grains	Dairy	Lean meats	Herbs and spices
• Asparagus • Celery • Peppers (multicolor) • Beets • Cucumber • Broccoli • Cauliflower • Eggplant • Spinach • Squash • Sweet potatoes • Onions (all types) • Kale	• Blueberries (fresh or frozen) • Apples • Oranges • Raspberries (fresh or frozen) • Strawberries (fresh or frozen) • Cantaloupe • Watermelon • Grapefruit • Peaches • Plums • Bananas • Mango • Coconut	• Almonds (no salt) • Cashews (no salt) • Walnuts • Pumpkin seeds • Sunflower seeds	• Brown rice • Wild rice • Millet • Oats • Quinoa (really a seed) • Whole-grain pasta	• Eggs (free range) • Low-fat cheese • Organic milk • Yogurt (Greek and plain)	• Grass-fed chicken, beef, lamb, and turkey	• Cinnamon • Turmeric • Cumin • Cilantro • Coriander • Peppermint • Rosemary • Thyme

* You can also get both seeds and nuts in a spread that is great on breads, wraps, and fruit.

To help make your food list, think about what meals you would like to prepare during the week. Start with Monday, keeping in mind the family's work and school commitments. Remember that dinner preparation is the best time to also prepare lunch for the next day. Leftover dinner makes a healthy and satiating lunch.

Include one whole food in each meal—breakfast, lunch, dinner, and snacks. This will help reduce the amount of processed foods your family consumes and ensure that a nutritious portion of whole food is included in every meal. For instance, breakfast on the run may include a granola bar with a banana or apple, and afternoon snack can be a cup of yogurt and a handful of homemade trail mix (cashews, almonds, sunflower seeds, and raisins). Adding whole foods to the three main meals of the day is easy once you get the hang of it. In fact, if you simply make the commitment to remove processed and prepackaged food and fast-food items, all you are left with is whole foods!

Whole foods require preparation time. Once you make your meal list, try to arrange sometime on the weekend for meal preparation. Wash all the fruit and place it in the refrigerator so the kids can easily access it. Buy fruits in season so you always have variety. Wash and prepare the vegetables and place them in containers so you can easily place them in the kids' lunch or toss them into a stir fry. Wash and cut the lean meats and marinate them in the refrigerator for a day or two so that you can simply place them in the oven or on the grill. Finally, if you take the time to make sauces or chili, make extra and freeze the leftovers. This will help during busy periods when you just don't have time to prepare a good meal and are tempted to pick up the phone and order a pepperoni pizza. We generally tell our athletes' parents to try to position themselves so that they go out for dinner or get takeout because they want to eat that particular food, not because of a lack of foresight in preparation.

You, the parent, are in charge, so make the list and stick to it. Try different recipes and various food combinations. If your kids just don't like vegetables, dress them up. If you have to use dips or a store-bought salad dressing they like, so be it. They are eating their vegetables and getting the necessary fiber and nutrients they need. More important, they are eating whole foods, which will slowly but surely change their palates to desire those types of foods. We don't have to follow a law of all or nothing—whole foods in and everything else out—when it comes to changing how we eat. What is important is that every meal has a whole-food component; that most meals are prepared at home; and that kids understand that eating vital fruits, vegetables, and lean proteins will help them get stronger, feel better, and improve their focus and concentration. If kids see your excitement about creating a new path for the entire family, they will also get excited about the results. It starts at home and it begins with the parents. You control the food supply.

If you are not much of a cook or if your kids have specific food allergies or intolerances and you feel it is difficult to prepare food for them, find an easy-to-follow cookbook that addresses their needs. Many books available in the marketplace address food allergies and specific food preferences, including vegetarian meals. Buying gluten-free snacks, prepackaged lean proteins, and sauces is an easy alternative, but unfortunately most of these foods are filled with additives and chemicals.

When possible, it is best for families to eat together so that both kids and teenagers understand the value of eating from a diverse menu and the importance of eating prepared food versus prepackaged or fast food. Also, the dinner table offers a good opportunity to discuss athletic goals and how proper eating can help build a stronger and healthier body. Taking control of the food supply is not about setting restrictive rules, which will most likely backfire. Rather, it is about demonstrating to your young athletes the inherent quality of real food and nature's intention in creating it.

Fueling Habit 3: Always Start With a Wholesome Breakfast

The word *breakfast* is a combination of two words, *break* and *fast*. Because you are sleeping and in essence fasting for 8 to 10 hours during the night (unless, of course, you get up to have a snack), the first food you place in your mouth is considered breaking the fast. Breakfast!

In adults, the importance of eating breakfast first thing in the morning has been challenged in the literature (Halberg et al., 2005; Karli et al., 2007) and in trade publications. A new wave of thought argues for extending the fast and possibly skipping breakfast altogether to further stimulate hormonal changes that elicit greater gains in lean muscle mass and improvements in body composition and health. We mention this only for the benefit of coaches and parents who may be aware of the current literature or theories on fasting and wonder whether they may be applicable to young athletes. The answer is no, they are not.

Young athletes require fuel upon rising and need to have a healthy, wholesome breakfast. Many studies have shown that nutritional deficiencies and poor eating habits established during adolescence can have detrimental consequences on health in adulthood (Daniels et al., 2002; Ogden et al., 2002). After 8 to 12 hours of sleep and fasting, a child's glycogen stores are very low. Without eating a proper breakfast she can feel lethargic, lack concentration, and not be able to keep up with the activity level required in school.

Of the many reasons children give for skipping breakfast, the main reasons are that they have no time or are not hungry when they wake up (Vanelli et al., 2005). Both reasons are legitimate because, once again, the busyness of life and the demands of work and school chisel away the time available to eat a proper breakfast in the morning. Also, kids may eat a late-night snack, which explains why they are not hungry when waking up. We suggest that parents omit the late-night snack and encourage their children to eat a well-balanced breakfast in the morning. This is important for two reasons: First, eating late at night can interrupt sleep patterns and prevent a restful sleep, and second, the snack may not be nutritionally dense or calorically balanced. In essence, the late-night snack may prevent the child from eating breakfast because he is still satiated upon waking, and when he gets hungry later in the morning he may grab a sugar- and fat-filled snack that is calorically dense, nutritionally empty (Nicklas et al., 2000), and void of the many vitamins and minerals that are required for growth and maturation.

Young athletes of all ages need to start the day with a healthy breakfast, and parents need to set the example. On weekends, or even during the week if time allows, parents are encouraged to sit down to eat with their children or simply create an environment in which breakfast is an important part of the day. The start needs to be nutritious!

When most people think of breakfast, the first thing that comes to mind is cereal. Breakfast can involve much more than sugary cereals, such as healthy smoothies, plain yogurt and fruit, eggs and toast, oatmeal, healthy granola bars, and some energy or protein bars. Also, fresh fruit is great first thing in the morning. Besides being packed with much-needed vitamins and minerals, bananas, blueberries, apples, cantaloupe, and watermelon are filled with fiber and provide immediate energy.

One study looked at the marketing and advertising messages of various cereal brands, which are energy dense and nutrient poor. Children viewed 1.7 cereal advertisements per day; 87 percent of these ads promoted high-sugar products, many of which are available at the local grocery store. Furthermore, 91 percent of these ads ascribed extraordinary attributes to these cereal products, and 67 percent showed both healthy and unhealthy eating patterns (LoDolce et al., 2013).

It is no wonder that children—even young athletes in the athletic formation stage—often ask for a particular high-sugar cereal for breakfast. Children who eat a breakfast that is low in sugar and higher in fiber show better memory and attention span and fewer signs of frustration two to three hours after eating (Benton et al., 2007). If an athlete wants cereal, look for one that has less than 10 grams of sugar and at least 4 grams of fiber per 1-cup or 8-ounce serving. Because these cereals lack the sugar content that gives them their palatable appeal (some breakfast cereals contain 19-24 grams of sugar per 1-cup serving!), athletes can use vanilla whey protein power or vanilla almond milk (sweetened or unsweetened) to add taste. If your child is lactose intolerant, you can choose a plant-based protein powder and dress the cereal with some coconut or nuts for taste.

Although it is always best to consume protein from whole foods, protein powders (in particular whey protein, a by-product of milk production) are great for increasing protein intake, helping the body recover from exercise, and strengthening the immune system (Krissansen, 2007). Because children tend to get enough protein from whole-food sources, protein powders can be used as supplements and added to shakes or cereals in small quantities. Parents and coaches should do research and choose a good-quality brand of protein powder to guarantee that the manufacturing standards meet or exceed the necessary guidelines of production and that the protein powders do not contain any chemicals or by-products that can elicit an allergic response.

You may also choose to make your own nutritionally dense, high-fiber, vitamin-packed cereal for the entire family to enjoy. Because the recipe is low in sugar, you may choose to add flavor by adding any of your favorite toppings, including fresh fruit, seeds, nuts, raisins, and coconut. Refer to table 10.2 for a healthy cereal recipe.

Make Breakfast a Priority

Make breakfast a habit for the young athlete. As with every meal or snack, the athlete does not need to gorge himself. This isn't about eating as much food as you can, regardless of its nutritional status, but rather about eating a balanced meal that includes foods from at least three of the five food groups (grains, fruits, vegetables, protein, and dairy)—real foods that are filled only with the sugar that nature intended! At least attempt to decrease the amount of added sugar by choosing breakfast items that are more nutritionally sound and packed with vitamins, minerals, and fiber. Taste is important, of course, so make better food choices and strive for balance.

Table 10.2 Cereal Recipe

Combine 1 c.* of each of the following:

- Organic quinoa puff or flakes
- Rolled oats
- Kasha
- Sliced almonds

Mix ingredients with 5 Tbsp. (75 ml) of olive oil in a large baking pan.
Roast in the oven at 350 °F for 20 min or until browned.
Before eating, add some of your favorite toppings: flax seed, chia, cinnamon, shaved coconut, dried cranberries, raisins, or fresh fruit (e.g., blueberries, bananas).
Add the cereal mixture to yogurt, milk, almond milk, or rice milk.

*Begin with 1 c. Once you find the correct mixture for you, add as many cups as you would like. Once cereal cools, place in mason jars or containers. Eat for breakfast or snack.

Start every morning with one or more of the following options:

A smoothie. Use 1 cup (236 ml) of water, skim milk, almond milk (sweetened or unsweetened), or fresh orange juice. Depending on the protein intake of the child and any dietary restriction such as dairy, nut, or legume allergies, you can also add a tablespoon of whey protein powder or a plant alternative. For example, a 12-year-old boy weighing 100 pounds (45 kg) would require approximately .45 gram of protein per pound of body weight per day; this equals approximately 45 grams of protein per day. If we assume that the boy eats three meals a day, he would require around 15 grams of protein per meal in order to fulfill his daily requirements. Therefore, a breakfast smoothie or shake would be an ideal way to incorporate a good-quality protein powder. Given that a scoop of commercial protein powder (around 23-26 grams of powder per scoop) contains approximately 18 grams of protein, using half a scoop of protein powder would yield around 7 to 9 grams of protein, which would complement a milk-, water-, or juice-based smoothie. Add fruit of your choice plus nuts, seeds, or a teaspoon of almond butter. The smoothie combinations are endless. It is not necessary that protein powders be added to smoothies. In fact, protein powders are useful to supplement a diet lacking in protein but need not become a general staple in a young athlete's daily diet. What is important is that all smoothies include a protein base (i.e., milk, yogurt, or whey protein powder), some fresh fruit, and a nut or seed butter for some essential fats. We have heard of many cases in which parents or athletes with good intentions made a smoothie that was too high in sugar and lacked the necessary fat and protein to create a well-balanced, slowly digestible meal. Avoid making a smoothie that includes only fruit and fruit juices and is void of any other nutritional component.

Eggs of your choice (e.g., scrambled, poached, boiled). Eggs are packed with protein and nutrients and are fairly inexpensive when compared with other proteins. Brown and white eggs look different, but they have the exact same nutritional content. You may choose free-range eggs, but know that the term *free range* means that the hens had access to a running area outdoors; it doesn't mean that the hens actually did run freely. If you live near a farm or farmers' market, buy local eggs and your eggs will be healthier and more nutrient dense. Compared with eggs from the grocery store, the yolks of eggs from local farmers tend to be larger, darker, and more orange. You may also choose to buy eggs that have a higher content of omega-3 fatty acids. Prepare the eggs any way you like and enjoy nature's goodness. Athletes can eat their eggs with a side of grains (e.g., oats, whole-wheat bread, or whatever bread they like). However, athletes should avoid white bread if possible or simply have it on rare occasions. As a rule of thumb, if you can roll a slice of bread into a ball and it retains its shape, it's probably not very healthful. Add some fruit or slices of tomato or avocado and you have a wonderful breakfast that is fast, easy to make, and filled with protein, vitamins, and minerals.

Oatmeal and fruit. Oatmeal is packed with fiber, antioxidants, and minerals such as magnesium, phosphorous, selenium, and copper. Try to stay away from instant oatmeal, which comes in flavors such as brown sugar, maple honey, and apple cinnamon. Although instant oatmeal tastes great, it is often packed with sugar, thus negating the true nutritional benefits of eating a wholesome bowl of oatmeal. Oatmeal can be cooked in water or milk and doesn't have to be dry and tasteless. Add cinnamon or a bit of natural maple sugar to sweeten it, or add some unsweetened applesauce or fresh berries. Pure oatmeal is gluten free, but sometimes oatmeal is made in facilities that also process wheat, so some cross-contamination may occur. Look for brands that are gluten free and make oatmeal a staple breakfast option. Use oats to make healthy muffins or use them in smoothies (just throw them in raw) to add texture.

It is very common these days to add protein powder to smoothies for a bit of a protein blast. Ever-popular smoothie and juice outlets offer to add a scoop of protein to any of their products. Protein powder is an easy and fast way to give your body a high-protein boost and is easily digestible. When preparing a protein smoothie for breakfast or as a snack for the young athlete, be aware of the athlete's total protein requirements based on their age and body weight. Too little protein can weaken the muscles and harm cell growth, whereas too much protein can place stress on the kidneys and be converted to fat. Although the effect of too much protein on the kidneys in adults is a contentious research issue, the effect of excess protein on young athletes is unclear. For this reason, a thoughtful balance is required. Once you have calculated the approximate amount of protein required per day for the young athlete, try to spread the protein intake among three meals and a couple snacks. Table 10.3 presents a recipe for a whey protein smoothie. This recipe is appropriate for some athletes in the late athletic formation stage and beyond. For younger athletes, modify the amount of protein to a half scoop and add or remove as needed. This will allow younger athletes to benefit from the wonderful nutritional value of this quick breakfast alternative.

A Word on Protein

Protein is found in many foods, including meats, dairy, legumes, grains, and some vegetables. We need protein to build muscles, strengthen the immune system, and help recovery. Since resistance training increases the body's demand for protein for recovery, regeneration, and muscle growth, protein supplements are hyped as a method for increasing the protein demand by making a good source of protein easily available. It can be a challenge to eat enough food to meet the body's demand for calories and protein or to find better food sources. Protein shakes have become very popular among athletes, bodybuilders, and recreational fitness enthusiasts because they are easy to digest and fulfill the athletes' protein requirements. Protein shakes are easy to make and come in many varieties. Whey protein powder is a high-quality protein that is easily absorbed except in those who are lactose intolerant or have a milk allergy. Whole food should always be the primary choice to guarantee intake of a range of amino acids (protein building blocks) and other nutritional components. However, for variety, taste, or simplicity, the young athlete can use whey protein powder or a plant-based protein as part of her nutrition plan. We recommended that young athletes eat whole foods to meet the bulk of their

Table 10.3 Whey Protein Smoothie

This whey protein smoothie is packed with dairy, fruit, and grains to provide the energy, protein, vitamins, and minerals the body needs to adequately grow and thrive in schoolwork, fun, and sport.

- 1 c. (236 ml) of skim milk, water, or almond milk (unsweetened or sweetened)
- 1 scoop of high-quality whey protein powder or 1 scoop of plant-based protein
- A few ice cubes (optional—gives the smoothie a thick texture)
- 1 small banana
- 1/2 c. (75 g) of blueberries or fruit of choice (frozen or fresh)
- 1 scoop (use of the protein scoop) of uncooked rolled oats (optional—gives the smoothie a nice texture)
- 1 tsp. (approximately 5 g) of flax seed (optional)

Place in blender and mix for 20 to 40 seconds or until desired texture is achieved. Enjoy!

nutritional needs and use protein powders sparingly as a way to add more protein to the overall diet or to supplement—not replace—a particular meal.

Before deciding on the protein needs of an athlete and how to meet those needs, it is important to take a look at the protein requirements for different age groups (see table 10.4). According to the Centers for Disease Control and Prevention (2015), protein requirements vary with age.

- Boy and girls aged 4 to 8 years (initiation stage) require 19 grams per day.
- Girls in the athletic formation stage and specialization stage require approximately 46 grams per day.
- Boys in the athletic formation stage and specialization stage require approximately 56 grams per day.

For a more specific calculation, you can calculate the recommended daily allowance (RDA) of protein according to the age and body weight of your young athlete (see How Much Protein Do I Need? at www.cdc.gov/nutrition/everyone/basics/protein.html). Protein requirements can then be matched to the approximate stage of athletic development (introduced in chapter 2).

The RDA provides a general guideline for protein consumption per pound of body weight. We suggest that you follow the recommendations for athletes in the initiation and athletic formation stages of development but allow for a higher total protein content for athletes in the specialization and high-performance stages of development. Studies have demonstrated that the protein requirements for young athletes who are involved in intensive training may be higher than those suggested by the RDA (Boisseau et al., 2002, 2007). Athletes in the specialization stage of development can increase the protein requirements to .55 gram per pound of body weight for strength sports and .45 gram per pound of body weight for endurance sports. Depending on the level of maturation, strength athletes in the late specialization stage and high performance stage can increase protein requirements to .75 gram per pound of body weight, whereas endurance athletes aim for .55 gram per pound of body weight.

For example, a strength athlete who weighs 180 pounds (81.6 kg) would require 135 grams of protein per day (180 × .75 = 135 grams). This may appear to be a large number. However, by spreading out the protein intake throughout the day, starting with a protein-rich breakfast and aiming for 20 to 30 grams of protein per meal, the athlete can meet the requirements needed for muscle growth, recovery, and performance improvements.

Table 10.4 Protein Needs by Stage of Athletic Development

Age (yr)	Protein (g/lb of body weight)	Stage of athletic development
4-7	.5	Initiation
8-14	.45	Initiation/athletic formation
15-18	.4	Specialization
18+	.36	High performance

Fueling Habit 4: Properly Fuel the Body Before and After Competition

Fueling the body both before and after a competition is no different than the normal balanced approach to eating. The foods are still high in wholesome carbohydrate, lean protein, and heart-healthy fats that occur naturally in nuts, seeds, fish such as salmon and tuna, and oils such as olive oil and coconut oil. What changes is when, where, and how to eat these foods.

Pregame Meal

We often get asked what a young athlete should eat before a game or competition. Regardless of the sport, all young athletes need to fuel their bodies with the right combination of carbohydrate, protein, and fats before a game. The athletes don't need to engage in "carbohydrate loading." Simply eating a balanced meal at least three hours before the game will top up the energy stores, allow time for digestion, and prepare the body for competition. Because a game places a lot of stress on the heart to pump blood to the working muscles, you don't want to slow down the body by diverting blood to the stomach for digestion.

Here are some tips for planning your pregame meal.

Between 50 percent and 60 percent of the meal should include high-carbohydrate foods such as whole-wheat or white pasta, whole-grain breads, brown or white rice, or quinoa. Pasta should not make up the entire meal—you need to include some vegetables and lean protein. A good pregame meal would include whole-wheat pasta with marinara sauce, four to six ounces (113-170 g) of grilled chicken breast, and broccoli or cauliflower on the side.

The athlete should eat as much food as he normally eats—no more and no less. Eat until satisfied and that is it. Game day is not a good time to eat more food than the body is accustomed to. Doing so can irritate the digestive system and cause stomach upset. After the pregame meal, simply have a piece of fruit and sip from a sport drink as game time approaches. Hunger is relatively at bay and the athlete is focused on the game.

Certain foods may need to be eliminated from the pregame meal, even if the foods are part of the athlete's daily nutrition plan. Foods that are high in fiber or fat should be avoided because they are slower to digest and can irritate the bowels, causing stomach upset. For instance, legumes such as chickpeas, lentils, or kidney beans are great sources of carbohydrate and protein but can cause gas and stomach distress. Similarly, high-fat foods such as a hamburger and fries, fried eggs and toast, or beef or pork should be avoided in the pregame meal. Table 10.5 lists foods that are good to eat before a game and foods you should avoid eating at least three hours before a game. The list is not exhaustive but rather is simply a reference tool. Each body reacts differently to various foods and food combinations regardless of nutritional value.

As a rule of thumb, remember these 10 basic steps to pregame meal planning:

1. Choose foods rich in carbohydrate, including pasta, whole-grain breads, cereals, and rice.
2. Include vegetables that you are accustomed to eating and generally cause little, if any, gas or bloating.

Table 10.5 Foods to Eat and Foods to Avoid Pregame

Eat*	Avoid
Whole-wheat or white pasta with marinara	Fruit juices (don't need the added sugar)
Brown or white rice	Processed luncheon meats (high in sodium)
Whole-grain bread or pitas	Fried foods of any kind
Grilled or baked chicken	High-fiber legumes: lentils, chickpeas, and kidney beans
Potatoes, sweet potatoes, or yams	
Poached, scrambled, or boiled eggs	Spices of any kind
Oatmeal	Soft drinks or carbonated drinks
Fresh fruit: bananas, apples, blueberries, strawberries, grapes	Red meat or pork
Fresh vegetables: broccoli, cauliflower, cucumber, fennel, zucchini	Protein bars or protein shakes (try to eat real food for the pregame meal)
Whole-wheat bagels	Candy or chocolate bars
Jams, almond butter, and peanut butter	Hamburger, fries, or pizza (homemade pizza or vegetable pizza with little cheese is fine)
Dairy: milk and plain yogurt	
Salmon and tuna	Cake, pie, and cookies

* Combine some of these foods to create a meal.

3. Avoid spices of any kind, especially hot spices such as curry, turmeric, or cayenne pepper.
4. Avoid fried foods of any kind, including fried eggs and meats.
5. Avoid soft drinks and carbonated drinks because these may cause abdominal distress and gas.
6. Avoid desserts of any kind.
7. Eat the same amount you are accustomed to eating at everyday meals.
8. Drink plenty of water.
9. If possible, avoid eating on the run or in the car. Try to take your time and eat while seated.
10. Eat real food and save the protein bars or snacks for postgame meals.

Questions: Food for Thought?

What foods are safe to eat immediately before a competition? Inevitably, some athletes will feel hungry an hour or two before the game. In this instance, athletes can have a light snack such as fruit or crackers with a tablespoon of peanut or almond butter. If an athlete ate a proper pregame meal at least three hours before the game, he should feel satiated. It is better to eat a bit more at the pregame meal and avoid the snack so that the body can focus on directing blood to the working muscles and not to digestion.

How Do You Properly Eat for an All-Day Tournament?

The pregame principles discussed earlier still apply. The athlete is encouraged to have a suitable and nutritious pregame meal at least three hours before the game. If the first game is at 9 a.m., it is best that the athlete have a meal that is lighter than normal around 6:30 or 7 a.m. Because the first game is relatively early in the day, the athlete needs to top up the fuel sources and rely on the energy stored from the previous day. A bagel with peanut butter or scrambled eggs and toast is enough to get him through the first game. Then, when the first game is complete, the athlete can eat a more suitable meal of carbohydrate, protein, and fat (as discussed earlier) to help fuel his body for the next game. Pack a few chicken or tuna wraps, some precut vegetables, and fresh fruit for the day. You can also pack some light snacks such as granola or protein bars, water, and sport drinks to help sustain energy throughout the tournament. It is important that the athlete eat carbohydrate-rich foods and continue to eat throughout the day—even if he is not hungry—to prevent a crash in energy. Remember that a high-protein, low-carbohydrate diet is not for young athletes. Young athletes need carbohydrate to sustain energy. If athletes venture to a restaurant between games, they should avoid fast food and fried meals and instead choose a meal that is high in carbohydrate. Choose pasta with chicken, pancakes, waffles, and other starchy foods that are easily digested and that quickly replenish energy stores.

Is It Important to Drink Sport Drinks During Competitions?

For games lasting 60 minutes or less, young athletes should continue to hydrate with water. It is important that athletes continue to sip water before and during the game to regulate body temperature and help the muscles work optimally. After spending hours training, you don't want fatigue or muscle cramps to negatively affect performance because the body is dehydrated. Drink plenty of water as part of a training lifestyle and continue to drink on game days.

If a game lasts for more than 60 minutes or the athlete is participating in a long-distance sport such as cross country or swimming, sport drinks can help replenish and balance electrolytes, including potassium and sodium, both of which are important for muscle function. Choose a brand that is relatively low in sugar and sip throughout the game. If you want to avoid giving the athlete a full bottle of a sport drink, simply dilute the drink by adding water so the athlete will be inclined to drink more of the fluid before, during, and after the game. During a day-long tournament consisting of multiple games, sport drinks can help prevent blood sugar levels from dipping and causing premature fatigue. Drink responsibly!

Eat a Postgame Snack Within 30 Minutes

The soccer match or hockey game is over. The kids are sweating and tired but fired up with excitement and adrenaline. They are still focused on the game and burning off steam by discussing certain plays, goals, and questionable calls by the referee. As they come off the ice or field they don't feel immediate hunger. However, they have depleted their energy stores and their muscles are ready for protein to help them recover. It is very common at the community-sport level, especially for athletes in the initiation stage and early years of the athletic formation stage, to be given snacks at the end of a sporting event. These snacks usually include some high fructose drink and dessert-type bar, cookie, or cake.

These items are high in sugar and will quickly absorb into the body. However, the body requires a good dose of protein within 30 minutes of the end of a game. Within this 30-minute window the body's ability to replenish energy stores and aid in muscle recovery is optimal, especially when carbohydrate is consumed along with protein. So, if your young athletes are given high-sugar treats, let them eat them to get the recovery process going, but instead of fruit juices or sugar-filled sodas, bring them a 250-milliliter (1-cup) container of skim or even chocolate milk to make sure that they are getting an adequate amount of protein immediately after the game. A 236-milliliter (1-cup) glass of milk contains approximately 8 grams of protein and a good amount of amino acids (building blocks of protein) to aid in muscle building. For a postgame treat, athletes in the initiation and athletic formation stages of development can eat a bagel with cream cheese or peanut butter, some dried fruit, and a glass of plain or chocolate milk. Young athletes in the late athletic formation and specialization stages of development can drink a protein shake similar to the one described in table 10.3, which provides a good dose of carbohydrate and protein. If you don't want to blend the protein drink before the game, simply pack some milk or orange juice in a cooler and place a scoop of protein powder in a container. After the game, mix the powder with the juice. You can also pack a bagel with peanut butter, some crackers, or fresh fruit to complement the protein shake. Athletes in the initiation stage of development can aim to consume between 8 and 10 grams of protein, such as a glass of milk or 1 cup (250 g) of Greek yogurt, after a game, whereas athletes in the athletic formation and specialization stages can aim for 10 to 20 grams of protein within 30 minutes after the game. As mentioned, all protein should be complemented with a good dose of carbohydrate.

Eat a Postgame Meal Within One to Two Hours After Competition

The athlete ate a small snack containing protein and carbohydrate after the game and now it is time to eat a more robust meal. Hours after a game, the body is still healing, replenishing, and growing. Proper care should be taken to ensure that a wholesome amount of carbohydrate, protein, and fats is eaten one to two hours after the game. If the ride home from the game is long, it is best to pack chicken or egg sandwiches or wraps for the car ride home in order to avoid having to stop at a fast-food restaurant because the athlete is famished. If there is time to eat a meal at home, the balanced approach to eating remains. A meal should include a grouping of complex carbohydrate such as rice or pasta, some grilled chicken or fish, and a good helping of vegetables. Like always, eat to the point of satiation and snack with nuts, seeds, dried fruit, and fresh fruit between meals.

Fueling Habit 5: Know Your Athlete

Hundreds of books and articles have been written about sport nutrition and about the need to properly fuel the young athlete with wholesome carbohydrate, lean proteins, and good fats. However, like most kids, these young athletes can be picky eaters and unfortunately have developed a palate for processed and fast-food items that provide a hefty amount of calories, chemicals, and sugars but very little in total-body nutrition. Of course parents want to provide a variety of foods for their children to eat and plan meals that include a balance of healthy carbohydrate, protein, and vegetables. But, more often than not, kids are determined to eat their own way and thus leave plates filled with good food and opt for chicken fingers and fries or frozen pizza. Growing bodies need good, sound nutrition. The question is how we as parents and coaches overcome these barriers and help athletes understand how eating well corresponds to growing well and, ultimately, performing well.

A study conducted in Australia (Odea, 2003) had students in grades 2 through 11 (ages 7-17 years) identify the perceived benefits of and barriers to healthy eating and physical activity and suggest strategies for overcoming barriers. Table 10.6 shows the results of this study.

Table 10.6 Perceived Benefits and Barriers to Healthy Eating and Physical Activity

Healthy eating		Physical activity	
Benefits	**Barriers**	**Benefits**	**Barriers**
Improvements in cognitive and physical performance	Convenience	Social benefits	Prefer indoor activities instead of outdoor activities
Improvements in fitness	Taste	Enhancement of psychological status	Lack of energy
Improvements in endurance	Social factors	Physical sensation	Lack of motivation
Psychological benefits		Sport performance	Time constraints
Feeling good physically			Social factors
Strategies for overcoming barriers			
Support from parents and school staff			
Better planning and time management			
Self-motivation			
Education			
Restructuring the physical environment			
Greater variety of physical activities			

Adapted from J.A. Odea, 2003, "Why do kids eat healthful food? Perceived benefits of and barriers to healthful eating and physical activity among children and adolescents," *Journal of the American Dietetic Association* 103(4): 497-501.

Although this study was conducted on Australian children, it provides a framework for understanding and acknowledging the benefits of eating well and physical activity. Children in this study understood the benefits of healthy eating, including feeling good physically and psychologically. However, although armed with an understanding of why certain foods are better for health than others, they cite convenience and taste as two barriers to eating well. As adults, we are expected to, and can, overlook the taste or texture of certain foods for the greater good of our health. We may dislike vegetables but eat them anyway. Some of us may even purchase a salad greens mixture or supplement with multivitamins to make sure we are getting our daily amounts of important vitamins and minerals. This may not be the case with children. Although kids understand the importance of eating whole-grain pasta and Brussels sprouts, unless the foods are prepared a certain way or smothered in a certain sauce they would rather starve than eat the food parents have prepared. But they are smart enough to know that they will not starve because the pantry is filled with delicious snacks that claim to be gluten free, fat free, lean, heart healthy, and, our favorite, filled with "wholesome goodness"—if you remove the 25 grams of sugar per serving, of course!

Table 10.6 lists time management, support from parents and school staff, and education as three of the six suggested strategies for overcoming barriers. All three strategies are pivotal to helping kids become better eaters and lovers of healthy foods. Life is hectic and is showing no signs of slowing down. Busyness has encroached on the household and has affected how families dine. After a busy day at work, neither Mom nor Dad want to spend time preparing and cooking a healthy meal. It is much more convenient and palatable to eat a charbroiled hamburger and fries than to grill some chicken and steam asparagus and sweet potatoes. After a long and stressful day, the burger sounds better!

But it isn't. A young athlete's body needs the proper nourishment that comes from lean protein and nature's multivitamins—numerous forms of vegetables that are filled with fiber and life-giving antioxidants.

How do we bridge the gap between knowing and doing? The first step is to take inventory of your young athlete. Ask yourself a few questions:

1. What does he or she like to eat?
2. What does he or she need to eat more of?
3. What is he or she eating too much of?
4. How can we work as a family to better prepare meals and snacks so that healthy eating becomes a priority?

Once you have answers to these questions you can better set a nutritional plan and help educate your young athlete about the importance of eating well. A few years ago we were coaching a group of 11-year-old soccer players. One of the fathers took a few moments at the end of practice to speak with us about proper nutrition for his son. His son was a typical 11-year-old boy who loved to play sports, was athletic, and detested vegetables or meat that he couldn't smother with ketchup. His father was having a tough time convincing him of the importance of eating better and decreasing the amount of sodas and prepared snacks he consumed on a daily basis. The problem was that this athlete was fit, healthy, and strong. How do you convince a boy who looks and feels healthy that he should be eating better when he is already experiencing exactly what healthy food is supposed to give you? The kid was reluctant to change his current diet. We asked the father to think about something extrinsic and tangible that would motivate his son to change. He later sent us an e-mail stating that he had found a video interview online in which one of his son's favorite European soccer players discussed what he eats before and after a game and how he eats very "clean." He shared the video with his son and was pleased by how receptive his son was to understanding the value of nutrition and performance. His son came to believe that the professionals eat well, and he wanted to be like them. Furthermore, his father kept emphasizing a major point to his son: "If you can be that fit and athletic by eating poorly, imagine how much better you will feel and perform if you begin to fuel your body with powerful foods."

You know your young athlete well. Take a moment to think about the changes she may need to make and consider some possible solutions. Remember, we are not looking for perfection in eating but rather the pursuit of perfection, and this can occur in small, subtle steps. Here are a few tips that have worked for some of our athletes and their families.

Discuss with the athlete the benefits of eating well, especially during training. Discuss how giving the body the proper nutrients to grow stronger and move faster will elevate her game.

If lack of time is the main issue with food preparation and you find yourself scrambling to put together a nutritious meal, then forward thinking is the key. Take one day a week to organize the meals for the upcoming week. Cook a batch of tomato sauce or chili and freeze it in mini containers so that you can easily defrost it when needed.

Grilling is a great way to incorporate vegetables and protein into meals. You can also grill chicken, beef, or other meat and freeze it in a vacuum pack for later use. Yes, even barbecued chicken can be prepared and frozen. That way, when you are in need of a healthy meal, you can simply defrost the meat and heat it when you get home from work.

Toss a lean meat and some vegetables in a slow cooker in the morning before you leave for work. Many good cookbooks containing recipes for both vegetarian and lean-meat dishes are available. Planning ahead and purchasing the ingredients are the vital steps.

Prepare great snacks that satiate your young athlete and provide the essential fats, protein, and vitamins that they need. In a large mason jar add equal amounts of unsalted almonds, cashews, walnuts, pecans, sunflower seeds, pumpkin seeds, and any other favorite nuts or seeds. Top it off with a good helping of your favorite dried fruit such as cranberries, raisins, apricots, apples, dates, and figs. For a bit of sweetness you can throw in some chocolate chips or carob. Purchase the items you need at a bulk-food store and simply mix together for a delicious and nutritious trail mix. The athlete can take this with him in a small container or can eat it at home. Many young athletes are allergic to nuts, including walnuts, almonds, hazelnuts, cashews, Brazil nuts, and pistachios. In this case, nuts can be substituted with seeds (given that no seed allergy exists), including pumpkin, sesame, and hemp seeds. Dried coconut and dried chickpeas are also wonderful alternatives and mix well with a variety of dried fruit. If you prefer a heartier snack, hummus or chickpea spread with a variety of raw vegetables packs a good vitamin punch and a healthy amount of plant-based protein. Parents should watch for cross-contamination before substituting a food for a child with allergies. For instance, oats do not contain gluten. However, if oats are processed in a factory that also processes wheat products, there is a possibility of cross-contamination, which could harm a young person with a gluten allergy. Many nutritional options are available for kids with food allergies. Once you determine the allergy, seek safe alternatives that provide similar nutritional benefits.

Lose the Battle, Win the War!

Seldom do we see a young athlete do a 180-degree turn when it comes to eating better. An athlete is not going to go from junk-food nut to health-food enthusiast. If your teenager didn't like your marinara sauce or the way you made chicken cutlets yesterday, the same will apply tomorrow. However, there are things you can do—or, shall we say, battles you can lose—in the hope that you will win the war on food. Here are a few examples.

If your child doesn't like to eat raw vegetables because she finds them boring or tasteless, find a dipping sauce that she likes. The dipping sauce may have more sugar, salt, or fat than you would like, but if it gets her to eat her raw vegetables, do it. Eventually she will develop a taste and appreciation for the power of eating pure foods.

You like to make healthy pizza at home instead of ordering out. You kill yourself to make spelt or whole-wheat dough and blend vegetables to make your own tomato sauce. The pizza is packed with nutrients. Your kids don't like the dough and don't care much about the sauce. Try this: Buy the dough they like and use your sauce on it. Another alternative, especially if they don't want to eat the sauce, is to buy or make the sauce that they do like to eat and simply mix the two sauces together. This way the taste of the sauce they like is not completely altered and you are able to get your nutrient-dense sauce into the mixture.

They want chicken fingers and fries. Of course they like the chicken fingers that come in a box. The fingers look like chicken and taste like chicken, but 13 chemicals that you can't pronounce are listed on the back of the box! As an alternative, make your own chicken fingers using a breading recipe that you find in a cookbook or online. You may need to add some mayonnaise or other ingredients to make the chicken more palatable, but at least you remove the majority of the chemicals that are present in the prepackaged form. As for the fries, simply cut up your own potatoes and season them for taste.

They don't eat salad. Chances are they like Caesar salad. So buy Caesar dressing and use it on the salad of your choice. Add your own grilled chicken and whatever vegetables you desire.

Kids are always looking for convenience, which is why the pantry always seems to need to be restocked. When they are hungry or between commercials, they simply scan the pantry and grab whatever is in their sight. If they open the fridge and have to wash the apple or cut the watermelon or peel the carrots—forget it! The Doritos, protein bars, or whatever dessert-like treat they find will do the trick. As arduous as it is, take time to prewash the fruits and vegetables so the kids can just open the fridge and grab a handful of carrots, celery, or fennel. Cut the watermelon and cantaloupe so they can simply reach for a piece.

This might sound like we are asking you to cater to your children's bad habits, but we are not. We are simply asking you to concede the battle and make it easy for them. Give them an opportunity to appreciate good food, a chance to feel the difference real food makes both physically and mentally, and in time you will win the war on food.

All young athletes should eat a balanced diet with wholesome carbohydrate, lean proteins, and fats, as well as a diet filled with plenty of vegetables, nuts, and seeds. What the young athlete eats before and after competition is just as important as what the athlete eats in the days, weeks, and months before competition. A healthy, vibrant, and strong body relies on good nutrition every day.

Young athletes must eat real foods to optimize energy, recovery, and muscle adaptations. An athlete is only as strong and efficient as his recovery, and recovery relies on adequate rest and a supercharged diet that takes advantage of nature's emporium. Don't be fooled by the promises of processed foods. Take the time to plan your meals, choose food sources that fuel the body with the necessary nutrients, and create an environment that positively affects the young athlete in sport and in life. A healthy young athlete will inevitably mature into a healthy adult.

chapter 11

Long-Term Training Plans

Compiling a long-term training model is necessary for anyone involved in children's training. Such a model gives a basic guideline to follow. Although it may undergo changes or additions, the basic plan will prevent rushing a children's program aimlessly, like a ship with no rudder.

To take a child from prepuberty to late postpuberty with a logical progression, you will need a long-term model, whether simple or complex. This chapter presents long-term training models for 11 sports. You can examine the one that interests you and either apply it as suggested or make changes to suit your athlete's needs or the environment in which you work. If the sport you are interested in is not present, create your own plan using a similar plan as a model.

The first plan is for a track sprinter. We explain this model so you can understand the process of compiling a training model. Ages (in years; from six to athletic maturation) are entered across the top of the chart. Training phases, skill acquisition, and physical-abilities training are listed down the left side of the chart. Competition levels are listed at the bottom of the chart, along with ages at which athletes enter each level.

The chart is divided by vertical lines that separate one type of activity from another. These activities which include coordination, speed, agility, strength training, aerobic training, etc. are either listed and thus important to the sport or blocked out signifying that specific skill acquisition or physical ability as being unnecessary for the sport. For instance, in the sprinting model, agility is blocked out during the athletic formation stage and beyond, because agility or speed in changing directions is not important for sprinting, since track sprinting is a linear event with no changes in direction.

The row showing skill acquisition refers to the progression of learning technical skills. In our example, the ultimate scope is to reach perfection. However, this will be impossible without first learning basic skills (ages 6-12 years) and then repeating parts of skills or full skills for automation (ages 12-16 years). For our purpose, automation means learning a skill so well that one can perform it automatically at a consistently high level.

Skill formation is not a quick fix—it takes time and occurs in several phases. In the early phase, a young athlete is exposed to the basic skills of the chosen sport. During this phase a skill is often performed with some rigidity. The child often appears awkward and lacks decent coordination because he is involuntarily involving some muscles that are not necessary for the particular action. Depending on the child's background and natural coordination, this phase could be relatively short or it could last up to two years.

After the first few years of technical teaching, athletes begin to feel familiar with the skills and start to perform them with ease. During skill automation, the athlete starts to automatically perform a skill—no matter how difficult—in a very natural way. Now only the prime movers (i.e., the muscles actually used in the performance of the skill) are contracted; therefore, the action is performed smoothly with ease.

During this skill automation stage, the instructor starts to work on skill perfection. Often called the highlight of athletic mastery, skill perfection is achieved when skills of high difficulty are performed fast with great finesse and maximum efficiency.

The acquisition of tactical skills, especially for team sports, also takes time because the skills are performed in a certain progression. As soon as an athlete is capable of performing the basic technical skills, she is progressively exposed to simple individual tactics. These skills are often position related, meaning that the child must learn and perform the tactics specific to a given position in a particular sport.

The next phase begins as soon as a child is comfortable with the tactical skills required for a given position. Here the coach teaches the athletes how to apply individual tactics to the team setting. Because team tactics change depending on the strategies applied by the opposition, the team's tactics must be applied with flexibility. Now the young athletes are required to adjust their own skills according to the specifics of the game and the game environment, such as weather, wind, temperature, and so on.

We advise all coaches to expose their players to different positions in the early years of training. The better a player can perform in other positions, the easier it will be for him to switch positions at a later date if he desires. Also, in the early years no one knows whether a player's best position is on offense or defense. Only in the late teens, during the years of specialization, should players be placed in a specific position where they have the highest effectiveness in the game.

A large part of the charts in this chapter refers to training the required physical abilities. This starts with coordination and performing simple skills at first, then progressing to more complex skills through the middle teens, and ultimately performing the skills as perfectly as possible.

Flexibility comes next. Children spend the early years of athletic involvement (ages 6-14 years) developing the best possible flexibility for all joints of the body. From the ages of 14 to 18 years, athletes emphasize sport-specific flexibility but must still maintain all-around flexibility. When children develop flexibility in this way, after age 18 years they can dedicate time to maintaining what they have achieved. It is always easier to maintain a given level than to develop it.

For agility, the focus is on developing agility during puberty and postpuberty and then maintaining it thereafter. Children can develop agility by performing specific exercises and drills, and they can influence it directly by repeating sport-specific exercises. Repeating many drills and exercises that develop speed and power also positively influences agility.

Speed training for sprinting consists of two elements: linear acceleration (i.e., straight speed) and starts. Athletes display linear acceleration immediately after the start and reach maximum velocity around 40 to 60 meters or yards. From 80 meters or yards on, the ability to maintain high velocity depends on how well speed endurance is trained. (Refer to the discussion of speed training in chapter 5.) A good start is a skill that must be learned, and it depends on one's reaction time. Good starts improve as a result of learning and practicing the skill. Strength training, on the other hand, starts with informal repetitions of simple exercises as suggested for prepuberty and is followed by periodization over the year. This starts with anatomical adaptation (ages 10-18 years), muscular endurance, power, and, finally, maximum strength. This sequence of strength training follows a progression from low to high loads; the highest load is for maximum strength (age 18 years onward). By the time a young athlete experiences heavy loads, he will have eight years of experience with lower loads. Such a progression ensures a good, long adaptation, resulting in an injury-free athlete.

The endurance component of training also follows a long-term progression from general endurance to aerobic training and, ultimately, anaerobic training. Anaerobic is the most taxing type of training for any athletes, especially young ones.

Finally, everybody involved in training young athletes should realize that competition should also increase progressively. For a child to enjoy sport, it is not important that she compete often and participate in stressful competitions. Winning at the age of 10 years does not guarantee that the same athlete will be winning at the age of maturation. Most often the opposite is true. Participation in competitions during the early years should have just one scope—enjoyment and fun! As the child grows older and becomes more skillful and better trained, she may progressively participate in local, state, and national competitions. Certainly some athletes who follow a long-term program will excel in a given sport and compete in international or professional sport.

Dominant Energy Systems and Physical Abilities for Specific Sports

Before you create a long-term training program for your athlete, you have to consider the dominant energy systems, or ergogenesis, and physical abilities used in your chosen sport. This is crucial information that will assist you in designing a long-term plan, especially the progression of the development of these abilities from initiation to high performance.

First, a quick review of the dominant energy systems of the body. In order for muscles to contract and for movement to occur, adenosine triphosphate (ATP) or energy must be present. ATP is produced and replenished by three main energy systems of the body:

1. ATP–creatine phosphate (CP) system
2. Glycolytic or lactic acid system
3. Aerobic system

We cannot turn any one system on or off. Each system is always turned on; however, the type of activity being performed determines which system dominates in executing or aiding the movement.

The ATP–CP system produces energy the most quickly. This energy system does not rely on carbohydrate or fats that are stored in the body for energy; it simply relies on a low amount of ATP already stored in the muscle and CP. The ATP–CP system can provide energy for very short and explosive movements lasting up to 12 seconds. This is the major energy system used in explosive sports such as sprinting and events such as the shotput and javelin throw. This system is applied in soccer and hockey, too; although both sports require a strong aerobic base, the ATP–CP system is required for producing quick, short bursts of power. The ATP–CP system is characterized as an anaerobic system (i.e., producing energy without the presence of oxygen).

The second anaerobic energy system, known as the glycolytic or lactic acid system, provides energy from 30 seconds to a maximum of 2 minutes. Both carbohydrate that is stored in the muscle (known as glycogen) and blood sugar are used to produce ATP.

The glycolytic system does not produce energy as quickly as the ATP–CP system, but it has a higher capacity to produce energy. As this system is taxed and the demand for ATP becomes too great, an athlete begins to feel a decrease in movement speed, an increase in fatigue, and a burning sensation in the muscles being used. The burning sensation is due to an increase in the acidity in the muscle, which is why this system is known as the lactic acid system.

The final system of energy, the aerobic energy system, produces energy slowly but produces much more energy than the other systems—approximately 18 times more energy than the glycolytic system. Because energy production in this system relies on the breakdown of carbohydrate and fats, energy production is slower but lasts much longer. This system can provide fuel for activities lasting two minutes to many hours.

Table 11.1 provides a review of the three energy systems of the body and the rate and capacity at which ATP can be produced.

As stated earlier, all three energy systems are always on. However, based on the activity or movement required, one energy system will dominate. For example, a coach may tell an athlete to sprint the length of a football field and not stop until completely fatigued. When the coach blows the whistle, the athlete will powerfully thrust his arms and legs for the first 10 seconds; here the ATP–CP system is dominant. Eventually, his legs will begin to feel heavy and the power in both his leg and arm swings will noticeably decrease; here the athlete is relying on the lactic acid system for energy. Eventually, the athlete's legs will feel too heavy to move, the burning sensation will become too great, and he will slow down to a slow jog or a walk while taking deep breaths; here the aerobic energy system is dominant. This example shows that all three energy systems play a role in movement and that the type of movement determines which system is used.

Why is this important? Information regarding energy systems can be overwhelming and technical at times, especially when describing the intricate details of energy metabolism. What is important is that coaches and parents understand which energy system dominates the sport and that they take care to plan a progressive program that challenges the athlete to grow and adapt to the needs of the sport. As with any system in the body, cumulative training sessions challenge the nervous, muscular, energy, and endocrine systems to get stronger and ward off fatigue. The sole purpose of training is to elicit a response or adaptation that helps the athlete run faster and longer, jump higher, throw farther, and fatigue slower. When an athlete trains the anaerobic system (ATP–CP and lactic acid), the body stores higher levels of ATP and CP, increases the levels of enzymes that aid in energy production, and enhances buffering capacity to ward off the accumulation of lactic acid. This does not occur overnight but rather happens as

Table 11.1 Energy Systems Used in Sport Performance

Energy system	Rate of ATP production	Capacity to produce ATP	Fuel used
ATP-CP	Extremely high	Very low	CP ATP in muscle
Lactic acid	High	Low	Blood glucose Stored glucose in liver and muscle (glycogen)
Aerobic system	Low	High	Blood glucose Stored glucose in liver and muscle Fat

ATP = adenosine triphosphate; CP = creatine phosphate.

a function of consistent and progressive training. The same holds true for the aerobic system, where the body uses a higher availability of carbohydrate and fat for fuel and improves capillary and mitochondrial density—all of which help with the efficiency of energy use. Thankfully, the body works as a cohesive unit that communicates, so when the athlete trains in accordance with the ergogenesis of the particular sport, all the important systems—neuromuscular, endocrine, and metabolic—equally adapt to the training stimulus. Plan your work and work your plan.

To assist you in creating your long-term plan, here we list specific information for several sports, including the dominant energy systems used, dominant physical abilities, energy suppliers, and anything else that is essential for success in that sport. Note that we use the term *ergogenesis* to refer to the proportion of each energy system used.

Baseball, Softball, and Cricket

- Ergogenesis: 95 percent alactic, 5 percent lactic
- Energy suppliers: CP, glycogen
- Dominant abilities: alactic and lactic acid endurance, throwing power, acceleration power, reaction power

Basketball

- Ergogenesis: 60 percent alactic, 20 percent lactic acid, 20 percent aerobic
- Energy suppliers: CP, glycogen
- Training objectives: alactic and lactic acid endurance, take-off power, acceleration power, power, maximum strength

Cycling: Road Racing

- Ergogenesis: 5 percent lactic acid, 95 percent aerobic
- Energy suppliers: glycogen, free fatty acids
- Training objectives: aerobic endurance, muscular endurance, acceleration power

Football

1. Linemen
   - Ergogenesis: 70 percent alactic, 30 percent lactic acid
   - Energy suppliers: CP, glycogen
   - Training objectives: alactic and lactic acid endurance, maximum strength, hypertrophy, starting power, reactive power
2. Wide receivers, defensive backs, tailbacks
   - Ergogenesis: 60 percent alactic, 30 percent lactic acid, 10 percent aerobic (cumulative)
   - Energy suppliers: CP, glycogen
   - Training objectives: alactic and lactic acid endurance, acceleration power, reactive power, starting power, maximum strength

Hockey

- Ergogenesis: 10 percent alactic, 40 percent lactic acid, 50 percent aerobic
- Energy suppliers: CP, glycogen
- Training objectives: alactic and lactic acid endurance, aerobic endurance, maximum strength, acceleration power, deceleration power

Figure Skating

- Ergogenesis: 40 percent alactic, 40 percent lactic acid, 20 percent aerobic
- Energy suppliers: CP, glycogen
- Training objectives: alactic and lactic acid endurance, takeoff power, landing power, maximum strength

Martial Arts

- Ergogenesis: 50 percent alactic, 30 percent lactic acid, 20 percent aerobic
- Energy suppliers: CP, glycogen
- Training objectives: alactic and lactic acid endurance, starting power, reactive power, maximum strength, power endurance

Racket Sports (tennis, badminton, squash, racquetball)

- Ergogenesis: 50 percent alactic, 30 percent lactic acid, 20 percent aerobic
- Energy suppliers: CP, glycogen
- Training objectives: alactic and lactic acid endurance, reactive power, acceleration power, deceleration power, power endurance

Rowing

- Ergogenesis: 20 percent lactic acid, 80 percent aerobic
- Energy suppliers: CP, glycogen
- Training objectives: aerobic endurance, lactic acid endurance, muscular endurance, power, maximum strength

Skiing

1. Alpine skiing
   - Ergogenesis: 40 percent alactic, 50 percent lactic acid, 10 percent aerobic
   - Energy suppliers: CP, glycogen
   - Training objectives: maximum strength, reactive power, power endurance
2. Cross-country skiing and biathlon
   - Ergogenesis: 5 percent lactic acid, 95 percent aerobic
   - Energy suppliers: glycogen, free fatty acids
   - Training objectives: aerobic endurance, lactic acid endurance, muscular endurance, power endurance

Soccer

- Ergogenesis: 15 percent alactic, 15 percent lactic acid, 70 percent aerobic
- Energy suppliers: CP, glycogen
- Training objectives: alactic and lactic acid endurance, aerobic endurance, acceleration power, deceleration power, power endurance, take-off power, maximum strength (>80 percent)

Swimming

1. Sprinting
   - Ergogenesis: 25 percent alactic, 50 percent lactic acid, 25 percent aerobic (for 100 meters)
   - Energy suppliers: CP, glycogen

- Training objectives: alactic and lactic acid endurance, power, power endurance, maximum strength, aerobic endurance

2. Long distance
   - Ergogenesis: 10 percent alactic, 30 percent lactic acid, 60 percent aerobic
   - Energy suppliers: glycogen, free fatty acids
   - Training objectives: aerobic endurance, lactic acid endurance, muscular endurance, power endurance

Track and Field (Athletics)

1. Sprinting
   - Ergogenesis: 80 percent alactic, 20 percent lactic acid
   - Energy supplier: CP
   - Training objectives: alactic and lactic acid endurance, starting power, reactive power, acceleration power, maximum strength, power endurance
2. Throwing events
   - Ergogenesis: 95 percent alactic, 5 percent lactic acid
   - Energy supplier: CP
   - Training objectives: throwing power, reactive power, maximum strength
3. Middle-distance running
   - Ergogenesis: 20 percent alactic, 30 percent lactic acid, 50 percent aerobic
   - Energy suppliers: CP, glycogen
   - Training objectives: alactic and lactic acid endurance, aerobic endurance, acceleration power, power endurance
4. Long-distance running
   - Ergogenesis (10K running): 5 percent lactic acid, 15 percent lactic acid, 80 percent aerobic
   - Energy suppliers: glycogen, free fatty acids
   - Training objectives: aerobic endurance, lactic acid endurance, muscular endurance

Volleyball

- Ergogenesis: 40 percent alactic, 20 percent lactic acid, 40 percent aerobic
- Energy suppliers: CP, glycogen
- Training objectives: alactic and lactic acid endurance, power, power endurance, maximum strength

Long-Term Training Models for Selected Sports

Any serious training program for young athletes has to start at early age and progress from initiation to high performance. The suggested models will help you have long-term vision and not fall into the trap of immediate results. Don't be influenced by the training programs created for high-performance athletes. Your child is just that—a child! He or she should be expected to achieve high performance from the late teens on. Have the patience to develop all the necessary abilities in a progressive way over several years of training. The suggested models are nothing else but a long-term progression from childhood to high performance.

Track and Field, Sprinting

			Age of Athlete: 6 7 8 9 10 11 12 13 14 15 16 17 18 19 20 21 22 25 30 35			
Training phase			**Initiation**	**Athletic formation**	**Special-ization**	**High performance**
Skill acquisition		Technical	Basic skills	Skill automation	Perfection	
Training	Coordination		Simple	Complex	Perfection	
	Flexibility		Overall	Specific	Maintain	
	Agility				Maintain	
	Speed	Linear				
		Reaction time	Starts		Perfection	
	Strength	Anatomical adaptation				
		Power				
		Maximum strength				
	Endurance	General				
		Anaerobic				
Competitions	Fun					
	Local					
	State/provincial					
	National					
	International/ professional					

Note: Shaded area shows the ages to start or end work on that ability.

Baseball

Training phase			Initiation	Athletic formation	Specialization	High performance	
Age of Athlete			6 7 8 9 10 11 12	13 14 15	16 17 18 19	20 21 22 25	30 35
Skill acquisition	Technical		Fundamentals	Fundamentals	Position-specific	Position- and game-specific	
	Tactical		Simple game strategy	Simple game strategy	Game strategy	Position and game strategy	
Training	Coordination		Simple	Complex	Perfection	Perfection	
	Flexibility		Overall	Overall / Specific	Specific / Maintain	Maintain	
	Agility					Maintain	
	Speed	Linear					
		Turns/ changes in direction					
		Reaction time					
	Strength	Anatomical adaptation					
		Power					
		Maximum strength					
	Endurance	General					
		Anaerobic					
Competitions	Fun						
	Local						
	State/provincial						
	National						
	International/professional						

Note: Shaded area shows the ages to start or end work on that ability.

Basketball

			Age of Athlete 6 7 8 9 10 11 12 13 14 15 16 17 18 19 20 21 22 25 30 35			
Training phase			**Initiation**	**Athletic formation**	**Specialization**	**High performance**
Skill acquisition	Technical		Basic skills	Skill automation		Perfection
	Tactical		Simple individual tactics	Foundation of team tactics		Perfection
Training	Coordination		Simple	Complex		Perfection
	Flexibility		Overall	Specific		Maintain
	Agility					
	Speed	Linear				
		Turns/changes in direction				
		Reaction time				
	Strength	Anatomical adaptation				
		Muscular endurance				
		Power				
		Maximum strength				
	Endurance	General				
		Aerobic				
		Anaerobic				
Competitions	Fun					
	Local					
	State/provincial					
	National					
	International/professional					

Note: Shaded area shows the ages to start or end work on that ability.

Football

Training phase			Age of Athlete: 6 7 8 9 10 11 12 13 14 15 16 17 18 19 20 21 22 25 30 35					
			Initiation		**Mini-football**	**High school**	**Specialization**	**High performance**
Skill acquisition		Technical		Fundamentals		Skill automation	Perfection of game-specific skills	
		Tactical		Simple rules		Game tactics	Position-specific tactics	
Training	Coordination		Simple		Complex	Perfection		
	Flexibility		Overall			Specific	Maintenance	
	Agility							
	Speed	Linear						
		Turns/changes in direction						
		Reaction time						
	Strength	Anatomical adaptation						
		Power						
		Maximum strength						
	Endurance	General						
		Aerobic						
		Anaerobic						
Competitions	Fun							
	Local							
	State/provincial							
	National							
	International/professional							

Note: Shaded area shows the ages to start or end work on that ability.

Gymnastics (Women)

			Age of Athlete														
			6	7	8	9	10	11	12	13	14	15	16	17	18	19	20
Training phase			**Initiation**			**Athletic formation**			**Specializa-tion**		**High performance**						
Skill acquisition		Technical	Skill formation				Skill auto-mation		Perfection								
Training	Coordination		Simple				Complex							Perfection			
	Flexibility		Over-all		Shoulders and hips			Maintenance									
	Agility					■	■	■	■	■	■	Maintain					
	Speed	Linear				■	■	■	■	■	■	■	■	■	■	■	■
	Strength	Anatomical adaptation				■	■	■	■								
		Power						■	■	■	■	■	■	■	■	■	■
		Maximum strength												■	■	■	■
	Endurance	Anaerobic				■	■	■	■	■	■	■	■	■	■	■	■
Competitions	Fun			■	■	■											
	Local						■										
	State/provincial							■	■	■							
	National										■	■	■	■	■	■	■
	International/professional										■	■	■	■	■	■	■

Note: Shaded area shows the ages to start or end work on that ability.

Ice Hockey

Training phase			Age of Athlete: 6 7 8 9 10 11 12 13	14 15 16	17 18	19 20 21 22 25 30 35
Training phase			**Initiation**	**Athletic formation**	**Specialization**	**High performance**
Skill acquisition	Technical		Fundamental	Skill automation	Perfection of game- and position-specific skills	
	Tactical		Simple individual tactics	Game tactics	Position-specific tactics	
Training	Coordination		Simple	Complex	Perfection	
	Flexibility		Overall	Specific	Maintenance	
	Agility					
	Speed	Linear				
		Turns/changes in direction				
		Reaction time				
	Strength	Anatomical adaptation				
		Power				
		Maximum strength				
	Endurance	General				
		Aerobic				
		Anaerobic				
Competitions	Fun					
	Local					
	State/provincial					
	National					
	International/professional					

Note: Shaded area shows the ages to start or end work on that ability.

Soccer

			Age of Athlete 6 7 8 9 10 11 12 13 14 15 16 17 18 19 20 21 22 25 30 35				
Training phase				**Mini-soccer**	**Novice**	**Junior**	**High performance**
Skill acquisition	Technical		Fundamentals			Skill automation	Perfection of game- and position-specific skills
	Tactical			Simple rules		Game tactics	Position-specific tactics
Training	Coordination			Simple		Complex	Perfection
	Flexibility		Overall			Specific	Maintenance
	Agility						
	Speed	Linear					
		Turns/ changes in direction					
		Reaction time					
	Strength	Anatomical adaptation					
		Muscular endurance					
		Power					
		Maximum strength					
	Endurance	General					
		Aerobic					
		Anaerobic					
Competitions	Fun						
	Local						
	State/provincial						
	National						
	International/ professional						

Note: Shaded area shows the ages to start or end work on that ability.

Swimming

Training phase			Age of Athlete: 6 7 8 9 10 11	12 13	14 15 16 17	18 19 20 21 22
Training phase			**Initiation**	**Athletic formation**	**Specialization**	**High performance**
Skill acquisition	Technical		Basic skills	Skill automation	Perfection	
	Tactical		Start		Even splits	
Training	Coordination		Simple	Complex coordination	Perfection	
	Flexibility		Overall	Specific	Maintenance	
	Agility					
	Speed	Linear				
		Turns/changes in direction				
		Reaction time	Starts		Perfection	
	Strength	Anatomical adaptation				
		Muscular endurance				
		Power				
		Maximum strength				
	Endurance	General				
		Aerobic				
		Anaerobic				
Competitions	Fun					
	Local					
	State/provincial					
	National					
	International/professional					

Note: Shaded area shows the ages to start or end work on that ability.

Tennis

Training phase			Age of Athlete: 6 7 8 9 10 11 12	13 14	15 16 17	18 19 20 21 22 25 30 35
			Initiation	**Athletic formation**	**Special-ization**	**High performance**
Skill acquisition		Technical	Basic skills		Skill automation	Perfection
		Tactical	Simple		Game tactics	Perfection
Training	Coordination		Simple		Complex	Perfection
	Flexibility		Overall		Specific	Maintenance
	Agility					
	Speed	Linear				
		Turns/ changes in direction				
		Reaction time				
	Strength	Anatomical adaptation				
		Muscular endurance				
		Power				
		Maximum strength				
	Endurance	General				
		Aerobic				
		Anaerobic				
Competitions	Fun					
	Local					
	State/provincial					
	National					
	International/ professional					

Note: Shaded area shows the ages to start or end work on that ability.

Track and Field, Throws and Jumps

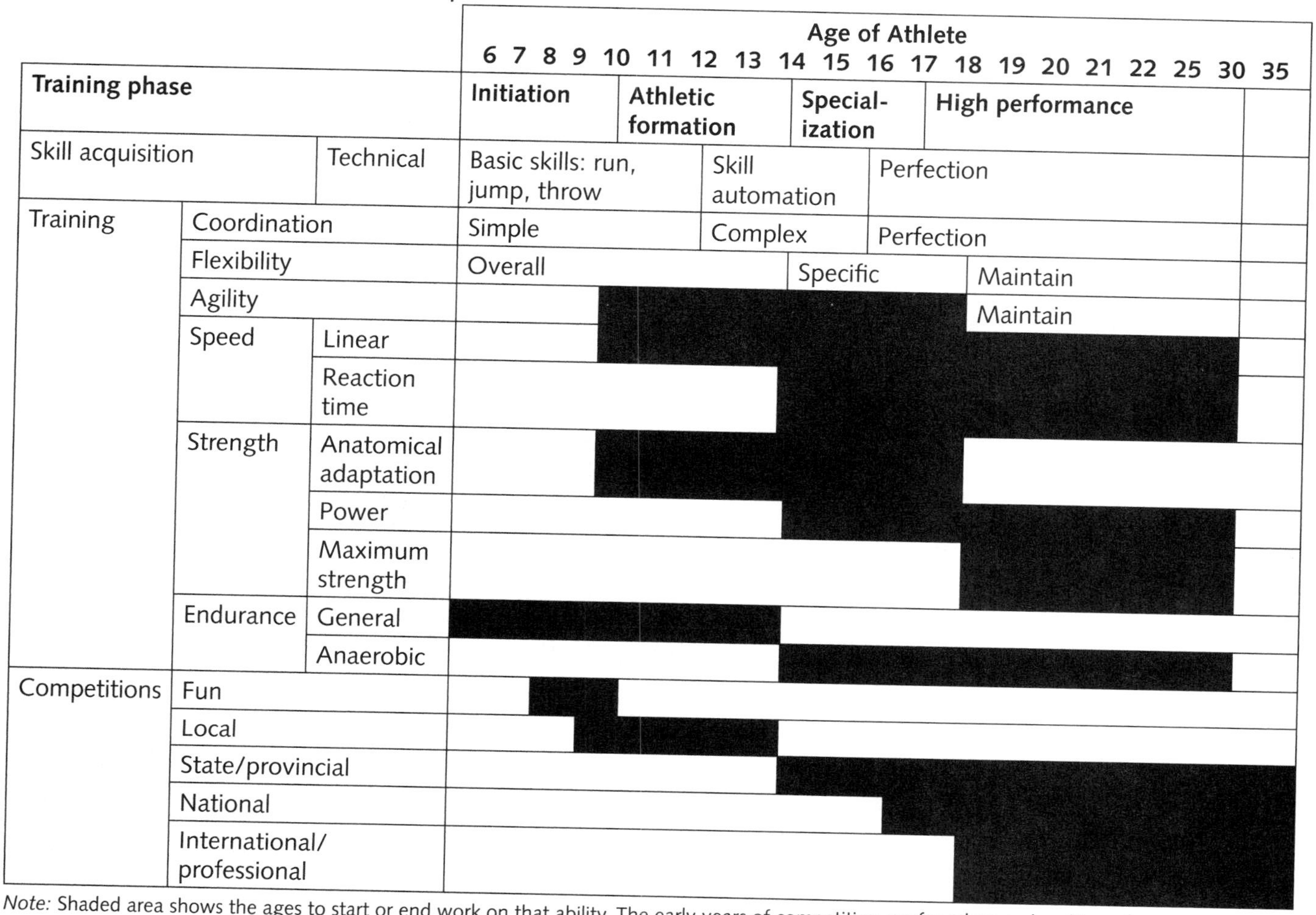

Training phase			Initiation	Athletic formation	Specialization	High performance	
Age of Athlete			6 7 8 9 10	11 12 13	14 15 16 17	18 19 20 21 22 25 30	35
Skill acquisition		Technical	Basic skills: run, jump, throw	Skill automation	Perfection		
Training	Coordination		Simple	Complex	Perfection		
	Flexibility		Overall		Specific	Maintain	
	Agility					Maintain	
	Speed	Linear					
		Reaction time					
	Strength	Anatomical adaptation					
		Power					
		Maximum strength					
	Endurance	General					
		Anaerobic					
Competitions	Fun						
	Local						
	State/provincial						
	National						
	International/ professional						

Note: Shaded area shows the ages to start or end work on that ability. The early years of competition are for relays and multievents.

Volleyball

			Age of Athlete 6 7	8 9 10 11	12 13 14	15 16 17	18 19 20	21 22 25 30 35
Training phase				**Initiation**		**Athletic formation**	**Special-ization**	**High performance**
Skill acquisition	Technical				Basic skills	Skill auto-mation	Perfection	
	Tactical				Simple tactics	Foun-dation of team tactics	Perfection	
Training	Coordination			Simple		Complex	Perfection	
	Flexibility			Overall		Specific	Maintenance	
	Agility							
	Speed	Linear						
		Turns/ changes in direction						
		Reaction time						
	Strength	Anatomical adaptation						
		Muscular endurance						
		Power						
		Maximum strength						
	Endurance	General						
		Aerobic						
		Anaerobic						
Competitions	Fun							
	Local							
	State/provincial							
	National							
	International/ professional							

Note: Shaded area shows the ages to start or end work on that ability.

chapter 12

Training Myths and Kids

Despite the lack of good methodological knowledge, physical training for most sports is not a novelty. Although some coaches still have confusion about when and how much to train and what type of equipment to use, the ancient Olympians didn't philosophize too much. They simply lifted heavy stones to improve the athletes' strength and, as a result, better their athletic performance.

In the late 1800s, physical training became an important part of the sport mostly in track and field, gymnastics, and rowing. Distance running, dumbbells, and medicine balls were the preferred methods for increasing endurance and strength.

The physical capabilities of team-sport athletes began to improve when coaches started to borrow exercises from track and field, such as drills for sprinting, jumping, and throwing. Exercises using medicine balls and dumbbells started to be used in the early 20th century. When athletes from Eastern Europe started to compete internationally in 1948, they used a large variety of fitness exercises to overcome the technical advantage of the Western countries. Exercises from Olympic weightlifting surfaced in the early 1950s. Rubber cords were first used in 1954 in Romania to train muscle endurance for rowing, kayaking, and canoeing.

Sport equipment companies realized that they could garner business by promoting varied training equipment. In the 1980s the market was invaded with training gadgets and equipment that are often not so effective. Every company claims that using their equipment will greatly improve athletic performance. Some of these training devices can be purchased online and are found in most sport-training facilities in North America.

It is one thing to attempt to improve an athlete's speed and strength using new equipment, but using such equipment on kids? Do children really need to use parachutes to improve speed or dumbbell chest presses on a stability ball to increase core strength? How about they instead master the push-up or chin-up or develop the strength needed to control the body? That is how core strength is built—not by performing a dumbbell press on a ball! Although there is a time and a place for stability balls, especially during the anatomical adaptation phase of training, this type of equipment is more useful for fitness than for preparing an athlete for competition—or, more importantly, for strengthening the body of a young athlete.

The proponents of these new exercise myths, such as parachutes to improve speed or the overuse of the stability ball to improve core strength, do not realize that the ideas they promote are often based on ignorance or a gross misunderstanding of sport science. Looking at these individuals, we cannot help but wonder whether their enthusiasm for different pieces of equipment is a result of dishonesty or of ignorance. Are these individuals seeking self-promotion and profit, or do they simply lack a fundamental knowledge of biomechanics and exercise physiology?

We do not entirely blame the producers of these gadgets. After all, they are merely trying to survive in a very competitive market. But college-educated individuals, training instructors who have taken courses in biomechanics and exercise physiology, are expected to have a better understanding of what works and what doesn't.

This is why we are taking a professional stance and unveiling the fallacies of some of these training ideas while recognizing the merits of others. We trust that we are not alone in this struggle to help coaches and instructors realize what works and what does not. Certainly, we are not too concerned for experienced coaches who can use their knowledge as a shield against many of these fallacies. But we are rather concerned for the thousands of novice personal trainers, junior coaches, parents, and university graduates who are more vulnerable to the promotion of new yet ineffective training equipment. Kids need to move their bodies and slowly adapt their training to work the primary movers in their sport. This means following a periodized training philosophy in which the body becomes the primary form of equipment, such as body-weight exercises, and later as the athlete physically matures, the use of external loads such as medicine balls and free weights should be added to the program. When the body is forced to run faster, jump higher, and lift heavier in natural body movements, the core muscles are worked extensively. You don't need fancy equipment—just exercises and methodologies that target the prime movers. This leads to two principles of understanding:

- **Principle 1:** Don't do what is new but rather what is applicable to your sport.
- **Principle 2:** Select only those training implements that clearly target the prime movers in your sport.

Exercise Versus Adaptation

For many training instructors and coaches, seminars are the preferred medium for being exposed to new ideas. In many instances the speakers promote new exercises, making it sound like the exercise per se will miraculously lead to substantial improvement. Not very often, however, do speakers cite anatomical and neuromuscular adaptation as the fundamental elements that improve athletic performance. We should remember that improvement in athletic performance will always depend on training methodology and applying superior physiological principles, not necessarily on the latest captivating exercises. Those who still are fascinated by elementary exercises and new training gadgets should keep in mind these laws of exercise selection.

1. The selected exercises must target the prime movers (i.e., the muscles performing the technical skills). The way you target the prime movers in training is essential; the gadgets you use are not. Select only exercises and gadgets that address the muscles involved in the selected sport.
2. Select exercises according to the phase of training. Because each training phase may have different objectives, such as strength versus speed, exercises have to address the physical quality you train.

3. Select exercises and training methodology according to the energy system dominant in your sport or training phase.

A good selection of exercises is certainly very important. However, don't forget that an exercise is essential only as it helps you target the prime movers! To continually discuss how to perform a bench press or whether one should use a simple bench or a stability ball is a great waste of time. For sport training the support you use for a bench press, as an example, is immaterial. The essential goal is to perform the exercise with a continuous acceleration through the range of motion. At the beginning of a bench press, fast-twitch (FT) muscle fibers are recruited to defeat inertia and the load of the barbell. As you continue to press the barbell upward, you should attempt to generate the highest acceleration possible. Under these conditions the discharge rate of the same FT muscle fibers is increased. Maximum acceleration, therefore, must be achieved toward the end of the action to coincide with the end of the bench press, or the moment of releasing a ball or other implement used in sport.

Anatomical and especially physiological adaptation are the essential adjustments of the human body in an athlete's quest to improve athletic or fitness capabilities. The training method you select, not the exercise, is the essential ingredient in achieving such adaptation.

Do you want to improve your athletes' potential? Learn more about training science, training methods, and methodology. In this chapter we describe eight general myths of training. We also briefly discuss the effectiveness of various products on the market. Although some do provide a minor benefit, most of the products that are intended to improve speed or power in particular are grossly misrepresented and in some cases, such as the parachute, can negatively affect the physical ability they are touted to improve – in this case that is speed!

Myth 1: Balance Training

Since the 1950s, it has been theorized—but never proven—that balance training is one of the abilities athletes need to successfully compete. Shortly after 1960, when East European nations finished testing whether balance training may have any effect on athletic results, balance training, as a separate entity in training was abandoned. However, since the late 1990s, sport equipment producers in the United States have promoted a variety of balance boards, BOSU balls, wobble boards, and so on as essential gadgets that have a positive effect on athletic performance.

On many occasions we have witnessed 10- to 12-year-olds standing on a wobble board and catching a medicine ball that has been tossed to them. The purpose of such an exercise is to improve balance. Balance will naturally improve as kids engage in various sporting activities and movement patterns. Trainers and coaches will argue that athletes trained on a BOSU ball show improved balance. Such improvement is not surprising given that the nervous system is very adaptable. Will the athletes be able to carry that balance to a stable environment (i.e., a field or floor) where competitions take place? No. In fact, the old speculation that training on an unstable surface engages greater core activation has been proven false (Willardson et al., 2009), as has the belief that such training elicits greater gains in strength (Drinkwater et al., 2007). Time would be better spent simply performing power exercises with the medicine ball. We once witnessed a young golfer performing squats while standing on a stability ball. Besides increasing the chance of injury, the exercise was ineffective. When questioned by his coach as to why we suggested the athlete get off the ball when squatting, we simply responded, "Unless golfing begins to be performed while standing on a stability ball, you are wasting your precious time." Our intention is simply to educate both coaches and athletes and help them use their training time wisely.

The importance of balance training in sport and fitness is more of an unfounded speculation than a certainty. There are, however, two sports in which balance training may play a determinant role: downhill skiing, and the balance beam in women's gymnastics.

With a width of only four inches (10 cm), the balance beam in women's gymnastics challenges the performer's ability to maintain good balance during a choreographed routine. Training for the development and improvement of balance has always been very specific and involves many repetitions of specific skills for one to two hours per day. Gymnastics coaches have observed for many years that some gymnasts have better natural balance than others. Therefore, natural selection has been working in gymnastics: Over time, gymnasts who lack natural balance have eliminated themselves from the elite groups.

Have you ever seen a gymnastics coach use a BOSU ball to improve the balance needed for the balance beam? Never! Any attempt to improve balance using any means other than specific work on the balance beam is ridiculed by gymnastics coaches. The use of equipment promoted by some as a means of improving balance is nonexistent in gymnastics.

Balance is important in skiing, especially during the turns performed in slalom or downhill races. Once again, coaches know that a fall in skiing is caused by loading the skis improperly. Simple biomechanics clearly states that if the leg force (i.e., the load) is applied on the downhill ski, the skier will adhere to the slope. If the force is applied at an angle that is more perpendicular to the slope, the skier will not fall. If, on the other hand, the load is on the uphill ski and the angle of force application is more tangential to the slope, the skier will fall. This occurs no matter how many repetitions one does on a wobble board.

The solution to balance problems in skiing is the correct application of forces during a race, not balance training on dry land. Therefore, the balance training equipment will have little, if any, effect on a skier's mechanics. Perhaps the best dry-land balance training for skiing is for the skier to stand in the back of a pickup truck that is moving over very difficult terrain, such as a hilly country road. The scope of such an exercise is for the skier to maintain a balanced downhill stance throughout the ride. However, most of the improvement in downhill skiing in the past has come not from using new equipment but rather from exposing skiers to a serious, well-periodized strength-training program focused on the core and the legs. With greater strength comes better sport-specific balance!

No other sports require the type of balance training some individuals are promoting in the United States, Canada, and, quite recently, Europe and other countries. In all other sports, balance is not and never has been considered a limiting factor for performance.

Despite the reality of biomechanics, some individuals still believe that balance training needs to be trained as a separate element in training like strength or flexibility. In actuality, balance is simply trained as a by-product of other training abilities such as strength, power, agility, and flexibility. As such, many so-called experts in balance training organize seminars that promote specific equipment and exercises as keys to future athletic improvement. Keep in mind, however, that companies selling such equipment are often the sponsors, or even the organizers, of these seminars! These promoters of balance training lack scientific understanding of sport training in general and basic sport biomechanics in particular. The same is often true for their hired instructors or speakers!

Figure 12.1 shows an athlete running in a curvilinear shape. Promoters of balance training claim that the player needs balance to run in an inclined, curvilinear position,

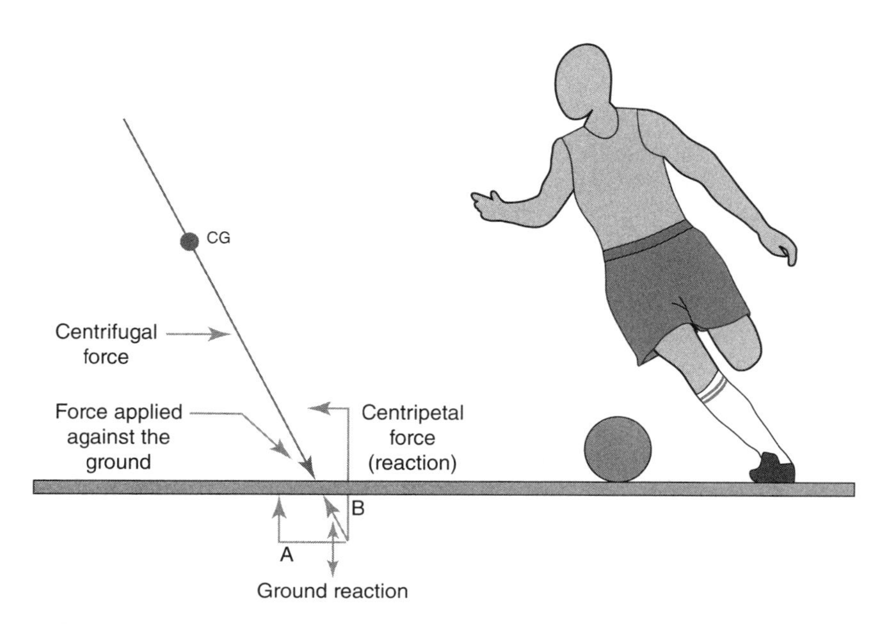

Figure 12.1 The parallelogram of vectors.

and, as such, that balance training will make the athlete capable of running in this inclined position without falling. However, maintaining an inclined position is not a problem of balance but rather of understanding simple rules of biomechanics.

As the player runs, centrifugal force is created, triggering a centripetal reaction of equal force in the opposite direction. Under this condition, force application is more perpendicular to the ground or in a state of dynamic equilibrium, making it impossible for the player to fall down (case A). If force application is more tangential to the ground (case B), the athlete cannot maintain a dynamic equilibrium and will fall regardless of whether he has performed any goofy balance training! This basic misunderstanding of sport science has triggered the present revival of balance training and the gross exaggeration of its benefits.

The equipment promoted as improving balance has little, if any, effect on an athlete's performance. Children in the initiation stage of development, such as kindergarten, might really enjoy some of these balance exercises. Maintaining balance on a balance board certainly involves some degree of difficulty. However, to claim that these exercises can positively affect sport training or that repeating some of these exercises will improve athletic performance is an insult to any good student of sport science.

Myth 2: Train the Stabilizer Muscles

Stabilizers are relatively small muscles that anchor or stabilize the position of bones to give prime movers a firm base from which to pull. For instance, during knee extension, the popliteus muscle (behind the knee joint) contracts isometrically to stabilize the thigh for effective movement of the calf. Similarly, during elbow flexion (e.g., a preacher curl), the shoulders, upper arms, and abdominal muscles contract isometrically to stabilize the shoulders and upper arms, giving the biceps brachii muscles a stable base from which to pull. Other similar muscles, often called fixators, are stimulated to stabilize part of a limb or body in order to facilitate better mechanical work.

For many years, some argued for the need to train the stabilizer muscles and believed that improper development of the stabilizers could limit the maximum mechanical efficiency of the prime movers. As with balance training, some individuals figured that stabilizer training could be another chance to gain fame, and sport equipment manufacturers welcomed another opportunity to create and promote new training gadgets. The most popular piece of equipment for training the stabilizers is probably the stability ball. People in North American fitness clubs rarely do the traditional bench press anymore. Worse, these stability balls have made their way into athlete-development programs. All of a sudden the old-fashioned bench, used for decades for bench press exercises, became a relic.

Many gadgets have been created in addition to the stability ball, and fashion influences the equipment in use. The use of new training gadgets is so exaggerated that you may ask yourself whether this is sport training or circus training! Exercises that require users to balance on top of a stability ball while performing various dumbbell exercises are constantly being invented. Although certain skill is required to perform these circus-like movements, the benefit of such exercises on athletic improvement is questionable at best. Improvements will occur, but the improvements will apply only to exercises performed on the stability ball, and very little transfer to the sporting arena will occur. More important, some exercises performed on stability balls are dangerous, especially for inexperienced lifters (see figure 12.2). Why use such exercises during the earlier stages of development? Injuries have occurred, and legal suits against instructors and the producers of stability balls may follow.

These exaggerations about the need for training the stabilizers are a waste of time and money. The human body is a perfect machine, the efficiency of which continues to marvel scientists everywhere. The body is very plastic and adapts to many environments—both good and bad. Once the prime movers of the sport have been identified, one can create a progressive program that strengthens all the muscles of the body by choosing movement patterns that are required in the sport. Neither coaches nor athletes need to worry about anything more, including specifically training the stabilizer muscles, thanks to a law of physiology called overflow of activation, or irradiation.

We can use a practical example to illustrate irradiation. As prime movers perform a training task, the muscles surrounding the joint are also activated. In other words, an overflow of activation involves not only the synergistic muscles but also the stabilizer muscles. For instance, the quadriceps muscles are stimulated to perform the task of leg extension. This action also arouses and activates other muscles, including a stabilizer called the popliteus (located on the back of the knee joint), ensuring stability and the transfer of power across the joint (Enoka, 2008; Howard and Enoka, 1991; Zijdewind and Kernell, 2001). This means that during knee extension the quadriceps contract to overcome resistance and, at the same time, the popliteus contracts to stabilize the knee joint.

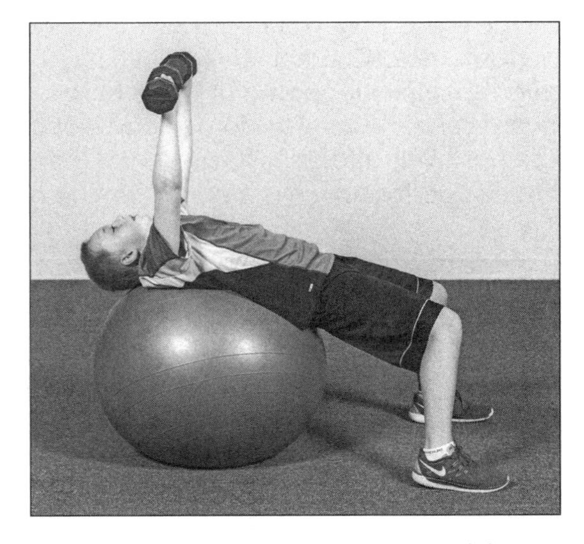

Figure 12.2 A press exercise on a stability ball may be dangerous for an inexperienced athlete.

This example shows that as the muscles in a region are stimulated to contract, so are the stabilizers. Consequently, contraction increases the strength of not only the targeted muscles, the prime movers (quadriceps), but also the irradiated muscles (popliteus). Therefore, any additional time spent training the stabilizers via new gadgets and circus-type exercises is a waste. Take the time to do what is necessary and not what is new! Do you want to improve your training efficiency? Be more careful with the exercises you use.

The promoters of the much-hyped new trends in stabilizer and core-strength training claim that the main benefit is injury prevention. Once again, this allegation is anecdotal. Well-informed individuals know that most sport and fitness injuries occur in the ligaments and tendons, not the muscles. A visit to a sport injury clinic will quickly prove this. Stabilizers are at the bottom of the list of frequently injured muscles. Why, then, waste so much time and money on something of very little concern?

Once again, the exaggerated need for exercises for the stabilizers comes at the expense of training adaptation. The more exercises you employ in training, the lower the number of sets per exercise. As a result, adaptation will be very low and training improvements will be more than questionable. Remember that it is not the number of exercises that is important but rather the movement patterns they elicit. So train the prime movers and train them well.

Myth 3: Focus on Core Strength

Core strength, or the strength of the midsection of the human body (i.e., abdomen, low-back muscles, and trunk), is also a preferred target of individuals who promote novel training concepts. The new ideas regarding core strength present nothing original except for some circus-like exercises of little consequence to athletic improvement. Most such exercises are recycled drills in which stability balls and a few other current gimmicks are used to justify the needs of core-strength training.

In *Periodization Training for Sports, Second Edition* (Bompa and Carrera 2005), we discuss the five basic laws of strength training. Considering its importance in many exercises and athletic actions, core strength is described as an important training element. The core area of the body is important in most athletic actions and exercises. The following examples illustrate the importance of strong core muscles.

- Perform an upright row while standing, feet apart, arms along the legs, holding a barbell or dumbbells. As the arm and shoulder muscles contract and the arms flex to lift the weight toward the chest, the abdominal muscles and back muscles (including the erector spinae) contract to stabilize the trunk so the arms can perform the action smoothly. The prime movers would not be able to perform the task without the support of the core muscles.
- One of the most dynamic athletic actions, a volleyball spike, could not be performed efficiently without the support of the core muscles. In spiking, the core muscles contract to stabilize the trunk so the legs can perform an explosive take-off and the arms can execute the spike.
- During running, jumping, quick-feet actions, throwing, medicine ball exercises, and so on, the trunk muscles invariably contract to stabilize the trunk so the legs and arms can perform the athletic tasks.

However, in referring to core strength, some individuals go too far off course and promote ridiculous and sometimes dangerous exercises. In doing so they undermine the area of athletic training and the importance of strength in sport. In one of the most laughable exercises promoted by some fitness instructors, the individual stands on one leg on an AirEx Pad, bends from the hips to reach forward to touch the floor, and returns to standing. The exercise is supposed to be beneficial to all sports in which change of direction is important. It is also purported to improve balance for skiers, surfers, and snowboarders. To propose that this exercise has athletic benefit is a gross embarrassment to all training professionals.

We do not wish to devote much space to exercises of no consequence to athletic improvement. We refer to the fallacy of balance training earlier. Balance can never be positively influenced in the previously mentioned sports unless the mechanics of force application and body-weight distribution are corrected. This is mechanics—not myths! These new exercises for core strength are not necessary because many traditional weight-training exercises take care of core strength via the overflow of activation, mentioned earlier (Enoka, 2002; Zijdewind and Kernell, 2001).

Myth 4: The Overspeed Treadmill

In the early 1990s, the fitness industry produced overspeed treadmills and claimed that they would improve an athlete's speed. Like most other treadmills, the overspeed treadmill has a belt, which can achieve a velocity of more than 26 miles (41.8 km) per hour. The athlete runs on the belt in an attempt to reach maximum velocity and match the mechanically imposed speed of the treadmill. The claim that this training device improves maximum velocity must be seriously questioned even though these devices are present in many sport-training facilities. Overspeed treadmills are marketed well to both parents and coaches, but do they actually improve speed? Because an important element for speed training in sport is agility, how does one combine this increase in speed with agility training?

The truth is that overspeed treadmills are not a practical way to improve sport-specific speed. When the treadmill is at top speed the athlete is simply skimming the belt, and foot contact and force production are required in order to increase speed. Speed is best improved on stable ground where ground reaction forces can be optimized during the contact phase. This can be achieved only in traditional speed training coupled with a long-term resistance-training program, which begins in childhood and continues throughout adolescence (Keiner et al., 2014).

A review of the three major elements of sprinting illustrates how overspeed treadmills are not useful in improving speed performance.

1. *Stride length.* The length of the runner's stride is directly proportional to the force of the propulsion phase (i.e., the push-off against the ground). A runner's stride lengthens as the athlete applies more powerful force against the ground, driving the thigh of the front leg to horizontal. At this point in running the stride length is maximal. During treadmill running, the belt speed exceeds the athlete's maximum speed capability. To keep up with the speed of the belt, the athlete has to increase running speed. To achieve this, something about the athlete's running behavior has to change. Because speed and propulsion are already at maximum, the only possibility is for the athlete to increase stride frequency—often beyond his capability. As a result, the athlete can increase stride frequency only at the expense of the force of propulsion. Thus, the athlete cannot achieve maximum speed without increasing the force of propulsion to maximum. Because the maximum speed of the belt is already beyond the athlete's capability, the athlete can increase nothing else to keep up with the speed of the belt. Therefore, the overspeed treadmill cannot improve stride length simply because the speed of the belt is so high that the athlete never has time to apply maximum force

against the ground (in this case, the running belt). The belt rotates faster than the athlete's capacity to apply maximum force against it. No maximum force, no maximum stride length!

2. *Propulsion phase.* The propulsion phase is the major element in making an athlete fast. As the force applied against the ground increases, the duration of the contact with the ground (i.e., the propulsion phase) decreases. Therefore, the critical element for improving speed is to shorten the duration of the contact phase. This is possible only by increasing leg power (i.e., the force generated by the triple extensor muscles: ankles, knees, and hips). However, the fast-moving belt is not propelled by the athlete's increased application of force. Rather, the speed of the belt is mechanically induced and is therefore not conducive to increased application of force against the ground. As such, the overspeed treadmill cannot improve an athlete's speed development. The only condition in which force application increases is when the ground is immobile. This is impossible when the belt is moving under the feet and away from the athlete. Under this condition the athlete never has time to apply force against the ground.

3. *Stride frequency.* Sprinting frequency depends, among other things, on the height of the athlete or the length of his legs. Shorter athletes always have a higher stride frequency, but short runners rarely become elite sprinters. Frequency is important but it is not the determinant element of speed. Because sprinting on a treadmill is not conducive to a powerful application of force against the belt, high frequency is artificially achieved at the expense of high force application during the propulsion phase. Because almost anyone, even a below-average sprinter, can move his legs quickly in the air (i.e., during the time between the propulsion phase and landing on the ground), frequency itself cannot compensate for the inability to apply strong force against the ground. To effectively increase stride frequency, one must reduce the duration of the contact phase. This is the only way to increase the force of the propulsion and improve speed. Because speed training on a treadmill cannot improve the force of propulsion, treadmill sprinting is a waste of time and money. The limited time that coaches have with their athletes for training should be spent on valuable skills that truly benefit the athlete and team dynamics.

Some fancy treadmills, sometimes called acceleration-training devices, pull the athlete forward using a harness and bungee cord. These new machines are even less effective than the traditional type of treadmill. Because the athlete is pulled forward faster than usual, he has even less time for increased application of force against the ground. Remember: No increased application of force against the ground, no shorter contact phase and, as a result, no increase in maximum speed!

Treadmill sprinting, in general, creates several other challenges. As a player is forced to adjust to an artificially created overspeed and increase frequency at the expense of strong propulsion, the mechanics of running change. The knee of the propulsion leg is not fully extended; the recovery leg does not swing up toward the buttocks as it should; the thigh of the driving leg does not have time to drive up to the horizontal position because the propulsion leg is not fully extended; and the trunk may lean slightly backward, therefore changing the vertical projection of the center of gravity. In addition, treadmill running alters the firing pattern and, more importantly, the recruitment of the FT fibers; this is not conducive to maximum velocity. As the propulsion phase is shortened and force application decreases, fewer FT fibers contract because maximum force is not applied. The end result is decreased rather than increased velocity and an increased chance of injury due to a sudden change in gait while running at overspeed on a belt surface. Do you want to improve your players' sprinting abilities? Improve their force of propulsion!

Myth 5: Sled and Harness Running for Increased Speed

Different forms of resistance training have been used for a long time, particularly since the early 1900s. Sled or harness running is one example. In this form of training, resistance is created as the athlete drags a sled on the ground. Athletes can use simple harnesses that are attached around the waist or more complex harnesses that the instructor disconnects after the athlete has traveled 10 to 20 meters or yards.

The purpose of sled or harness running is to increase leg strength by defeating drag or resistance. More force is applied during the propulsion phase of the running step. There are benefits to using these two training devices, but some important doubts exist about whether the assumed training purpose is ever achieved.

As the athlete attempts to overcome resistance, she experiences physical challenges in the form of increased application of force against the ground, metabolic difficulties (e.g., lactic acid buildup), or both. The speed and power benefits of this exercise are questionable, especially if the load is high. Overall leg strength can be improved, but athletes who are expecting improvements in maximum velocity should be ready for some disappointment (Whelan et al., 2014). Maximum velocity increases only when the athlete is able to apply force very quickly. The application of force during the propulsion phase of the running step is simply far too slow to benefit maximum speed, agility, and explosiveness.

Harness running does have some merit, but it does not totally create the conditions needed to increase maximum speed. Harness running can be used in two main ways:

1. *Running to overcome resistance.* As the athlete attempts to run as fast as possible, more FT fibers are recruited to overcome the resistance. Therefore, it has some benefit for the development of leg strength. However, the expectation of increasing maximum speed is unrealistic because the application of force against the ground is far too slow.
2. *Fast running after the harness is disconnected.* After the coach releases the harness, the athlete has the impression of running with a velocity that is higher than that achieved under normal running conditions. However, this is just an illusion. In order to generate higher velocity, the player must apply greater force against the ground. Otherwise the release of the harness simply creates momentum for two to four steps. The momentum the runner experiences is the result of
   - the elimination of the resistance (i.e., the disconnection of the harness) and
   - the fact that the vertical projection of the center of gravity is ahead of the base of support, forcing the athlete to quickly accelerate to avoid losing balance and falling forward.

The momentum created after the harness is released is not an expression of maximum speed but rather a prolongation of the momentum produced after disconnecting the harness. As already discussed, the most important element in developing higher velocity is the quick application of force during the propulsion phase. Any artificially created illusion of quickness has no speed benefit at all!

Sled or harness running does, however, have training benefits that most proponents of this training device do not consider. As a form of interval training, it can be useful in developing anaerobic endurance. Use short repetitions (5-10 seconds) to improve alactic endurance, or use longer repetitions (20-45 seconds) to improve tolerance to the buildup of lactic acid. Do you want to increase your players' speed? Work on leg power without using unproven myths.

Myth 6: The Chute and Speed Development

The chute, often called the power fitness chute (with or without adjustable resistance), is meant to increase speed or overspeed. The runner starts the exercise with the chute hooked around the waist. The early part of running is performed against increased air resistance (i.e., the air captured by the chute). After 20 to 40 meters or yards, the chute is released and the athlete is supposed to experience a sudden burst of speed or overspeed.

Several elements can be discussed regarding the benefits of using a chute. The early part of the exercise—running against the resistance provided by the chute—can have some positive effect because more FT muscle fibers must be recruited to defeat increased resistance. Like the harness, using the chute can improve leg strength because the resistance of the chute forces the athlete to increase force output. This assumption may be true only if the chute is not moving behind the athlete. However, because most chutes are not stable (i.e., they move sideways or vertically), any gains from running against increased air resistance are deterred by a destabilized body. Unfortunately, some people see the negative effect of an unstable chute as an opportunity for improving balance and, of course, core strength! Once again, this is fine for fitness but it has no place in sport. Use the chute to improve leg strength or alactic endurance but not speed or high velocity. The effect is the same as that achieved with any overspeed training device: an increase in the foot contact phase and a resulting decrease in the athlete's velocity. Have you ever seen a top sprinter using the chute?

As with sled or harness running, the sudden burst of speed that follows the release of the chute is nothing but a momentary illusion. Do you want to increase your athletes' maximum velocity? Forget about this myth and work to increase leg power and, consequently, decrease the duration of the contact phase.

Myth 7: Hill Running for Increased Strength and Power

Hill running on both incline and decline slopes is very popular in sport training and in team-sport training in particular. Strength- and power-training programs for teams can be difficult to plan given the number of athletes, equipment required, and facilities available for use. Running outdoors, either up or down a hill, is an easy and inexpensive way to improve an athlete's fitness. Hill running can be easily implemented in a training program, and an entire team can train at once, thus making efficient use of time—especially the time devoted to conditioning athletes.

However, an effective plan has a specified goal and a set of objectives that can be attained by using various forms of training. In the case of uphill running, the objective is often an increase in explosive power. However, the slope of the hill used in training can often negate improvements in power and simply result in improvements in overall fitness—which is fine if general fitness and cardiovascular health are the primary objectives. The following sections discuss the benefits of various forms of hill running and how to best use them in training.

Incline Slopes

If you have ever asked someone why he is doing uphill running, the answer is always the same: to improve leg strength and power. The early promoters of incline running were track and field coaches who specialized in middle- and long-distance running.

The audience has increased lately, especially for the early preparatory phase, to include some team-sport athletes, mostly from soccer, rugby, lacrosse, and field hockey.

In incline running, the players run uphill for 25 to 50 meters or yards in a specified length of time and then jog back to the starting point. The athletes take a rest interval of one to two minutes between repetitions. Training demand depends on the distance of a repetition, the time it takes to perform the repetition, and the degree of inclination of the slope. A slope of more than 10 degrees is very challenging.

Incline running can be very beneficial for an athlete, but not in the way that is often professed. To develop leg strength from uphill running, the athlete must perform the propulsion phase of the running step much faster than usual. As for power, see the discussion on power training in myths 4 and 5. Any action performed for the development of power should be fast and explosive. In the case of uphill running, the propulsion phase should be very dynamic—quite similar to plyometric actions. For such an action to be beneficial for power development, the propulsion phase must be around or below 200 milliseconds. The push-off in uphill running is at best around 300 milliseconds. Therefore, the idea that uphill running will increase strength and power is merely a training anecdote.

Uphill running does, however, benefit the cardiorespiratory system. When an athlete runs uphill the heart rate can be around 160 or 170 beats per minute. This demonstrates that uphill running strengthens the heart by engaging it to pump higher amounts of blood to the working muscles.

The best time to begin using incline running to develop the cardiorespiratory system is the middle of the preparatory phase, following initial aerobic training. Training can be organized based on the interval-training methodology: several repetitions of a given distance, with a specified completion time and rest interval (e.g., 8 repetitions of 30 meters or yards × 7-8 seconds; rest interval = 1 minute). From a planning perspective, you may use incline running during the second part of the preparatory phase, after aerobic or long-tempo training.

Incline-running programs can best be organized to train a specific energy system.

- Alactic repetitions on a slope of less than 15 degrees inclination, performed as fast as realistically possible: 6 to 15 repetitions × 5 to 8 seconds; rest interval = up to 3 minutes
- Lactic acid repetitions on a slope of less than 10 degrees inclination, performed at a fast but steady speed: 6 to 10 repetitions × 15 to 30 seconds; rest interval = 1 to 2 minutes

The slope of a hill is designed by nature and sometimes coaches are at the mercy of what is available to them at parks or open fields. Be creative and find a hill or slope that best serves the cardiovascular needs of your athletes. Our experience shows that hill running is also a better deterrent or form of punishment than running laps!

Decline Slopes of Less Than 3 Degrees

Although hill or incline running is quite popular, decline running is not widely known and is therefore rarely used. More research has investigated decline running than incline running, especially in the former East Germany. (East German female sprinters dominated sprinting events from the late 1960s to the late 1980s.) In an attempt to further the methodology of sprint training and especially to break the speed barrier, sport scientists in that country tested whether decline sprinting has any merit. The East German researchers concluded that decline running has positive effects in increasing acceleration if the slope is not greater than 3 degrees (i.e., 3 degrees below the horizontal line). To improve acceleration and break the speed barrier, short tracks of 30 to 50 meters or yards with a slope of 3 degrees have been built in some German training centers (see figure 12.3).

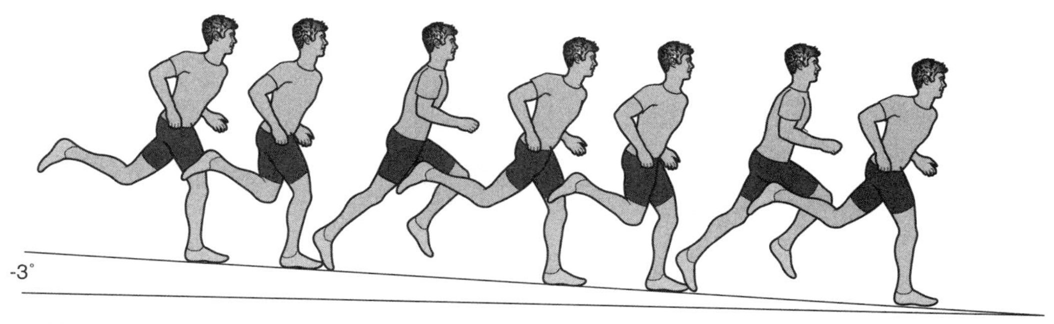

Figure 12.3 Decline sprinting on a slope of 3 degrees.

Using slopes of greater than 3 degrees (e.g., 5 to 7 degrees below the horizontal line) negatively affects the mechanics of running, resulting in a decrease of maximum velocity due to a prolonged contact phase. This has the same effect as overspeed training. When a sprinter runs on a decline track of more than 3 degrees, the contact phase is prolonged because the athlete experiences an unknown environment. The proprioceptors (specialized nerve cells that detect new stimuli) send nerve impulses via the afferent neurons to the central nervous system. The central nervous system analyzes the new conditions the athlete is experiencing, and nerve impulses are sent from the central nervous system to the working muscles via efferent neurons with the message to stabilize the body. The propulsion phase is then performed. During all these nerve transmissions to and from the muscles, passing time delay occurs because of the prolonged contact and thus in prolonging the duration of the contact phase. running velocity decreases as a result.

Decline Slopes of Greater Than 5 Degrees

Decline running beyond 5 degrees potentially has a positive effect, mainly in improved eccentric leg strength. As an athlete runs on a downhill slope inclined 7 to 15 degrees below horizontal, the quadriceps muscles must overcome the pull of gravity. The greater a slope's inclination, the higher the muscles must contract to overcome the force of gravity. As the slope's inclination increases so does the duration of the contract phase, thus prolonging the duration of muscle tension. Increased muscle tension translates into an improvement in eccentric force. Whether muscle tension comes from concentric or eccentric contraction is immaterial because each type of contraction results in improved muscle strength.

Coaches can use decline running as a form of strength development, especially during the middle to late preparatory phase. Once again, coaches can find a suitable hill on which to perform runs and teach their athletes proper running and deceleration techniques in order to avoid injury and fully achieve the eccentric muscular benefits of downhill running. Downhill running is different from incline running and can provide a fun and effective environment for training, learning, and variety.

Myth 8: Running and Walking Drills For Increasing Arm Drive

An arm swing drill with the athlete holding a dumbbell in each hand is supposed to increase the power of the arm drive with the scope of developing the frequency and speed of arm movements, thereby increasing running speed. As is the case with many other training myths, the proponents of this exercise fail to understand how muscles work and that an effective arm drive is performed by the latissimus dorsi, not the biceps brachii.

- The power and frequency of the arms' drive lead the quickness and frequency of the legs' forward drive.
- The force of the backward pull of the arm dictates the force and quickness of the opposite leg's forward drive.
- The force of the arm's pull dictates the speed of the arm's backward pull. Therefore, the quickness of the arm drive and the subsequent forward action of the opposite leg depend on the power of contraction of the latissimus dorsi.
- Holding resistance instruments or weights in the hands, contracts the biceps brachii, not the latissimus dorsi. The action of the latissimus dorsi is minimal and therefore does not result in a powerful arm drive. Consequently, there is no positive effect on running speed.
- This exercise should be reserved for the world of fitness, not sport training.

The arm swing drill with dumbbells in each hand completely misrepresents sprinting action, is misleading, and demonstrates complete ignorance on the part of its proponents.

Important Points to Consider

It would be impossible for us to comment on all the products available on the market. One can claim that any product is useful if it improves performance. Although this may be true in the world of fitness and health, where the main goal is to increase fitness or general strength and power and where variety in exercise is marketed as the spice of life, this is not the case in sport training. Today, coaches have very little time to devote to sport-specific training, particularly strength and speed training. The little time they have should be devoted to following a plan that will harness the greatest potential and athletic development in their athletes. Time should not be wasted on myths and gimmicks and on using new, ineffective equipment that does not live up to the marketing hype. Coaches are better off sticking with traditional methods of improving strength, power, speed, and endurance and leaving the use of these products to the fitness industry. The following sections discuss the potential benefits and, more importantly, the uselessness of some products on the market today.

Ankle Flexion–Extension Roller

There is no need to argue that flexibility training is important. However, we can argue against several inappropriate techniques that are used to improve players' flexibility. Similarly, we can argue that team-sport athletes have the worst ankle flexibility among most athletes.

The ankle is the joint that is most neglected by team-sport athletes. The ankle flexion–extension roller (see figure 12.4) is a good product that athletes can use to effectively develop ankle flexibility. Ankle flexibility, specifically plantar flexion (i.e., lowering the toes away from the tibia) and dorsiflexion (i.e., bringing the toes toward the

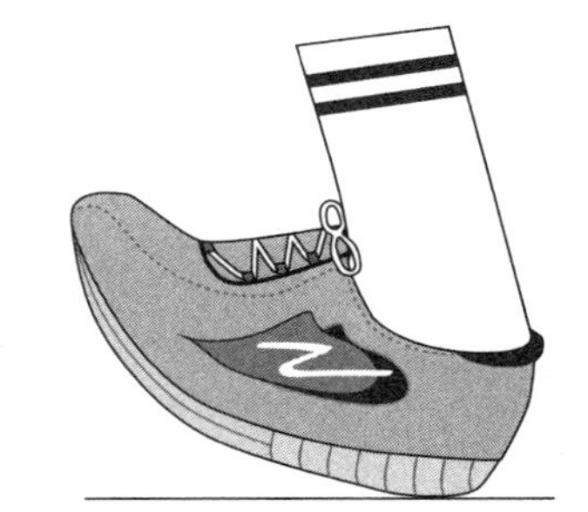

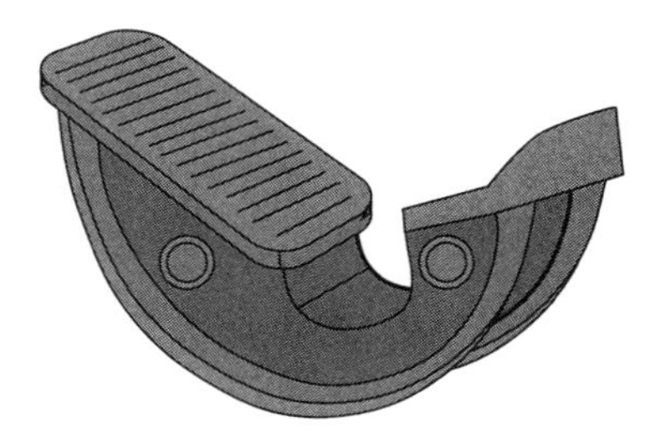

Figure 12.4 Ankle flexion–extension roller.

tibia), is very important in team sports because many movements—performing a takeoff, crouching down, reaching forward to catch a ball without moving the legs, kicking a soccer ball to fly low—require good ankle flexibility. However, most teams and players spend very little time stretching the ankle either passively or actively.

Jump Soles

Jump soles, or rounded sole shoes, are promoted as an effective way to improve jump power. The athlete wears the shoes and repeatedly performs countermovement jumps, jumping up and down for a certain amount of time or repetitions. The contact occurs at the thick part of the shoe's sole. The jump soles are made of an elastic material that gives the athlete the feeling of jumping higher. We had a great deal of suspicion regarding the effectiveness of these shoes when they were introduced because the jump the athlete performs is the result of the elasticity of the material, not of muscle activity. The same holds true for any shoes or boots that have a coil or spring. These types of shoes do not improve jumping capacity or speed (Salinero et al., 2014).

The jumps performed with jump soles are typical reactive jumps (i.e., jumping repeatedly on the balls of the feet without touching the heels to the ground) used in plyometrics training. However, typical reactive jumps that rely on muscle action and not on artificial products involve the soleus and gastrocnemius muscles. When the ball of the foot makes contact with the ground, it stretches these two muscles and stimulates a response from the stretch reflex, which elicits the contraction of the muscles.

The primary sensory receptor responsible for detecting rapid elongation or stretching of the muscle fibers is the muscle spindle, a muscle receptor that is capable of responding to both the magnitude and the rate of change in muscle fibers. Sensory impulses from the spindle are sent to the spinal cord, which in turn sends a nerve impulse that stimulates the muscle to contract. However, any jumps that rely on artificial means do not change the length of the skeletal muscles. As such, the stretch reflex is not stimulated and the activity is not effective or beneficial for improving leg power or jump power.

There is another reason why such artificial means do not improve jump power. As a jump is performed with artificial means, the inhibitory motor neurons of the antagonistic muscles lower the excitability of the agonistic muscles. Because the net muscle activity about a joint results from the difference in activity between pairs of agonistic and antagonistic muscles, the reciprocal inhibition reflex (Enoka, 2002) lowers the excitability of the antagonistic muscles and in turn increases the inhibition of the agonistic muscles. As a result, little contraction is evoked by these artificial means, meaning that the jump soles or boots have little effect on jump power.

Resistance Bands or Cords

Resistance bands and rubber cords have been used in training since 1954. Romania was the first country to apply these simple training tools. Today, resistance bands are used in fitness and sport training to improve health and strength and in rehabilitation settings. Individuals perform exercises using resistance bands or cords because it is very easy to target selected prime movers. Because it is very easy to anchor the bands or cords to a support, this simple and inexpensive training equipment can be used for a variety of exercises and muscle groups.

The resistance of the band or cord comes from stretching it; the more you stretch it, the higher the resistance. The progression of a resistance band program is based on the elasticity of the band and the number of bands an athlete uses. If one band does not provide enough resistance, the athlete can use more than one. Consider the following when using bands:

- Because the band's resistance increases with the amplitude of the stretch, strength-training benefits are achieved only at the end of the stretch.
- When strength training using free weights, the resistance comes at the beginning of the action, where the highest force is required to defeat the inertia of the barbell or dumbbell. Comparatively less force is used toward the end of the action. As such, free weights and elastic bands can be used to complement each other.
- Elastic bands are best used in endurance training for individual sports, such as swimming, rowing, or canoeing, where a high number of repetitions can result in the development of muscle endurance specific to the sport.
- Because the resistance of elastic cords and bands is relatively low, bands are not effective for mature athletes or athletes with a good strength-training background. However, for the same reason, elastic cords or bands are useful for children and young athletes. Resistance increases as the elastic cord is stretched. As resistance increases, the strain in the joint increases. This strain may overstretch the ligaments, resulting in an increased risk of injuries.
- In any action performed with the goal of developing power, acceleration has to continually increase throughout the range of motion and maximum speed must be achieved at the instant of release (i.e., in any throws of balls or athletic implements). Without constant acceleration, the discharge rate of the FT muscle fibers is low and the development of power is quite impossible.

Therefore, resistance bands and cords cannot improve sport-specific power or strength. A variety of so-called sport-specific exercises using resistance bands have appeared on the market, each claiming to improve maximum speed, footwork, and jump power. Keep one point in mind: If you want to increase your athletes' strength and power, use sport-specific exercises with traditional strength-training equipment!

Overspeed Training Bands

Since the late 1980s, a variety of pulling devices have been manufactured for the purpose of increasing speed. The creators of these devices speculate that using elastic bands or cables to pull an athlete forward will stimulate the neuromuscular system more than natural sprinting and as a result will improve maximum speed. As previously discussed, some of these devices, such as sleds or harnesses, have limited benefit. However, most others (including the one illustrated in figure 12.5) simply fail to complement the mechanics or physiology of muscle contraction during sprinting and thus are useless when it comes to improving speed.

Maximum acceleration is generated not by artificially pulling the body forward but rather by pushing it forward. In high-velocity running the body is propelled forward by the power the foot applies against the ground during the propulsion phase (e.g., the push-off in ice hockey or the pulling–pushing against water resistance in swimming and water polo). The more powerful the propulsion, the shorter the duration of the contact phase. As a result, the athlete will run forward faster.

One of the first researchers to measure the duration of the contact phase was Dietmar Schmidtbleicher (1984). He found that the best sprinters have a short (100-200 milliseconds) contact phase. The duration of foot contact with the ground for mediocre sprinters is well over 200 milliseconds. Therefore, high velocity is the result of a powerful and fast force applied against the ground (propulsion phase), not the outcome of a pulling force produced by artificial means. Therefore, the shorter the duration of the contact phase, the faster the force application. As a result, the player develops a higher velocity. Also,

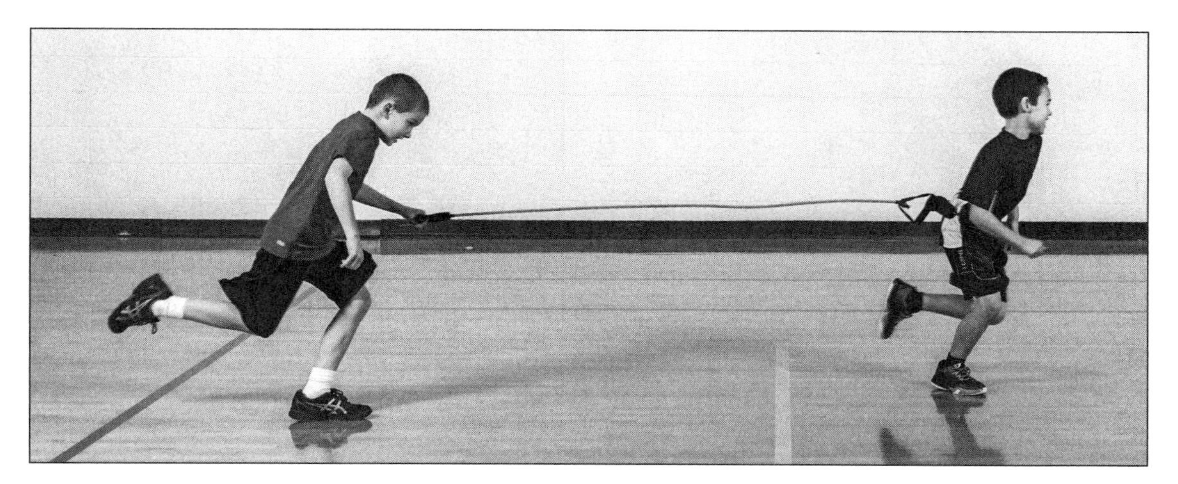

Figure 12.5 In doubleman overspeed exercises, the front runner stretches the elastic band. When maximum stretch is achieved, the back runner is artificially pulled forward and encouraged to continue to run at top speed. The promoters claim that this artificial fast pull forward will increase maximum velocity.

one has to wonder how the athlete will display high velocity when the pulling device is missing. Pulling an athlete forward with elastic bands to improve speed is simply wrong.

Furthermore, as a cable or elastic band pulls a player forward, velocity is decreased rather than increased. The artificial forward pull places the landing leg in an unknown, disturbed neuromuscular condition. As the foot touches the ground in a biomechanically unnatural movement the proprioceptors (specialized nerve cells that detect an increased response to stimuli) detect that the leg is pulled over the landing phase far too quickly compared with normal running, thus destabilizing the steadiness of foot contact in landing and running mechanics. The proprioceptors send information about this new condition to the central nervous system, telling it to monitor the status of the neuromuscular system (Enoka, 2002). These neural actions work to correct the disturbing factors and stabilize the leg before the athlete once again performs a strong propulsion action. The time necessary to relay these neural signals and stabilize the body is a few milliseconds—just long enough to prolong the duration of the contact phase. A longer contact phase means a decrease in sprinting velocity, thus negating the exact benefit the exercise is intended to accomplish: an increase in speed! Figure 12.6 shows proper running technique, including the propulsion, leg drive, recovery, and landing phases.

The forward pull of an artificial pulling device also affects the force of propulsion. As the coach or partner pulls the athlete forward, the propulsion leg does not have enough time to powerfully apply force against the ground. Consequently, a strong propulsion phase is impossible. As the force of propulsion decreases, the duration of the contact phase increases and the player's velocity decreases. The conclusion, therefore, is that overspeed training decreases an athlete's speed rather than improving it!

This artificial pull also changes the mechanics of running. During stabilization of the landing leg (see earlier definition), the trunk leans backward slightly, moving the center of gravity to behind the support leg. This is a typical position for deceleration, not for acceleration, and is not a favorable position for a strong forward push. In reaction to the backward lean of the trunk, the forward driving leg is lifted over the horizontal line, thus lengthening the duration of this leg's action and slowing running velocity.

Sprinting coaches are arguably the most knowledgeable individuals in sprinting training and technique. Have you ever seen a sprinting coach use overspeed bands?

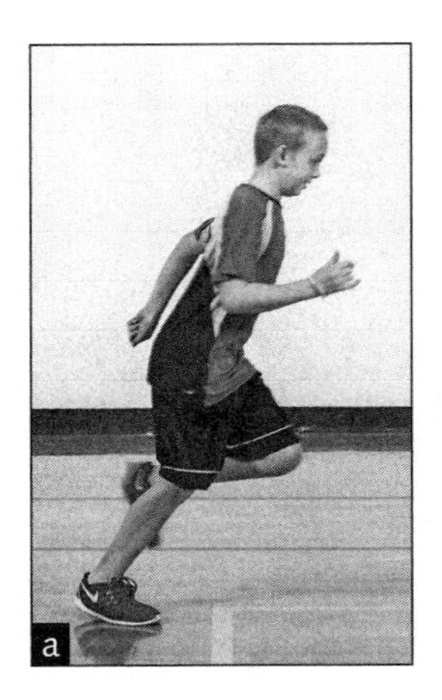
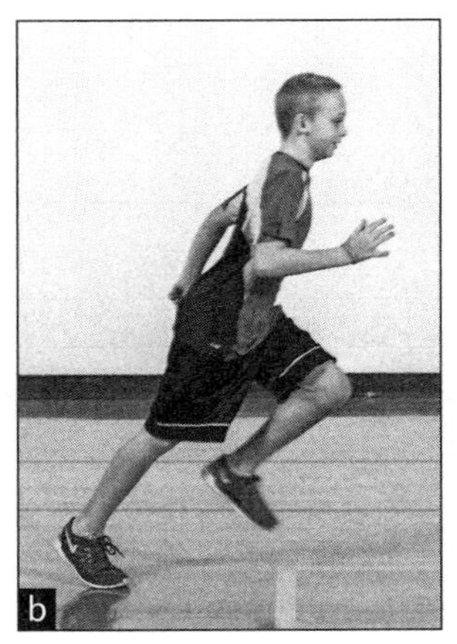
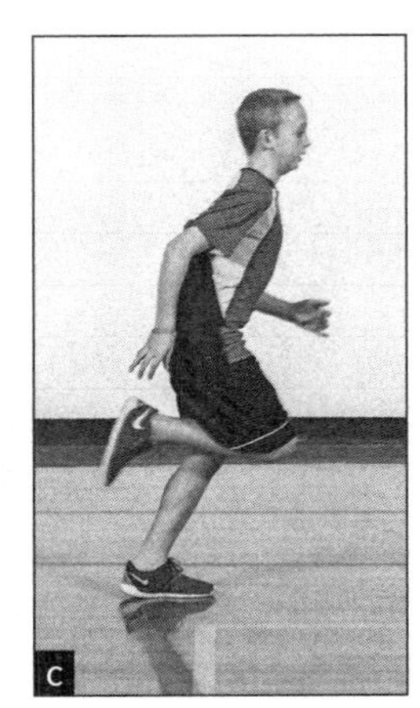
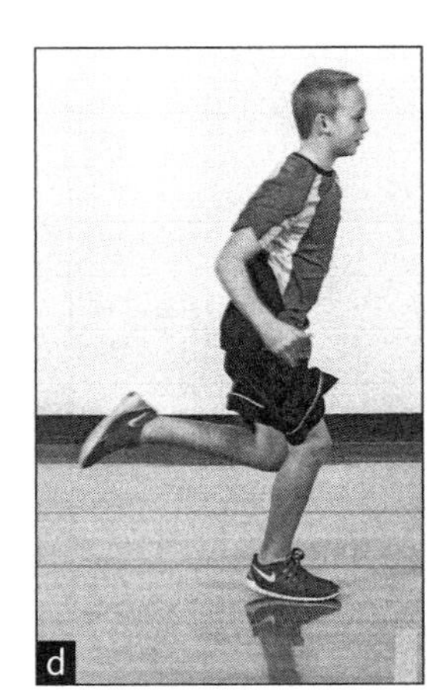

Figure 12.6 The four phases of running: *(a)* propulsion (right leg); *(b)* leg drive (left leg); *(c)* recovery (right leg); and *(d)* landing (right leg).

Overspeed elastic bands have also been used in swimming. One end of the cord is hooked around the waist of the swimmer and the other is attached to the opposite end of the pool. The swimmer stretches the cord to its limit and then allows the cord to pull his body forward. As the cord pulls the swimmer forward, he has to swim as fast as possible to keep up with the force and speed of pulling. When the artificial pulling stops, so does the speed of the swimmer. In other words, the velocity of the swimmer is not produced by the athlete but rather by artificial means—the elastic property of the cord. A swimmer can increase maximum speed only as a result of applying force against the water resistance. To overcome water resistance and as a result increase maximum velocity, the swimmer has only one option: increase the application of force against the water. And this can be achieved using only one method: Increase muscle strength via strength training using heavier loads!

Side Stepper

The promoters of the side stepper (a device which requires movement against resistance provided by an elastic band; see figure 12.7)—claim that the device develops lateral speed. However, this exercise does not correctly take into account what generates a fast lateral action. The dominant leg in any fast lateral action is not necessarily the lead leg; rather, it is the leg on the ground (i.e., the trail leg). The quickness of any lateral movement depends on the force of propulsion (push-off) applied against the ground by the trail leg. Furthermore, the quickness of the lead leg depends directly on how quickly the opposite arm initiates a short, fast movement in the intended direction of travel, not on the resistance it encounters from an elastic band looped around the ankles. Remember that the quick action of the arm results in an equally fast movement of the lead leg. Therefore, the elastic band has no substantial role in any lateral movement.

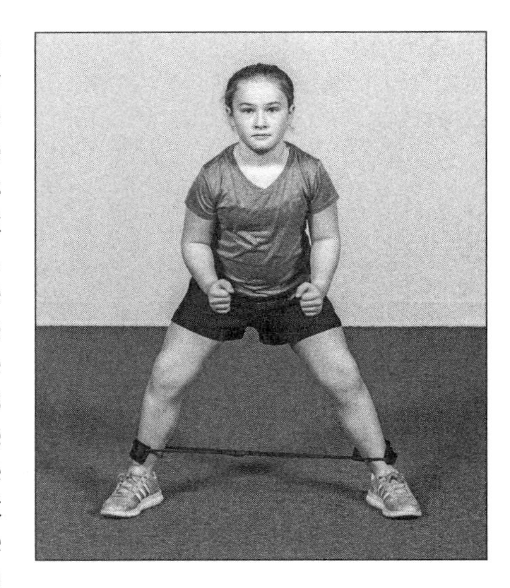

Figure 12.7 A modified elastic band is used to improve lateral stepping and takeoff power.

The same comments are valid for any variation of the carioca drill intended to generate quick feet. The coordination between lead arm and push-off leg are once again the dominant elements in quick-feet drills. Do you want to improve your players' fast lateral movements? Improve the power of the push-off leg!

Power Dunks

Power dunks, or jumps performed against the resistance provided by an elastic band (figure 12.8), claim to increase jump power. However, as with any other jumps performed against an elastic cord or band, the resistance is at a minimum (i.e., the cord is not stretched) exactly when it is necessary—at the moment of take-off. By the time the elastic cord creates the most resistance (i.e., when the cord is stretched to maximum), the athlete is already airborne and incapable of applying strength against the ground. Because the athlete cannot apply force against the ground, the device has no training effect on power development. The power dunk is, in fact, an exercise in futility!

Band Motion Products

It is claimed that various resistance bands products, such as a wrist rocket, develop strength and speed for throwing balls or other athletic implements or for batting. To achieve the goal of improving arm speed and strength, the athlete performs the arm action against the resistance of an elastic band or cable. Not only does this exercise not assist the athlete in achieving this goal, it is even dangerous! Why? Resistance increases as the band is stretched. The more power the athlete applies against the elastic cable, the higher the strain in the shoulders. As a result, the ligaments of the shoulder are exposed to high levels of strain, thus increasing the risk of injury.

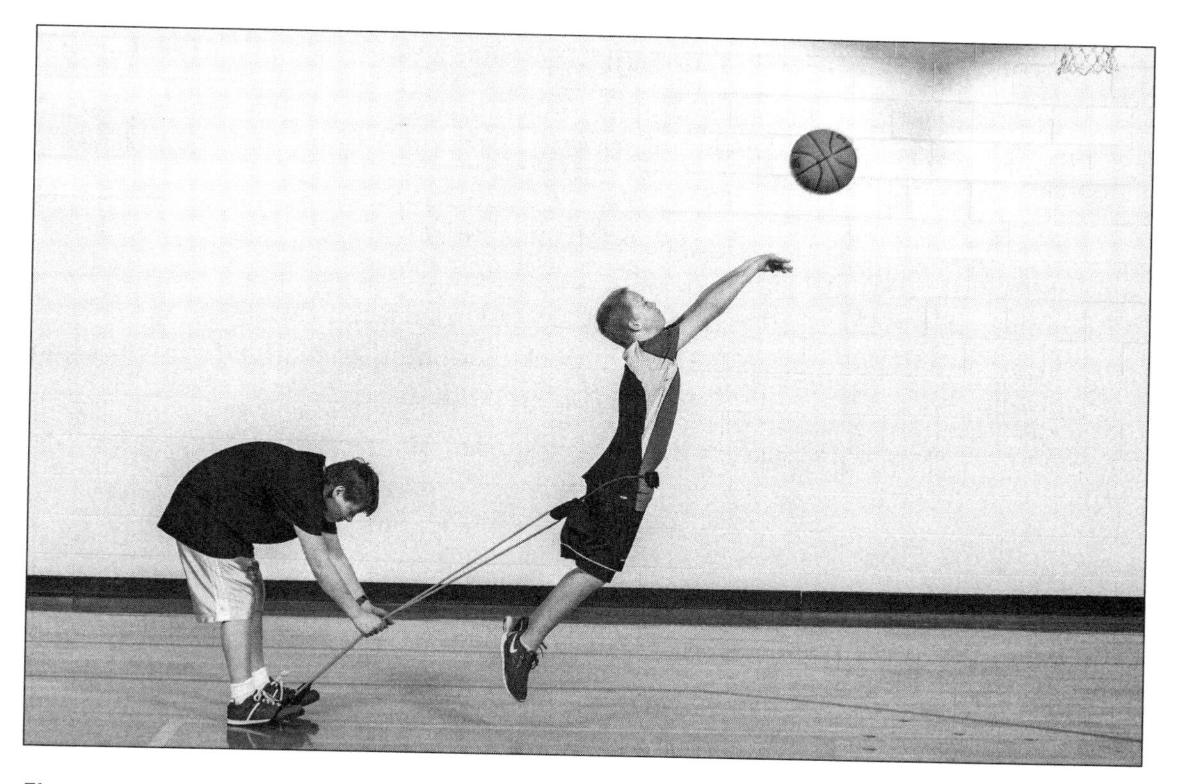

Figure 12.8 A power dunk performed against the resistance of an elastic band.

Sprint Trainer

The sprint trainer or power sprinter is a typical device that misjudges the mechanics of running, the relationship between the arms and legs during speed running, and how the muscles of the two sets of limbs work together to generate maximum speed. The marketing material for this training device claims that a set of cables can increase maximum speed because the resistance is placed directly on the athlete's muscles!

A set of elastic cables is placed on the arms and legs with the intent of creating resistance on specific muscles. However, the cables are hooked onto the wrong parts of the limbs, therefore not targeting the working muscles (i.e., prime movers). A short analysis of the mechanics of running helps demonstrate our claim.

Arms. The bands are hooked onto the upper arms and the resistance comes from behind the athlete. To overcome the resistance of the cables, the arms have to move forward—an action exactly opposite to what happens during running. As explained earlier, the arms' drive backward (not forward) generates the frequency and power of the legs' actions. Without this powerful arm drive, the athlete won't be able to have high leg frequency and perform powerful running steps. A powerful arm drive, therefore, is not performed by the biceps and anterior deltoids but rather by the latissimus dorsi. This powerful muscle is the engine of fast running. As such, the proposed sprint trainer (and other similar devices) misjudges the actions of the arms during running and misrepresents the muscles involved during a powerful running step.

Legs. When using this device, four main muscle groups are not targeted at all: gluteus maximus (for hips extension), biceps femoris (for knee flexion during the recovery phase of the running step), quadriceps (for knee extension during the push-off), and gastrocnemius and soleus (the extremely important calf muscles that perform the push-off). The straps placed below the knees are ineffective in stimulating a powerful running step. A calf drive forward is not performed against any resistance—just the air, which is nonexistent! There is a saying in sprinting: "Anybody can move a limb fast in the air!"

This type of device fails to train the prime movers that are involved in running. Speed training should target the dominant muscles that perform the powerful and quick running step:

- Latissimus dorsi (the main engine of the arms' drive)
- Gluteus maximus (for hip extension)
- Quadriceps (one of the engines of the propulsion phase)
- Gastrocnemius and soleus (the extremely essential muscles that perform quick and powerful calf action during the propulsion phase)

The sprint trainer or any similar product has little if any significance in training fast and quick athletes.

The Ladder

A highly utilized training device, the ladder has been around for many years. It originated in football, where tires have also been used to enhance quickness and agility. Athletes using the ladder can move their feet and legs forward, laterally, and even backward.

The ladder is an effective device, but mostly for children. In fact, if used by children the ladder should be incorporated as part of a strength-training program. Recent research has validated the use of strength training for children as an effective way of improving agility or rather change-of-direction speed (Keiner et. al. 2014). It is ineffective for adult athletes who have a good background in strength and power training. To increase the efficiency of ladder exercises for good athletes, the feet must be pounded against the ground with power (see figure 12.9). This properly stimulates the reactivity of the neuromuscular system, and the athletes can still benefit from ladder exercises. If the athlete doesn't pound the feet against the ground with force, the device has no positive benefit for the development of quick legs and feet, muscle reactivity, or agility. This is also true for similar devices that utilize floor rings or dotted mats. Again, these products are useful for improving speed and agility (especially footwork and coordination) in younger athletes but are ineffective for advanced athletes who have a solid background in both strength and power training.

Remember: Improvement in power, agility, quick feet, and reactivity is obtained when you use higher force.

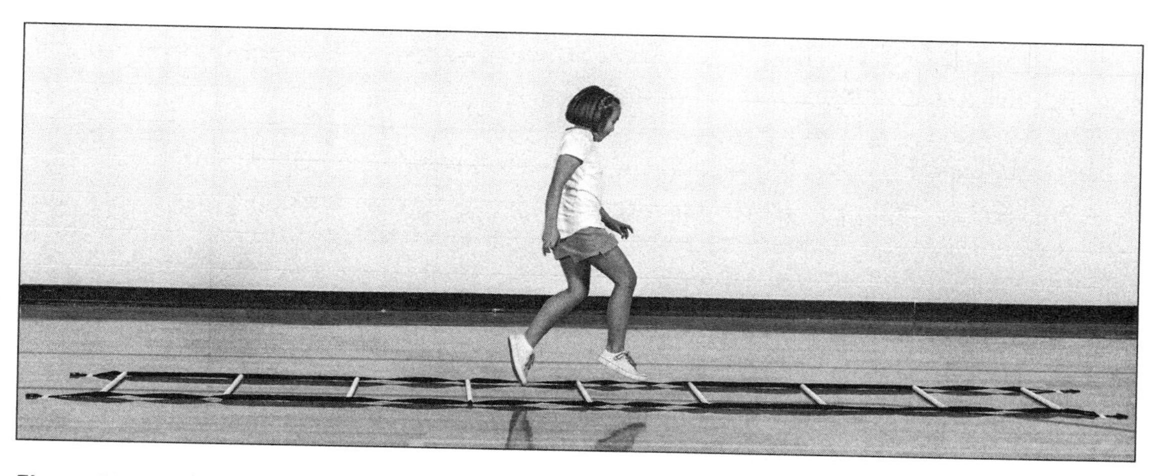

Figure 12.9 The agility ladder can be used to improve foot speed and reaction for younger athletes.

Reaction Ball

The reaction ball or agility ball is one of the most successful agility and reaction devices put forth by the industry. Because the ball, which is the size of a tennis ball, has four or more bumps on its surface, one cannot predict where the ball might rebound after it is thrown against the floor or wall (see figure 12.10).

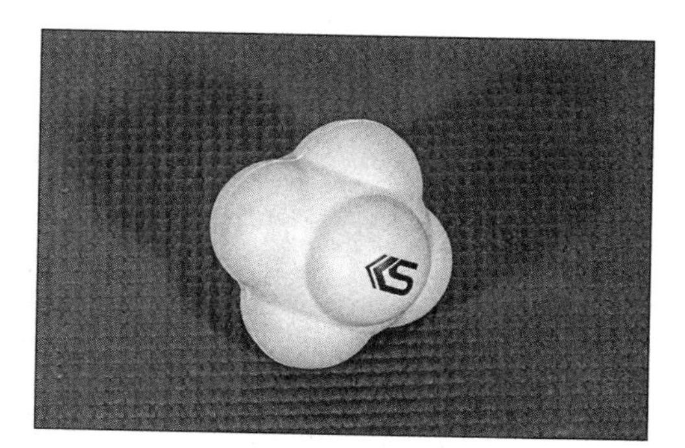

Figure 12.10 The reaction ball is an effective ball for training an athlete's reaction.

By creating different drills using the reaction ball, you can train movement time (i.e., moving the limbs quickly in different directions) and reaction time. The following are a few examples:

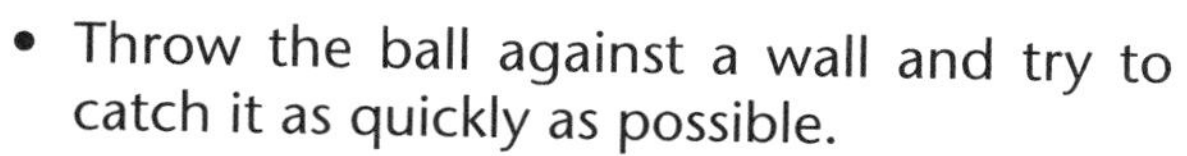

- Throw the ball against a wall and try to catch it as quickly as possible.
- Throw the ball against the floor. From the floor the ball should hit a wall. When it returns, try to catch it.
- Face a corner formed by two walls. Throw the ball against one of the walls so that the ball hits the other wall and eventually the floor. Try to catch the ball as quickly as possible.

The unpredictability of the bounce forces the athlete to focus on the movement and explode as quickly as possible toward the ball. This is a relatively inexpensive piece of equipment that can be used for individual or group play and is effective for all age groups.

Summary

Practitioners, coaches, and instructors are often the targets of so-called new breakthroughs in training. As you attempt to distinguish between training myths and products and techniques that will benefit your athletes, keep the following points in mind:

- Use common sense! The body has not changed much over the past few thousand years. Although supplements and drugs allow the body to go harder and longer and recover faster, the movements of the muscles remain the same. Don't concentrate on exercises so much; rather, focus on movements! That is where an athlete's potential strength and power reside.
- Be selective of whom you listen to. Just because something is new doesn't mean it is necessary or, more importantly, useful in training.
- Research a new product to see whether it works in reality. Equally important, test your knowledge in biomechanics and exercise physiology against that of those preaching untested training novelties. Challenge the promoters of these gimmicks to demonstrate scientifically why the product works.
- Simplify rather than complicate your training. Ask yourself in what specific training situations a given piece of equipment may be applicable.
- There are far too many "incredibly effective" new exercises and training gadgets and not enough training time to use them all.
- The more exercises you use in training, the fewer repetitions you can do. As a result, training adaptation and benefits will be low. Remember that only a strong adaptation of the major prime movers and movement patterns will lead to improvements. There is no other way!
- Do only what is important! Define the limiting factors in your sport and train your athletes using a simple but effective training methodology.

Finally, if you want your athletes to be powerful, fast, reactive, and agile, expose them to traditional strength training. None of the novelties available on the market will be as effective as strength training using medium and heavy loads. In the early years, have fun and expose the children to all kinds of movement patterns. As young athletes mature, focus on the needs of the sport and apply sound training principles in strength, power, speed, and endurance. Don't fall prey to the many myths that surface on the Internet or in print. Focus on what works: Training methodology—not gimmicks or training myths—results in performance improvement!

References

Alaranta, H., H. Hurri, M. Heliovaara, A. Soukka, and R. Harju. 1994. Flexibility of the spine: Normative values of goniometric and tape measurements. *Scand. J. Rehab. Med.* 26:147-154.

American Academy of Pediatrics. Council on Sports Medicine and Fitness. 2008. Strength Training for Children and Adolescence. *Pediatrics,* 4, 835-840.

Anshel, M.H., P. Freedman, J. Hamill, K. Haywood, M. Horvat, and S.A. Plowman. 1991. *Dictionary of the sport and exercise sciences.* Champaign, IL: Human Kinetics.

Bailey, D.A., R.M. Malina, and R.L. Mirwald. 1985. The child, physical activity and growth. In *Human growth,* Vol. 2, 2nd ed., ed. F. Falkner and J.M. Tanner, 147-170. New York: Plenum.

Barbieri, D., and L. Zaccagni. 2013. Strength training for children and adolescents: Benefits and risks. *Coll. Anthrop.* Suppl. no. 2:219-225.

Bar-Or, O., and B. Goldberg. 1989. Trainability of the prepubescent child. *Physician Sportsmed.* 17:64-66, 75-78, 80-82.

Baxter-Jones, G., and N. Maffulli. 2003. Endurance in young athletes: It can be trained. *Br. J. Sports Med.* 37:96-97.

Behm, D.G., A.D. Faigenbaum, B. Falk, and P. Klentrou. 2008. Canadian Society for Exercise Physiology position paper: Resistance training in children and adolescents. *Appl. Physiol. Nutr. Metab.* 33(3):547-561.

Behringer, M., A. vom Heed, Z. Yue, and J. Mester. 2010. Effects of resistance training in children and adolescents: A meta-analysis. *Pediatrics* 126:e1199-e1210.

Benson, A.C., M.E. Torode, and M.A.F. Singh. 2007. A rationale and method for high-intensity progressive resistance training with children and adolescents. *Contemporary Clinical Trials.* 4: 442-450.

Benton, D., A. Maconie, and C. Williams. 2007. The influence of the glycaemic load of breakfast on the behaviour of children in school. *Physiol. Behav.* 92(4):717-724.

Berstein, A. 2002. Is it time for a victory lap? Changes in the media coverage of women in sport. *International Review for the Sociology of Sport* 37(3-4): 415-428.

Bigelow, B. 2000. Is your child too young for youth sports or is your adult too old? In *Sports in school: The future of an institution,* ed. J.R. Gerdy, 11-18. New York: Teachers College Press, Columbia University.

Blimkie, C.J. 1993. Resistance training during preadolescence. *Sports Medicine.* 15:389-407.

Boisseau, N., C. Le Creff, M. Loyens, and J.R. Poortmans. 2002. Protein intake and nitrogen balance in male non-active adolescents and soccer players. *Eur. J. Appl. Physiol.* 88(3):288-293.

Boisseau, N., M. Vermorel, M. Rance, P. Duché, and P. Patureau-Mirand. 2007. Protein requirements in male adolescent soccer players. *Eur. J. Appl. Physiol.* 100(1):27-33.

Bompa, T. 1993. *Periodization of strength: The new wave in strength training.* Toronto: Veritas.

Bompa, T.O and C. Buzzichelli, 2015. *Periodization training for sports,* 3rd ed. Champaign IL: Human Kinetics.

Bompa, T.O. and M. Carrera. 2005. *Periodization training for sports,* 2nd ed. Champaign, IL: Human Kinetics.

Borms, J., and M. Hebbelinck. 1984. Review of studies on Olympic athletes. In *Physical structure of Olympic athletes, Part II, Kinanthropometry of Olympic athletes,* ed. J.E.L. Carter, 7-27. Basel, Switzerland: Karger.

Bouchard, C., G. Lortie, J.A. Simoneau, C. Leblanc, G. Thériault, and A. Tremblay. 1984. Submaximal power output in adopted and biological siblings. *Ann. Hum. Biol.* 11(4):303-309.

Bowman, S.A., S.L. Gortmaker, C.B. Ebbeling, M.A. Pereira, and D.S. Ludwig. 2004. Effects of fast-food consumption on energy intake and diet quality among children in a national household survey. *Pediatrics* 113(1):112-118.

Bray, G.A., S.J. Nielsen, and B.M. Popkin. 2004. Consumption of high-fructose corn syrup in beverages may play a role in the epidemic of obesity. *Am. J. Clin. Nutr.* 79(4):537-543.

Bray, M.S., J.M. Hagberg, L. Pérusse, T. Rankinen, S.M. Roth, B. Wolfarth, and C. Bouchard. 2009. The human gene map for performance and health-related fitness phenotypes: The 2006-2007 update. *Med. Sci. Sports Exerc.* 41(1):35-73.

Cahill, B.R. 1998. *American Orthopaedic Society for Sports Medicine: Proceedings of the Conference on Strength Training and the Prepubescent.* Chicago: American Orthopaedic Society for Sports Medicine.

Caine, D., J. Difiori, and N. Maffulli. 2006. Physeal injuries in children's and youth sports: Reasons for concern? *Br. J. Sports Med.* 40:749-760.

Caine, D.J. and N. Maffulli. 2005. Epidemiology of children's individual sports injuries. An important area of medicine and sport science research. *Med. Sport Sci.* 48:1-7

Capranica, L., and M.L. Millard-Stafford. 2011. Youth sport specialization: How to manage competition and training? *Int. J. Sports Physiol. Perform.* 6(4):572-579.

Carpinelli, R.N., R.M. Otto, R.A. Winett. 2004. A critical analysis of the ACSM position stand on resistance training: Insufficient evidence to support recommended training protocols. *J. Exerc. Physiol.* 7:1.

Centers for Disease Control and Prevention. 2015. Nutrition for everyone: nutrition basics—protein. Retrieved from http://www.cdc.gov/nutrition/everyone/basics/protein.html.

Cooper, D.M. 1996. Cardiorespiratory and metabolic responses to exercise: Maturation and growth. In *The child and the adolescent athlete*, ed. O. Bar-Or, 54-73. Oxford: Blackwell Scientific.

Cupisti, A., C. D'Alessandro, I. Evangelisti, M. Piazza, F. Galetta, and E. Morelli. 2004. Low back pain in competitive rhythmic gymnasts. *J. Sports Med. Phys. Fitness* 44(1):49-53.

Dahab, K., and T. McCambridge. 2009. Strength training in children and adolescents: Raising the bar for young athletes? *Sports Health* 1(3):223-226.

Daniels, S.R., D.K. Arnett, R.H. Eckel, H. Robert, S.S. Gidding, S. Samuel, L.L. Hayman, S. Kumanyika, L.L. Shiriki, T.N. Robinson, B.J. Scott, S. St. Jeor, and C.L. Williams. 2002. Overweight in children and adolescents: Pathophysiology, consequences, prevention, and treatment. *J. Am. Med. Assoc.* 288(14):1728-1732.

Dotan, R., C. Mitchell, R. Cohen, P. Klentrou, D. Gabriel, and B. Falk. 2012. Child–adult differences in muscle activation—A review. *Ped. Exerc. Sci.* 24(1):2-21.

Drinkwater, E.J., E.J. Pritchett, and D.G. Behm. 2007. Effect of instability and resistance on unintentional squat-lifting kinetics. *Int. J. Sports Physiol. Perform.* 2(4):400-413.

Duda, M. 1986. Prepubescent strength training gains support. *Physician Sportsmed.* 14(2):157-161.

Duffey, K.J., and B.M. Popkin. 2008. High fructose corn syrup. Is this what's for dinner? *Am. J. Clin. Nutr.* 88:1722S-1732S.

Ebbeling, C.B., D.B. Pawlak, and D.S. Ludwig. 2002. Childhood obesity: Public-health crisis, common sense cure. *Lancet* 360(9331):473-482.

Enoka, R. 2008. *Neuromechanics of human movement.* 4th ed. Champaign, IL: Human Kinetics.

Enoka, R. 2002. *Neuromechanics of human movement.* 3rd ed. Champaign IL: Human Kinetics.

Faigenbaum, A. 2000. Strength training for children and adolescents. *Clinics Sports Med.* 19(4):593-619.

Faigenbaum, A.D., M. Bellucci, A. Bernieri, B. Bakker, and K. Hoorens. 2005. Acute effects of different warm-up protocols on fitness performance in children. *J. Strength Cond. Res.* 19:376-381.

Faigenbaum, A.D., W.J. Kraemer, C.J. Blimkie, I. Jeffreys, L.J. Micheli, M. Nitka, and T.W. Rowland. 2009. Youth resistance training: Updated position statement paper from the National Strength and Conditioning Association. *J. Strength Cond. Res.* 23(Suppl. no. 5):S60-S79.

Faigenbaum, A. D., R.S. Lloyd, & G.D. Myer. 2013. Youth resistance training: Past practices, new perspectives, and future directions. *Pediatric Exercise Science,* 25, 591-604.

Faigenbaum, A.D., R.L. Loud, J. O'Connell, S. Glover, J. O'Connell, and W.L. Westcott. 2001. Effects of different resistance training protocols on upper-body strength and endurance development in children. *J. Strength Cond. Res.* 15(4):459-465.

Faigenbaum, A.D., L.A. Milliken, R.L. Loud, B.T. Burak, C.L. Doherty, and W.L. Westcott. 2002. Comparison of 1 and 2 days per week of strength training in children. *Res. Q. Exerc. Sport* 73(4):416-424.

Flatters, I., L.J. Hill, J.H. Williams, S.E. Barber, and M. Mon-Williams. 2014. Manual control age and sex differences in 4 to 11 year old children. *PLoS One* 9(2):e88692.

Fleck, S.J., and J.E. Falkel. 1986. Value of resistance training for the reduction of sports injuries. *Sports Med.* 3:61-68.

Fox, E.L., R.W. Bowers, and M.L. Foss. 1989. *The physiological basis of physical education and athletics.* Dubuque, IA: Brown.

Gidding, S., B. Dennison, L. Birch, S. Daniels, M. Gilman, A. Lichtenstein, R.T. Rattay, J. Steinberger, N. Stettler, and L. Van Horn. 2005. American Heart Association scientific statement: Dietary recommendations for children and adolescents. A guide for practitioners: Consensus statement from the American Heart Association. *Circulation* 112:2061-2075.

Gillis, C. 2014. Did a missed pull-up cost Bennett the No. 1 NHL draft spot? Charles Gillis on Samuel Bennett and the strange psychology of the NHL draft. Retrieved from http://www.macleans.ca/society/life/the-strange-psychology-of-an-nhl-draft/

Halberg, N., M. Henriksen, N. Söderhamn, B. Stallknecht, T. Ploug, P. Schjerling, and F. Dela. 2005. Effect of intermittent fasting and refeeding on insulin action in healthy men. *J. Appl. Physiol.* 99:2128-2136.

Hansen, L., J. Bangsbo, J. Twisk, and K. Klausen. 1999. Development of muscle strength in relation to training level and testosterone in young male soccer players. *J. Appl. Physiol.* 87:1141-1147.

Harre, D. 1982. *Trainingslehre.* Berlin: Sportverlag.

Hebbelinck, M. 1989. Development and motor performance. Roma, Scuola dello Sport VIII: 16.

Herbert, R.D., and M. Gabriel. 2002. Effects of stretching before and after exercising on muscle soreness and risk of injury: A systematic review. *Br. Med. J.* 325:468-470.

Howard J.D., and R.M. Enoka. 1991. Maximum bilateral contractions are modified by neurally mediated interlimb effects. *J Appl Physiol.* 70(1):306-316.

Hughson, R. 1986. Children in competitive sports: A multi-disciplinary approach. *Can. J. Appl. Sport Sci.* 11(4):162-172.

Hulthén, L., B.A. Bengtsson, K.S. Sunnerhagen, L. Hallberg, G. Grimby, and G. Johannsson. 2001. GH is needed for the maturation of muscle mass and strength in adolescents. *J. Clin. Endocrinol. Metab.* 86(10):4765-4770.

Ingraham, S.J. 2003. The role of flexibility in injury prevention and athletic performance: Have we stretched the truth? *Minnesota Med.* 86(5):58-61.

Iwasaki, K., R. Zhang, J.H. Zuckerman, and B.D. Levine. 2003. Dose-response relationship of the cardiovascular adaptation to endurance training in healthy adults: How much training for what benefit? *J. Appl. Physiol.* 95:1575-1583.

Kakebeeke, T.H., I. Locatelli, V. Rousson, J. Caflisch, and O.G. Jenni. 2012. Improvement in gross motor performance between 3 and 5 years of age. *Percept. Mot. Skills* 114(3):795-806.

Karli, U., A. Guvenc, A. Aslan, T. Hazir, and C. Acikada. 2007. Influence of Ramadan fasting on anaerobic performance and recovery following short time high intensity exercise. *J. Sports Sci. Med.* 6(4):490-497.

Kavey, R.E., S.R. Daniels, R.M. Lauer, D.L. Atkins, L.L. Hayman, and K. Taubert. 2003. American Heart Association guidelines for primary prevention of atherosclerotic cardiovascular disease beginning in childhood. *Circulation* 107:1562-1566.

Kavey, R.E., S.R. Daniels, R.M. Lauer, D.L. Atkins, L.L. Hayman, and K. Taubert. 2003. American Heart Association guidelines for primary prevention of atherosclerotic cardiovascular disease beginning in childhood. *Journal of Pediatrics.* 142(4):368-372.

Keiner, M., A. Sander, K. Wirth, and D. Schmidtbleicher. 2014. Long-term strength training effects on change-of-direction sprint performance. *J. Strength Cond. Res.* 28(1):223-231.

Kenney, L., J. Willmore, and D. Costill. 2011. *Physiology of sport and exercise*. 5th ed. Champaign, IL: Human Kinetics.

Kimmons, J., C. Gillespie, J. Seymour, M. Serdula, and H.M. Blanck. 2009. Fruit and vegetable intake among adolescents and adults in the United States: Percentage meeting individualized recommendations. *Medscape J. Med.* 11(1):26.

Kohl, H.W. III, and H.D. Cook, eds. 2013. *Educating the student body: Taking physical activity and physical education to school.* Washington, D.C.: National Academic Press.

Kraemer, W.L., and S.J. Fleck. 1993. *Strength training for young athletes*. Champaign, IL: Human Kinetics.

Krissansen, G. 2007. Emerging health properties of whey proteins and their clinical implications. *J. Am. College Nutr.* 26(6):713S-723S.

Laemmle, J., and B. Martin. 2013. Children at play: Learning gender in the early years. *J. Youth Adolesc.* 42(2):305-307.

Lim, S., J.M. Zoellner, J.M. Lee, B.A. Burt, A.M. Sandretto, W. Sohn, A.I. Ismail, and J.M. Lepkowski. 2009. Obesity and sugar-sweetened beverages in African-American preschool children: A longitudinal study. *Obesity* 17(6):1262-1268.

LoDolce, M.E., J.L. Harris, and M.B. Schwartz. 2013. Sugar as part of a balanced breakfast? What cereal advertisements teach children about healthy eating. *J. Health Commun.* 18(11):1293-1309.

Ludwig, D.S., K.E. Peterson, and S.L. Gortmaker. 2001. Relation between consumption of sugar-sweetened drinks and childhood obesity: A prospective, observational analysis. *Lancet* 357(9255):505-508.

MacDonald, J., and P. D'Hemecourt. 2007. Back pain in the adolescent athlete. *Pediatr. Ann.* 36(11):703-712.

Machado, F.A., and B.S. Denadai. 2011. Validity of maximum heart rate prediction equations for children and adolescents. *Arq. Bras. Cardiol.* 97(2):136-140.

MacPhail, A., T. Gorely, and D. Kirk. 2003. Young people's socialization into sport: A case study of an athletics club. *Sport Edu. Soc.* 8:251-267.

Mahon, A.D., A.D. Marjerrison, J.D. Lee, M.E. Woodruff, and L.E. Hanna. 2010. Evaluating the prediction of maximal heart rate in children and adolescents. *Res. Q. Exerc. Sport* 81(4):466-471.

Malina, R. 2006. Weight training in youth—Growth, maturation, and safety: An evidence-based review. *Clin. J. Sports Med.* 16(6):478-487.

Malina, R.M. 1984. Physical growth and maturation. In *Motor development during childhood and adolescence*, ed. J.R. Thomas, 3-40. Minneapolis: Burgess.

Mariscalco, M.W., and P. Salvan. 2011. Upper extremity injuries in the adolescent athlete. *Sports Med. Arthrosc.* 19(1):17-26.

Matsui, H. 1983. Discovery of hereditary ability for junior athletes. *Asian Stud. Phys. Educ.* 6(1):50-56.

Mei, Z., L.M. Grummer-Strawn, A. Pietrobelli, A. Goulding, M.I. Goran, and W.H. Dietz. 2002. Validity of body mass index compared with other body-composition screening indexes for the assessment of body fatness in children and adolescents. Am. J. Clin. Nutr. 75:978-985.

Merkel, D.L. 2013. Youth sport: Positive and negative impact on young athletes. *J. Sports Med.* 4:151-160.

Micheli, L.J. 1988. Strength training in the young athlete. In *Competitive sports for children and youth*, ed. E.W. Brown and C.E. Brants, 99-105. Champaign, IL: Human Kinetics.

Miller, P.E., R.A. McKinnon, S.M. Krebs-Smith, A.F. Subar, J. Chriqui, L. Kahle, and J. Reedy. 2013. Sugar-sweetened beverage consumption in the U.S.: Novel assessment methodology. *Am. J. Prev. Med.* 45(4):416-421.

Miyaguchi, K., S. Demura, H. Sugiura, M. Uchiyama, and M. Noda. 2013. Development of various reaction abilities and their relationships with favorite play activities in preschool children. *J. Strength Cond. Res.* 27(10):2791-2799.

Morgan, R.E. 2013. Does consumption of high-fructose corn syrup beverages cause obesity in children? *Pediatr. Obes.* 8(4):249-254.

Mostafavifar, A.M., T.M. Best, and G.D. Myer. 2013. Early sport specialisation, does it lead to long-term problems? *Br. J. Sports Med.* 47(17):1060-1061.

Mulvihill, C., K. Rivers, and P. Aggleton. 2000. Physical activity "at our time": Qualitative research among young people aged 5 to 15 years and parents. London: Health Education Authority.

Nagorni, M.F. 1978. Facts and fiction regarding junior's training. *Fizkulturai Sport* 6.

Nettle, H., and E. Sprogis. 2011. Pediatric exercise: Truth and/or consequences. *Sports Med. Arthrosc.* 19(1):75-80.

Nicklas, T.A., C. Reger, L. Myers, and C. O'Neil. 2000. Breakfast consumption with and without vitamin-mineral supplement use favourably impacts daily nutrient intake of ninth-grade students. *J. Adolesc. Health* 27:314-321.

Odea, J.A. 2003. Why do kids eat healthful food? Perceived benefits of and barriers to healthful eating and physical activity among children and adolescents. *J. Am. Dietetic Assoc.* 103(4):497-501.

Ogden, C.L., G.S. Connor, J. Rivera Dommarco, M.D. Carroll, M. Shields, and K.M. Flegal. 2010. The epidemiology of childhood obesity in Canada, Mexico and the United States. In Epidemiology of obesity in children and adolescents—Prevalence and etiology, ed. L. Moreno, I. Pigeot, and W. Ahrens. New York: Springer.

Ogden, C.L., K.M. Flegal, M.D. Carroll, and C.L. Johnson. 2002. Prevalence and trends in overweight among U.S. children and adolescents, 1999-2000. *J. Am. Med. Assoc.* 288(14):1728-1732.

Ostojic, S.M., C. Castagna, J. Calleja-González, I. Jukic, K. Idrizovic, and M. Stojanovic. 2014. The biological age of 14-year-old boys and success in adult soccer: Do early maturers predominate in the top-level game? *Res. Sports Med.* 22(4):398-407.

Papaiakovou, G., A. Giannakos, C. Michailidis, D. Patikas, E. Bassa, V. Kalopisis, N. Anthrakidis, and C. Kotzamanidis. 2009. The effect of chronological age and gender on the development of sprint performance during childhood and puberty. *J. Strength Cond. Res.* 23(9):2568-2573.

Passer, M.W. 1988. Determinants and consequences of children's competitive stress. In *Children in sport*, 3rd ed., ed. F.L. Smoll, R.A. Magill, and M.J. Ash, 135-148. Champaign, IL: Human Kinetics.

Passer, M.W., and B.J. Wilson. 2002. At what age are kids ready to compete? In *Children and youth in sport: A biopsychosocial perspective*, ed. F.L. Smoll and R.E. Smith, 211-231. Dubuque, IA: Kendall/Hunt.

Prasad, D.C., and B.C. Das. 2009. Physical inactivity: A cardiovascular risk factor. *Indian J. Med. Sci.* 63(1):33-42.

Rader, R.K., K.B. Mullen, R. Sterkel, R.C. Strunk, and J.M. Garbutt. 2014. Opportunities to reduce children's excessive consumption of calories from beverages. *Clin. Pediatr. (Phila).* 53:1047-1054.

Ramsey, J., C. Blimkie, K. Smith, S. Garner, D. Macdougall, and D. Sale. 1990. Strength training effects in prepubescent boys. *Med. Sci. Sport Exerc.* 22(5):605-614.

Ratel, S. 2011. High-intensity and resistance training and elite young athletes. *Med. Sport Sci.* 56:84-96.

Raudsepp, L., and M. Pääsuke. 1995. Gender differences in fundamental movement patterns, motor performances, and strength measurements of prepubertal children. *Pediatr. Exerc. Sci.* 7(3):294-304.

Reider, B. 2011. Kids will be kids. *Am. J. Sports Med.* 39(5):923-925.

Richmond, E.J., and A.D. Rogol. 2007. Male pubertal development and the role of androgen therapy. *Nat. Clin. Pract. Endocrinol. Metab.* 3(4):338-344.

Roberts, D., A. Norton, A. Sinclair, and P. Lavkins. 1987. Children and long distance running. *New Stud. Athlet.* 1:7-8.

Rogol, A.D., J.N. Roemmich, and P.A. Clark. 2002. Growth at puberty. *J. Adolesc. Health* 31(Suppl. no. 6):192-200.

Rotella, R.J., T. Hanson, and R.H. Coop. 1991. Burnout in youth and sports. *Elem. School J.* 91(5):421-428.

Round, J.M. 1999. Hormonal factors in the development of differences in strength between boys and girls during adolescence: A longitudinal study. *Ann. Human Biol.* 26(1):49-62.

Rovere, G.D. 1988. Low back pain in athletes. *Physician Sportsmed.* 15:105-117.

Rowland, T.W., and A. Boyajian. 1995. Aerobic response to endurance exercise training in children. *Pediatrics* 96:654-658.

Sale, D.G. 1986. Neural adaptation in strength and power training. In *Human muscle power*, ed. N.L. Jones, N. McCartney, and A.J. McComs, 281-305. Champaign, IL: Human Kinetics.

Salinero, J.J., J. Abian-Vicen, J. Del Coso, and C. González-Millán. 2014. The influence of ankle dorsiflexion on jumping capacity and the modified agility t-test performance. *Eur. J. Sport Sci.* 14(2):137-143.

Schmidtbleicher, D. 1984. *Sportliches Krafttraining.* Berlin: Jung, Haltong, and Bewegung bie Menchen.

Sebastian, R.S., C. Wilkinson Enns, and J.D. Goldman. 2009. U.S. adolescents and MyPyramid: Associations between fast-food consumption and lower likelihood of meeting recommendations. *J. Am. Dietetic Assoc.* 109:226-235.

Seger, J.Y., and A. Thorstensson. 2000. Muscle strength and electromyogram in boys and girls followed through puberty. *Eur. J. Appl. Physiol.* 81(1-2):54-61.

Sharma, K.D., and P. Hirtz. 1991. The relationship between coordination quality and biological age. *Med. Sport* 31:3-4.

Shephard, R.J. 1982. *Physical activity and growth.* Chicago: Yearbook Medical.

Shrier, I. 2004. Does stretching improve performance? A systematic and critical review of the literature. *Clin. J. Sport Med.* 14(5):267-273.

Skinner, R.A., and J.P. Piek. 2001. Psychosocial implications of poor motor coordination in children and adolescents. *Hum Mov Sci.* 20(1-2): 73-94.

Smith, T.K. 1984. Preadolescent strength training. Some considerations. *J. Phys. Educ. Rec. Dance* 55:43-44,80.

Tomkinson, G. American Heart Association's Scientific Sessions 2013: "Global Changes in Cardiovascular Endurance of Children and Youth since 1964." Systematic Analysis of 25 million Fitness Test Results from 28 countries.

U.S. Department of Agriculture. Food and Nutrition Service. 2015. School meals. Child nutrition programs. Retrieved from http://www.fns.usda.gov/school-meals/child-nutrition-programs.

Valovich McLeod, T., L.C. Decoster, K.J. Loud, L.J. Micheli, J.T. Parker, M.A. Sandrey, and C. White. 2011. National Athletic Trainers' Association Position Statement: Prevention of Pediatric Overuse Injuries. *J Athl Train* 46(2): 206-220.

Vanelli, M., B. Iovane, A. Bernardini, G. Chiari, M.K. Errico, C. Gelmetti, M. Corchia, A. Ruggerini, E. Volta, and S. Rossetti. 2005. Breakfast habits of 1,202 northern Italian children admitted to a summer sport school. Breakfast skipping is associated with overweight and obesity. *Acta Biomed.* 76(2):79-85.

Wang, Y., and M.A. Beydoun. 2007. The obesity epidemic in the United States—Gender, age, socioeconomic, racial/ethnic, and geographic characteristics: A systematic review and meta-regression analysis. *Epidemiol. Rev.* 29:6-28.

Whelan, N., C. O'Regan, and A.J. Harrison. 2014. Resisted sprints do not acutely enhance sprinting performance. *J. Strength Cond. Res.* 28(7):1858-1866.

Wild, C.Y., J.R. Steele, and B.J. Munro. 2013. Musculoskeletal and estrogen changes during the adolescent growth spurt in girls. *Med. Sci. Sports Exerc.* 45(1):138-145.

Willardson, J.M., F.E. Fontana, and E. Bressel. 2009. Effect of surface stability on core muscle activity for dynamic resistance exercises. *Int. J. Sports Physiol. Perform.* 4(1):97-109.

Wilson J.M., J.P. Loenneke, E. Jo, G. J. Wilson, M.C. Zourdos, J.S. Kim. 2012. The effects of endurance, strength, and power training on muscle fiber type shifting. *J Strength Cond Res.* 26(6):1724-1729.

Wingfield, K. 2013. Neuromuscular training to prevent knee injuries in adolescent female soccer players. *Clin. J. Sport Med.* 23(5):407-408.

Young, D.R., D.S. Sharp, and J.D. Curb. 1995. Associations among baseline physical activity and subsequent cardiovascular risk factors. *Med. Sci. Sports Exerc.* 27:1646-1654.

Zijdewind, I., and D. Kernell. 2001. Bilateral interactions during contractions of intrinsic hand muscles. *J. Neurophysiol.* 85(5):1907-1913.

Index

Note: The italicized *f* and *t* following page numbers refer to figures and tables, respectively.

About the Authors

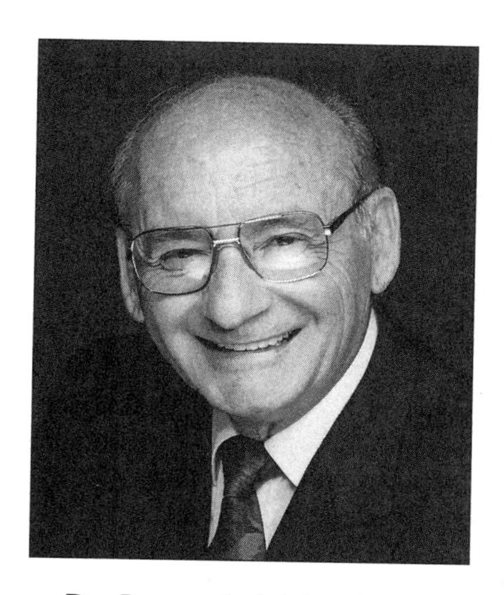

Tudor O. Bompa, PhD, revolutionized Western training methodology and methods when he introduced his groundbreaking theory of periodization of motor abilities (periodization of strength and power) in Romania in 1963. After adopting his training system, the Eastern Bloc countries dominated international sports through the 1970s and 1980s. In the 1970s Dr. Bompa developed periodization endurance, and in the early 1980s he applied this theory to speed and agility training. One of his most successful training concepts is in short- and long-term planning. Dr. Bompa has personally trained 11 Olympic and world championship medalists (including four gold medalists) and has served as a consultant to coaches and athletes worldwide.

Dr. Bompa's 14 books on training methods, including *Theory and Methodology of Training: The Key to Athletic Performance and Periodization of Training for Sports,* have been translated into 19 languages and used in more than 180 countries for training athletes and educating and certifying coaches. Dr. Bompa has been invited to speak about training in more than 40 countries and has been awarded certificates of honor and appreciation from 23 prestigious organizations, including the Argentinean Ministry of Culture, the Australian Sports Council, the Spanish Olympic Committee, the International Olympic Committee, and the National Strength and Conditioning Association (NSCA). In 2014 Dr. Bompa received the Lifelong Achievement Award from the NSCA.

Dr. Bompa is a professor emeritus at York University in Toronto, Ontario, where he taught training theories since 1974. He and his wife, Tamara, live in Sharon, Ontario.

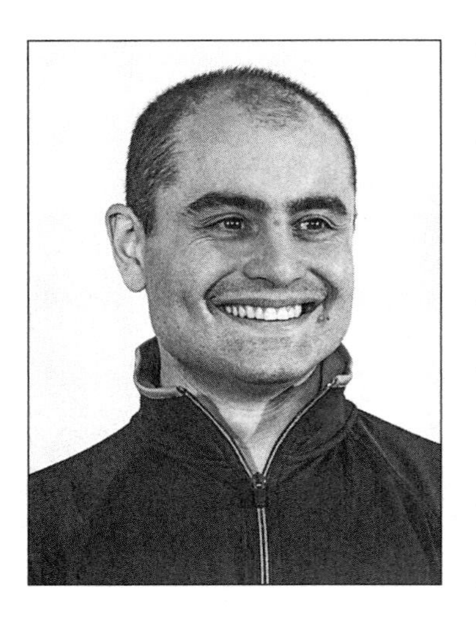

Michael Carrera is a certified exercise physiologist and personal trainer with vast experience as a health, fitness, and sports conditioning expert. He holds a master's degree in exercise science and has trained elite athletes, including national-level swimmers and professional hockey players. His education and experience have qualified him to create and administer strength test protocols for athletes in ice hockey, soccer, figure skating, lacrosse, and swimming at the provincial and national levels.

Carrera has contributed to numerous scientific journals, articles, chapters, and manuals in the areas of fitness, health, and sport conditioning. He has published three books and produced DVDs integrating spirituality with weight training and fitness. He coauthored the second edition of *Periodization Training for Sports* (Human Kinetics, 2005).

Carrera is widely recognized in the media, having appeared as an expert on numerous radio and television programs, including morning shows and specialty channels. He has been a contributor to national publications such as *Men's Health, Canadian Living, Alive,* and the *National Post*.

Carrera created and implemented corporate wellness programs and health management strategies for top Canadian companies. He has also created more than 14,000 exercise programs for health and fitness websites and has overseen fitness and weight-loss centers catering to women across Canada.